Nutrition, Immunity and Infection

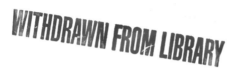

For Nandini
No need to say anything. She knows.

Nutrition, Immunity and Infection

Prakash Shetty

School of Medicine
University of Southampton, UK

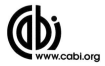
www.cabi.org

CABI is a trading name of CAB International

CABI Head Office
Nosworthy Way
Wallingford
Oxfordshire OX10 8DE
UK

Tel: +44 (0)1491 832111
Fax: +44 (0)1491 833508
E-mail: cabi@cabi.org
Website: www.cabi.org

CABI North American Office
875 Massachusetts Avenue
7th Floor
Cambridge, MA 02139
USA

Tel: +1 617 395 4056
Fax: +1 617 354 6875
E-mail: cabi-nao@cabi.org

A catalogue record for this book is available from the British Library, London, UK.

Library of Congress Cataloging-in-Publication Data

Shetty, Prakash S.
  Nutrition, immunity, and infection / Prakash Shetty.
     p. ; cm. -- (Modular texts)
  Includes bibliographical references and index.
  ISBN 978-0-85199-531-1 (alk. paper)
1. Malnutrition--Immunological aspects. 2. Communicable diseases--Nutritional aspects.
3. Immunity--Nutritional aspects. I. Title. II. Series: Modular texts.
  [DNLM: 1. Malnutrition--complications. 2. Communicable Diseases--complications. 3. Communicable Diseases--immunology. 4. Immunity. 5. Malnutrition--immunology. WD 100 S554n 2010]

RA645.N87S54 2010
616.3'9079--dc22

                                        2009051405

ISBN: 978 0 85199 531 1

Commissioning Editor: Sarah Mellor
Production Editor: Shankari Wilford

Typeset by SPi, Pondicherry, India.
Printed and bound in the UK by Cambridge University Press, Cambridge.

Contents

Preface

This modular textbook *Nutrition, Immunity and Infection* has had a long gestation! For someone who has barely made any significant contribution to this specific field, accepting the invitation to develop a module on 'Nutrition and Infection' for the new Masters Course in Infectious Diseases at the London School of Hygiene & Tropical Medicine for London University's Distance Learning Programme, required some considerable arm twisting. Once I started working on the module it was apparent that an understanding of the interactions of nutrition and infection could not be accomplished without integration with immunity and immune function. For someone who was not overwhelmed by intimate association and deep involvement with any one of the aspects of the three corners of this interesting and interacting triad, it was apparent that there was a lacuna in the form of a book that could cater to the needs of the student from any one of the disciplines contributing to this triad without overburdening them with too much technical and scientific information related to the other disciplines involved. Interest expressed by CABI to publish a book on this topic meant I had to get clearance from London University's Distance Learning Programme and I am grateful to Professor Bo Drasar who not only encouraged me in this venture but also facilitated my receiving the required clearance.

My subsequent move to work for the United Nations in Rome soon thereafter meant I had to put this on the backburner for several years. It was my earlier intent to produce a small textbook which would be a beefed up version of the distance learning module and which I was particularly keen to be made available as an inexpensive paperback catering to the demands of students from developing countries. However, the passage of time meant that CABI, who had re-activated their interest in my book on my return to the UK, had decided that it would be one of a series of modular textbooks they would be producing. This has meant the current book is much bigger and more technical than was originally conceived. I hope it has the necessary balance and the right amount of information, and addresses the needs of a wide range of students. Graduate or postgraduate programmes cater to a wide range of students from diverse backgrounds, and a fair proportion of them are exposed to these disciplines for the first time. There are epidemiologists, statisticians and public health workers who have a barely passable knowledge of nutritional sciences or of the biology of human immune function. They need to obtain enough knowledge and information to appreciate the close interactions in the three legs of the triad of nutrition, immune function and infection.

I would like to express my gratitude to Professor Nevin Scrimshaw whom I have had the privilege to know for nearly three decades, and I am indeed honoured that he wrote a Foreword to this book. He is a pioneer in this field of interactions such as synergism and antagonism between nutrition and infection and published the first, most exhaustive review on the subject in 1959 (*American Journal of Medical Sciences* 237, 367), which then culminated in the World Health Organization's monograph of 1968 (*Interactions of Nutrition and Infection*). We need to salute Scrimshaw and his colleagues, who in their 1959 review made several important observations which are true to this day, 50 years hence. I quote from their review:

> Many of the important infections of human populations are rendered more serious in their consequences by the presence of malnutrition; that few infections are indeed less severe when associated with nutritional deficiency; and that many infections themselves precipitate nutritional disturbances.

It was written at a time when microbiological research continued to identify new infectious agents and when nutritional scientists identified increasing numbers of specific nutrients and the scientific basis of nutrition was being established. This was also a period when our understanding of immunology was nascent and the discipline was not exalted by terms so familiar to us now such as cell-mediated immunity and cytokines. The only measure of 'resistance' to infection in laboratory experimental studies was 'almost exclusively by the ability of the host to produce antibodies'. However, it was also recognized that resistance to infection was 'the sum total of body mechanisms which impose barriers to the progress of invasion by infectious agents' – at a time when nutritional immunology was not even a speck on the horizon. According to these authors, reports in the literature as early as 1949 indicated that 'the relationship of each nutrient to each infectious agent in each host would need to be worked out individually'. We are only beginning to appreciate and understand this, and I hope this book illustrates some of that new knowledge.

This important review by Scrimshaw and colleagues published 50 years ago provided a working generalization that 'in human populations interactions between nutrition and infection are probably more important than laboratory investigations would indicate'. They concluded so presciently, 'Where both malnutrition and infection are serious, as they are in most tropical and technically underdeveloped countries, success in control of either condition commonly depends on the other'. How true and how evident it is, in our current global public health strategies.

Events, progress and time change perspectives. One cannot discuss the topic of nutrition and immunity without recognizing and saluting the yeoman contribution of Ranjit Chandra in the then new and emerging field of nutritional immunology, which he strode like a colossus for decades since his early contribution in the 1970s. Chandra deserves much of the credit for the growth of this scientific area in the pre-AIDS era, during much of which he ploughed a lone furrow, with his singular contributions showing impaired immune response and immunocompetence in protein–energy malnutrition.

In more recent years several technical and scientific monographs have highlighted the importance of nutrition on immune function and I owe a debt of gratitude to several contributors to many of these excellent volumes, which I have depended on and draw heavily upon in putting together this modular student textbook. Writing a textbook is different from writing a scientific manuscript or review, and enabling easy readability means compromising the need to cite all statements and all the evidence. Only crucial ones are outlined for further reading while all others are listed under sources. To the numerous authors and editors from whom I have learnt so much and whose ideas, information and evidence I have adapted and used so freely, I express my gratitude. A few specific mentions of my colleagues in Southampton whose edited volumes and books have provided much help would not be out of place here and they include Penny Nestel, Philip Calder and Barrie Margetts.

It would not have been possible to write this book without access to the various libraries and their most helpful staff – these include the University of Southampton Medical School library and the excellent libraries in London at the Royal Society of Medicine (RSM), University College, London (UCL) and London School of Hygiene & Tropical Medicine (LSHTM). I would like to place on record my thanks to Alan Dangour of LSHTM for his prompt help on several occasions to obtain crucial publications and books, which has been invaluable.

I would be failing in my duty if I did not record my gratitude to Sarah Mellor at CABI, whose constant support and faith in my ability to deliver the manuscript more than compensated for the occasional reminder of the deadline! I would like to thank Nigel Farrar, Rachel Cutts and Shankari Wilford, the Publishing and Production team at CABI. To have a good copy editor is to be fortunate, and I have been well looked after by Gill Watling. Numerous other staff of CABI have been responsible for the illustrations and in producing this book. Thank you all very much.

Prakash Shetty

Foreword

It is difficult to believe that as recently as the 1950s the relationship between nutrition and infection was unrecognized except for limited references to tuberculosis. With only minor exceptions, the textbooks on nutrition made no reference to infection, and those on infectious disease were similarly lacking mention of nutrition. The relationship first received attention as a result of the recognition in the 1950s that kwashiorkor, then common in almost all developing countries, was precipitated by infections in young children whose diets were already inadequate.

Extensive studies at the Institute of Nutrition of Central America and Panama (INCAP) in Guatemala plus research in Ghana, Chile, Brazil, South Africa and a few other developing countries confirmed that kwashiorkor in young children, characterized by a severe deficiency of protein relative to energy, rarely occurred without the adverse metabolic effects of diarrhoeal or respiratory infections or the common communicable diseases of childhood, particularly measles and whooping cough.

Field studies of the relationship between infection and malnutrition soon led to the recognition that the high mortality rates in poorly nourished young children could not be ascribed to either malnutrition or infection alone. A two-year INCAP study of all deaths in children below 5 years of age in four Guatemalan villages found that about 40% at that time were due to kwashiorkor. However, all of these cases were precipitated by a preceding infection and probably none of the deaths attributed to diarrhoeal or respiratory infections would have occurred if the children had been better nourished.

Sceptical of such sweeping conclusions, the Pan-American Health Organization sent an epidemiologist and a statistician to investigate the causes of child deaths in eight Public General Hospitals in Latin American cities. Despite the limitations of the hospital records they reported that at least half of the deaths were due to a combination of malnutrition and infectious disease. Evidence for nutrition and infection interactions began accumulating in the world literature. However, it was not until these were brought together in the 1968 World Health Organization (WHO) Monograph on *Interactions of Nutrition and Infection*, with nearly 900 supporting references, that both workers in nutrition and those concerned with infectious disease began to appreciate the synergistic interrelationship of the two types of disease: infections worsen nutritional status and poor nutrition weakens immunity to infections.

By the time the WHO monograph was published, the mechanisms by which even subclinical infections had an adverse effect on nutritional status had been well worked out and described. However, those by which the various types of undernutrition and malnutrition were associated with increases in the prevalence and severity of infections were not understood. The principal potential mechanism known at that time was humoral immunity, i.e. antibody formation. However, in field studies, poorly nourished children with high morbidity and mortality usually did not have impaired antibody response to common antigens.

Immunology was then in its infancy! Cell-mediated immunity, its complex control by cytokines and the contribution of immunoglobulins to resistance to infections were almost entirely unknown. The WHO monograph established beyond doubt that malnourished individuals were more susceptible to infection, but it was not until the virtual explosion of research in the field of immunology that the reason for this was fully explained. Soon delayed cutaneous hypersensitivity, T-cell numbers, immunoglobulins and secretory antibodies were being described as affected by even mild malnutrition.

The first nine chapters of this textbook cover comprehensively and in a well-organized manner the great amount of new knowledge on the synergistic interactions of nutrition, immunology and infectious disease that has been developing rapidly in recent decades. The last of these deals with specific diseases of global importance: HIV/AIDS, malaria, tuberculosis and systemic helminthic infections. However, knowledge of nutrition and immune functions in man now goes far beyond their relationship to infectious diseases. This textbook appropriately includes a chapter on immunity in chronic diseases. Micronutrients that affect the immune system can also play a role in chronic inflammatory responses and in cancer. Mild immune impairment may even be a feature of human obesity. A chapter deals with the complex effects of ageing on immune function and another with the rapidly growing field of probiotics, prebiotics and synbiotics. These compounds reduce the incidence and duration of acute diarrhoeal episodes in infants and children by exploiting the normal role of the intestinal microflora in modulating immune function and reducing the risk of infection. The final chapter discusses the growing problem of food allergies.

This book is authoritatively and clearly written. The summary points at the beginning of each chapter are particularly helpful and the references have been carefully selected for the material to which they refer without being excessive. It is written to be equally useful for students and researchers in developing and industrialized countries. Students who use this textbook will acquire a good basic understanding of the relationships among nutrition, immunity, infectious diseases and chronic diseases. This book is a valuable contribution to the training of students and researchers in nutrition, immunology, infectious disease, paediatrics, general medicine and public health.

Nevin S. Scrimshaw PhD, MD, MPH
Institute Professor Emeritus, Massachusetts Institute of Technology
President Emeritus, International Nutrition Foundation
Visiting Professor, Tufts University

Glossary

Achlorhydria A condition where the acid production in the stomach is abnormally low.

Acquired immunity or adaptive immunity Antigen-specific immunity that increases during infection. It is composed of highly specialized mechanisms that eliminate pathogens and has the ability to recognize and remember them, to mount stronger attacks each time the pathogen is encountered.

Allergen A non-parasitic or common environmental antigen capable of inducing a hypersensitivity reaction in an atopic individual.

Allogenic From different individuals of the same species.

Amoebiasis Infection caused by the pathogenic amoeba *Entamoeba histolytica*.

Anergy Lack of reaction by the body's defence mechanisms to foreign substances.

Angioedema Recurring attacks of oedema of the skin and mucous membrane, which suddenly appears.

Anorexia Loss of appetite leading to a reduction in food intake.

Antibodies Proteins (i.e. immunoglobulins) produced on exposure to an antigen that neutralize the activity of the antigen.

Antigen A molecule that induces a specific antibody or cell-mediated immune response.

Atopy or atopic syndrome A condition characterized by allergic hypersensitivity affecting parts of the body not in direct contact with the allergen.

Attributable risk The difference in the rate of a condition or disease between an exposed population and an unexposed population.

Autoantibody An antibody produced by the immune system that is directed against one or more of the individual's own proteins or cells.

Autoimmune disease A disease caused by an overactive immune response of the body against substances and tissues normally present in the body and where the body actually attacks its own cells, mistaking them for pathogens.

Bactericide A substance that can kill bacteria.

Body mass index (BMI) An index for assessing the appropriateness of weight-for-height in adults and children. It is weight (in kilograms) divided by the height (in metres) squared.

Candidiasis Also known as 'thrush'. A fungal infection which may vary from a superficial infection like oral thrush to a systemic and potentially life-threatening infection.

Cell-mediated immunity A defence mechanism directly mediated by cells, i.e. T lymphocytes.

Cephalo-pelvic disproportion A condition that exists when the capacity of the pelvis is inadequate to allow the fetus to negotiate the birth canal and may lead to obstructed labour.

Cheilosis An inflammatory lesion at the corner of the mouth, and often occurs bilaterally. Also referred to as angular stomatitis.

Chelator An agent that detoxifies poisonous and heavy metals, like mercury and arsenic, by converting them to a chemically inert form that can be excreted without further interaction with the body.

Chemokine A protein secreted by cells, which induces directed chemotaxis or chemical attraction in responsive cells.

Chemotaxis A process which causes cells, to direct their movements due to the presence of certain chemicals in the environment.

Colostrum The first milk produced by the mammary gland in late pregnancy, which is rich in antibodies.

Commensal An organism that exhibits commensalism, i.e. a relationship between two organisms where one organism benefits but the other is unharmed. Unlike mutualism where both organisms benefit and parasitism where one benefits and the other is harmed.

Complement system A biochemical cascade that amplifies the effects that result in helping to clear a pathogen from the body.

Complementary feeding The provision of foods and liquids along with continued breastfeeding of infants.

Cytokine A chemical that mediates communication between cells of the immune system.

Delayed cutaneous hypersensitivity (DCH) test A direct functional measure of cell-mediated immune response.

Eclampsia An acute and life-threatening complication of pregnancy, characterized by the appearance of seizures.

Endocytosis A process by which cells absorb molecules and nutrients from outside the cell by engulfing with their cell membrane.

Endotoxin Unlike an exotoxin, an endotoxin is not secreted in soluble form by live pathogens but is a structural component of the pathogenic cell and is released mainly when a pathogenic cell is lysed.

Epitope or antigenic determinant Part of the macromolecule (antigen) recognized by the immune system, more specifically by antibodies or by T and B lymphocytes. The part of the antibody that recognizes the epitope is referred to as the paratope.

Exclusive breastfeeding The provision of nothing but breast milk to an infant for the first 6 months of life.

Exotoxin A substance excreted by a pathogen that can cause major damage to the host by destroying cells, disrupting normal cellular metabolism. Exotoxins may be secreted or released like endotoxins following the death and lysis of the pathogenic cell.

Exposure The contact over time and space between the individual and one or more biological, chemical or physical agents.

Food allergy An adverse immune response to a food protein.

Food intolerance or non-allergic food hypersensitivity A delayed, negative reaction to a food, beverage or food additive that may produce symptoms in one or more body organs and systems.

Furunculosis Commonly referred to as a 'boil'. A skin disease caused by the infection of hair follicles and localized accumulation of pus and dead tissue. Individual boils can cluster together and form an interconnected network, called a carbuncle. Infection of the hair follicle of the skin is also referred to as folliculitis.

Gluconeogenesis Metabolic pathway through which glucose is produced from non-carbohydrate sources such as amino acids.

Gut-associated lymphoid tissue (GALT) The immune system within the gastrointestinal tract located in the lymphoid tissue.

Haptens A small molecule that can elicit an immune response only when attached to a large carrier protein, while the carrier may be incapable of eliciting an immune response by itself.

Helminth A parasitic worm which lives and feeds off a living host and may cause disease in the host.

Humoral immunity Defence mechanisms mediated indirectly by the production of antibodies by B lymphocytes.

Hyperkeratosis Thickening and keratinization of the skin.

Idiotype A shared characteristic between a group of immunoglobulin or T-cell-receptor molecules based on the antigen-binding specificity and the structure of their variable region.

Immunoglobulins A group of proteins categorized as gamma globulins that act as antibodies and come in different varieties known as isotype classes.

Immunomodulator A substance that modulates the immune response.

Immunosurveillance Immune cells that act as sentinels in recognizing and eliminating continuously arising, nascent transformed or abnormal cells.

Incidence A measure of the risk of developing a disease within a specified period of time. Often expressed simply as the number of new cases during a specific time period.

Incidence proportion or cumulative incidence The number of cases within a specified time period divided by the size of the population at risk.

Infant mortality rate The number of infant deaths (1 year of age or younger) per 1000 live births.

Inflammation Local changes that characterize the tissue response to the entry of a foreign body or pathogenic agent. It is a protective response to remove the injurious stimulus as well as to initiate the healing process.

Innate immunity or natural immunity Provides defence against infective agents and comprises mechanisms that defend the host in a non-specific manner. It does not confer long-lasting or protective immunity to the host.

Interferon A protein released in response to the presence of a pathogen or tumour cell which allows for the communication between cells, to trigger the immune system to respond to eradicate the pathogen or tumour cell.

Intrauterine growth restriction or retardation (IUGR) A condition that may result in a low-birth-weight or small-for-gestational-age infant.

Kwashiorkor Severe undernutrition in young children, characterized by oedema.

Leishmaniasis A disease caused by a protozoan parasite that is transmitted by the bite of certain species of sand fly.

Low birth weight (LBW) A full-term infant with a birth weight below 2500 g.

Lymphopaenia Abnormally low level of lymphocytes in the blood.

Lysozome A spherical organelle in the cell that contains enzymes to digest worn-out cell components, food particles, and engulfed and phagocytosed pathogens.

Marasmus Severe undernutrition in young children, characterized by severe muscle wasting.

Meta-analysis A statistical analysis that combines the results of several studies that address a set of related research hypotheses.

Metalloprotein A generic term for a protein that contains a metal ion as a cofactor. A metalloprotein fulfils several functions; when it acts as an enzyme it is referred to as a metalloenzyme.

Mitogen A protein that encourages a cell to commence division by triggering mitosis.

Multigravida A woman who has been pregnant more than one time.

Odds ratio The ratio of the odds of an event occurring in one group compared with the odds of it occurring in another group.

Opportunistic infection An infection caused by a pathogen that usually does not cause disease in a healthy host with a healthy immune system. A compromised immune system, however, presents an 'opportunity' for the pathogen to infect the host.

Opsonin A molecule that acts as a binding enhancer to facilitate phagocytosis.

Outcome The occurrence of disease, event or health related state.

Parasitaemia The quantitative content of parasites in blood, used as a measurement of parasite load in the organism and an indication of the degree of an active infection.

Partial breastfeeding The provision to the infant of other liquids and solids in addition to breast milk.

Pathogen Any foreign agent (worm or helminth, fungus, protozoan, bacterium, virus, prion) that gets into the human body and does harm of some kind.

Perinatal mortality Refers to the death of a fetus or neonate. The definition by the World Health Organization for perinatal mortality is 'deaths occurring during late pregnancy (at 22 completed weeks gestation and over), during childbirth and up to seven completed days of life'. Perinatal mortality thus includes the sum of both fetal and neonatal mortality.

Pertussis Also known as whooping cough. A highly infectious disease caused by the bacterium *Bordetella pertussis*.

Phagocytosis A cellular process which involves the engulfing and ingestion of solid particles or bacteria.

Population attributable risk The reduction in incidence that may be observed if the population were entirely unexposed, compared with its current exposure pattern.

Prebiotic A food ingredient that stimulates the growth and activity of bacteria in the gut which are beneficial to the health of the body.

Predominant breastfeeding The provision to the infant only of liquids, like water, in addition to breast milk.

Prevalence The total number of cases of the disease in the population at a given time, or the total number of cases in the population, divided by the number of individuals in the population.

Primigravida A woman who is pregnant for the first time or has been pregnant one time.

Prion An infectious agent composed solely of protein.

Probiotic Live organisms which when administered in adequate amounts confer health benefits to the host.

Prostaglandin A lipid mediator that acts on platelets and mast cells and is derived from essential fatty acids.

Protozoa Unicellular organisms, some of which may cause human disease like *Entamoeba* and *Giardia*.

Pyrogen Any fever-producing compound or substance.

Relative risk The risk of a nutritionally deficient child getting infection compared with the risk of a healthy child getting infection.

Retrovirus An RNA virus that is replicated in a host cell to produce DNA from its RNA genome; the DNA is then incorporated into the host's genome and the virus replicates as part of the host cell's DNA.

Rhinitis Irritation and inflammation of the inner mucosal surface of the nose.

Saccharolytic A form of fermentation of carbohydrate precursors by bacterial flora that results in the production of short-chain fatty acids.

Sarcopaenia The degenerative loss of skeletal muscle mass and strength associated with ageing.

SGA infant A full-term infant that is small for its gestational age due to intrauterine growth restriction.

Short-chain fatty acids (SCFA) A subgroup of fatty acids produced in the large intestine following the digestion of fibre and other carbohydrates by the microbial flora of the colon.

Stunting Undernutrition in children, characterized by growth faltering, which leads to short stature and a diagnosis of 'below acceptable range of height-for-age'.

Supplementary feeding The provision of extra foods to infants and children over and above the normal ration of their daily diets.

Synbiotic Nutritional supplements combining both prebiotics and probiotics.

Thalassaemia An inherited blood disease, which results in reduced synthesis of one of the globin chains of haemoglobin and causes the formation of abnormal haemoglobin molecules, thus leading to anaemia.

Vertical transmission Also known as mother-to-child transmission. The transmission of an infection from mother to child immediately before and after birth during the perinatal period.

Xerophthalmia Also known as keratomalacia. The eye signs associated with and characteristic of mild vitamin A deficiency in children, which may show as clouding of the cornea. It is a condition with pathologic dryness of the conjunctiva and cornea which, if untreated, may lead to corneal ulceration and blindness.

1 Nutrition, Immunity and Infection

- The global problem of undernutrition is linked both to poor access to adequate quantity and quality of food and to a poor environment which increases the risk of infectious diseases.
- Both generalized undernutrition and specific nutrient deficiencies are associated with increased frequency and severity of infections.
- Poor nutritional status has a synergistic association with infectious disease – infection predisposes to undernutrition and the undernourished state is susceptible to the risk of infection.
- In some instances nutrient deficiencies demonstrate an antagonistic relationship with infection.
- A historical analysis shows that the interactions of nutrition and infection are grounded in a good evidence base.

1.1 Introduction

The problem of undernutrition worldwide is one of enormous public health significance. Despite the major advances in agriculture and food production, over 900 million people are food insecure and nearly 2 billion are at risk of micronutrient deficiencies. They are at risk of inadequate access to and thus intake of adequate food which provides energy and protein. The poor quality of the diet further deprives them of the ability to meet their needs for a wide range of micronutrients like vitamins and minerals. The overall state of the poor environment they live in and the limited access to good health care impose a further burden of infectious disease risk. The complex interaction between the food they eat, the environment they live in and the overall state of their health perpetuates the undernutrition which is an invariant companion of poverty.

Undernutrition casts a long shadow, affecting about 20% of people in the developing world. It affects all ages although the most vulnerable are infants and children, women in the reproductive age range and the elderly in any population. It is estimated that over 148 million children are undernourished despite decades of efforts to reduce the problem. Undernutrition is responsible for premature mortality and plays a major role in the over 9 million deaths annually of children under 5 years

of age. Undernutrition contributes more than a third of these childhood deaths, while infections of the respiratory tract and diarrhoeal illness cause another third. In spite of major advances in universal immunization, measles still accounts for about 5% of these deaths and the other causes include malaria and HIV/AIDS. Undernutrition not only kills but causes disability such as blindness. Undernutrition not only affects intellectual and cognitive development but also affects work output and economic productivity, thus compromising economic development and human resource development of nations. Poor nutrition is not merely a medical problem but an economic and social problem rooted in poverty, discrimination and social inequalities.

1.2 Interaction and Synergism of Nutrition, Immunity and Infection

The suggestion that the relationship between undernutrition and infection is synergistic was made in the late 1950s. Collation of the extensive evidence published until that time demonstrated both the adverse effects of infective episodes on the nutritional status of the individual and the increased susceptibility to infection of the undernourished condition of the individual. Critical examination of this evidence suggested that each interacted to worsen the other and revealed that the effects of infection and under-nutrition combined were greater than the sum of the two. With our increasing understanding of the biology of the immune system and how it functions to protect the host from infections, the part played by the nutritional status of the individual generally and the role of specific nutrients in this process are now increasingly well recognized. The growth in our understanding of this interaction and synergism has resulted in the development of nutrition interventions and strategies to address public health issues such as the reduction of maternal and child morbidity and mortality in developing countries.

The functional impact of undernutrition on increased susceptibility to infections may result in mild morbidity to life-threatening infections and death. This results from undernutrition causing immunodeficiency and the compromise in immune function due to undernutrition, which is often referred to as 'nutritional immunodeficiency'. A range of host factors, which include non-specific barriers that prevent entry of pathogens and innate and acquired immune mechanisms, operate in the human body to prevent infections. Undernutrition compromises several of these functions, increasing the susceptibility to the infective agent. In addition to generalized undernutrition lowering the function of the immune systems, deficiencies of micronutrients like vitamins and minerals tend to specifically affect one or more components of the immune mechanisms and increase the risk of infections. Deficiencies in vitamin A and zinc are good examples of micronutrients that compromise immune function in man. It is important to know that micronutrient deficiencies are a much bigger public health problem, affecting nearly 2 billion people worldwide. In addition to compromising immune function, increasing susceptibility to infections and increasing the risk of morbidity and mortality, micronutrient deficiencies also impair physical and intellectual growth and reduce human capital. Repeated infective episodes in children reduce catch-up growth and result in growth faltering, thus contributing to forms of childhood undernutrition described as stunting and underweight.

The problems of overweight and obesity are increasing globally and now appearing increasingly alongside undernutrition in developing countries, posing a double burden of malnutrition. Overnutrition states like obesity may also compromise immune function and increase the risk of infections. This area has not been well studied, although evidence is now available to suggest that obesity increases the incidence of cutaneous infections like candidiasis, furunculosis and folliculitis. However, whether this is the result of overnutrition per se or due to possibly poor peripheral circulation or other problems relevant to the physiology of the skin is not clear.

A review of the early literature on the interactions of nutrition and infections illustrates the terminology that evolved to explain the effects, associations and interactions that were observed (see Box 1.1). The relationship between nutrition and infection in man is not always synergistic. In some instances, some nutrients like iron show an antagonistic interaction with infection. This paradoxical situation is exemplified by a nutrient deficiency favouring the host and providing a protective advantage to the host. The nutrient that typifies this type of response is iron. Iron deficiency favours the host by restricting the availability of this specific nutrient to the invasive pathogen. Excess iron or iron overload manifests with an antagonistic interaction as seen in Bantu tribesman who are at risk of fulminant amoebiasis as a result of excess of iron in their body from the consumption of an iron-laden brew. Malaria is another example where supplementation with iron increases malarial infection. In Zanzibar increased hospitalization and excess mortality were observed in children who were receiving iron supplements.

1.3 Historical Background to the Study of the Interactions of Nutrition and Infection

The simultaneous advances made in microbiological sciences and in the identification and functions of specific nutrients in the early years of the 20th century resulted in scientific exchanges between our understanding of infectious diseases and the nutritional sciences. It was soon becoming evident that the outcome of an infection was determined by the interaction of the infectious agent and the response of the host; the latter largely influenced by the host's nutritional status among other factors. These interactions provided not only a scientific basis for how infections impact on the nutritional status of an individual and worsen it, but also highlighted the role of poor nutrition in increasing the individual's susceptibility to a wide range of infections to which he or she is exposed. It needs to be pointed out that in the early years of our understanding of this interaction between infection and nutrition, more was

Box 1.1. Terminology Used in Interactions of Nutrition and Infection.

In the early years during the critical review of the literature on the interactions of nutrition and infection, terminology evolved in this field to summarize the effects, associations and interactions observed. Some of these terminologies are explained here.

- *Synergism* is when poor nutritional status or a specific nutritional deficiency promotes the frequency and severity of an infection. When infection aggravates undernutrition or undernutrition lowers resistance to infection, the relationship between the two is called 'synergistic'. The mutual interaction of the infectious disease and the undernutrition may act as a vicious cycle resulting in a fatal outcome. Synergism may result from a reduction in the capability of the host defence mechanisms to deal adequately with the infectious agent and may affect any component of the host's defence and immune systems.
- *Antagonism* is seen when a nutritional deficiency results in decreased frequency and severity of an infection. There are some instances where a

specific nutrient deficiency may favour the host and the interaction is then termed as being 'antagonistic'. The main determinant of this antagonistic interaction is attributed to the specific nutrient deficiency affecting the metabolic needs of the infectious agent and thus compromising the ability of the agent to promote the infection. The principal mechanism appears to be related to the lack of adequate amounts of that nutrient to meet the metabolic demands of the infectious agent in order for it to multiply and proliferate in the host's tissues. Good examples of antagonistic interactions are seen in iron deficiency states and malarial infection.

These terms imply an interaction of the host with the infectious agent. Synergism usually results when the nutritional deficiency acts mainly on the host to compromise the host's defence mechanisms, while in antagonism the main impact is on the infectious agent. They also imply a decrease or an increase respectively in the resistance to the infectious agent offered by the host.

---

known of the former than of the latter; it is only in more recent times, in the latter half of the last century, that the role of specific nutrients in influencing the susceptibility of the host to infectious agents has been better understood.

It was evident from a careful review of the literature carried out 50 years ago that the interactions of most infections with nutritional deficiencies in man were almost always synergistic. The risk of infection was higher among those with poor nutrition, the consequences of infection were likely to be more serious in the undernourished person, and the infectious disease in turn nearly always worsened coexisting undernutrition. This implied that the synergistic interaction between infection and nutrition may create a vicious cycle which often results in a fatal outcome. Thus the synergistic interactions of infection and undernutrition would contribute not only to morbidity but also to mortality.

Evidence for synergistic interactions of nutrition and infection are numerous in the historical literature. During World War I, the mortality due to tuberculosis (TB) in Denmark rose when the diet lacked meat and fish but decreased markedly when local consumption of meat increased as a result of the German blockade. Between the World War

years, naval cadets in Norway showed a dramatic reduction in morbidity due to TB when the quality of their diets improved. During World War II death rates from TB doubled in Germany and the prevalence of TB was high among Russians prisoners of war who had poor diets, compared with British prisoners of war. Post-war, among US recruits to the Navy, those who were underweight had four times as much TB as those with normal weight. All these are instances of a synergism between the nutrition of individuals and their susceptibility to bacterial infections like TB. There are innumerable examples illustrating this synergism in the literature since those times, which include observations from developing countries that measles was more severe in poorly nourished children and that moderate to severe malnutrition was often precipitated in infants and children following episodes of infectious illnesses.

That undernutrition increases susceptibility to infectious diseases and that they in turn have an adverse effect on the nutritional state was recognized by the World Health Organization (WHO) soon after it was founded at the end of World War II. A Joint Food and Agriculture Organization/WHO Expert Committee on Nutrition recommended in

1950 that the relationship between nutritional status and infections be studied. From a historical perspective, a systematic approach to examine this complex interaction between nutrition and infection apparently began with a review published by Scrimshaw, Taylor and Gordon in 1959 in *The American Journal of Medical Sciences*. They were further supported by investigations carried out in developing countries which showed that acute infectious diseases, both bacterial and viral, were a main contributing factor to the development of protein–energy malnutrition in infants and children. Other studies demonstrated the interactions between nutritional deficiencies and acute diarrhoeal disease, while health programmes aimed at the control of infectious diseases suggested that episodes of infections were often closely associated with undernutrition. All these developments culminated in the WHO convening a meeting of experts in 1965. This WHO Expert Committee on Nutrition and Infection examined the interrelationships between undernutrition and infectious diseases and put forward suggestions for a comprehensive programme of research in this area. The authors of the 1959 review (Scrimshaw, Taylor and Gordon) were given the task to collate, examine and sift the vast amount of epidemiological, clinical and experimental evidence, which resulted in the seminal publication in this area in 1968 in the form of a WHO Monograph entitled *Interactions of Nutrition and Infection*. The paradigm outlined in this important monograph has endured and enlightened this field of interdisciplinary science for at least the last 40 years.

One of the important outcomes of the focus of interest in this area of interactions of nutrition and infection was the initiation and conduct of a classic prospective study carried out in the Guatemalan highlands between the years 1964 to 1972. The most important publication that resulted from this 9-year prospective incidence observation study on the interactions of infection and nutrition is the classic book by Leonarda Mata entitled *The Children of Santa Maria Cauque: A Prospective Field Study of Health and Growth*. Figure 5.1 (in Chapter 5) from Mata's book is one example that demonstrates how a child growing normally shows growth faltering and deterioration in nutritional status occurring at the onset of weaning from repeated infections and poor supplementary feeding.

From a historical perspective, distinctions between generalized undernutrition or inanition (from a reduction in the intakes of all nutrients) and the relative deficiency of one or more specific nutrients (specific nutrient deficiencies) became important as our understanding of this interaction developed over time. The role of specific nutrients such as vitamin A manifesting both as an increase in mortality due to infections in mild deficiency states and a positive impact following supplementation in children in Indonesia elaborated the latter aspect of this interaction. It also coincided with the tremendous growth in our appreciation of the science of immunology over the years. And in the last two decades, the advent of new and emerging infections like HIV has once again fuelled interest in the need to understand the intimate relationship that nutrition has with human immune function and infection.

The HIV/AIDS global epidemic has highlighted once again the importance of the intimate relationship that nutrition has with human immune function and infection. Several research studies and nutrition interventions being undertaken in Africa and Asia alongside clinical trials of antiretroviral drugs emphasize the crucial role of the interplay between nutrition and immunity in human infection. These programmes not merely aim to assess the effectiveness of enhancing nutritional status of the host in improving the immune responsiveness, but also evaluate an adjuvant role for nutritional supplements during the therapeutic treatment for the infection. While the HIV/AIDS problem captures current interest in this interaction between nutrition, immunity and infections, it is important to remind ourselves of the long historical background to this nutrition–immunity relationship, that the interactions of nutrition and infection have much to do with the persisting global problem of undernutrition and that intervention strategies are needed to address these huge global public health problems. Interest in the clinical management of hospitalized patients who are at risk of undernutrition has also contributed to the growth in this field of nutrition and infection. All of these aspects will be covered in more detail in this book.

1.4 Rationale for the Book

Nutrition is both a scientific discipline and an applied science. It is a broad church that is open to and has benefited from the contributions of a wide range of academic disciplines and sciences – from archaeology and anthropology to public health – and by the end of the 20th century was occupied quite legitimately by journalists and activists. The truth is that we all eat and enjoy food and hence believe that we know a lot about food and nutrition. The field of nutrition is now a vast and diverse terrain. Anyone who is involved in and has the responsibility to impart information knows that graduate programmes in the area of nutrition cater to a wide range of students, a fair proportion of whom are learning about the subject for the first time. There are epidemiologists, statisticians and public health workers who have a barely passable knowledge of nutritional sciences or of the biology of human immune function. They need to know enough to appreciate the close interactions in both nutrition and infection for an understanding of the literature, which perhaps pertains to a double-blind placebo-controlled clinical trial with a nutrient supplement in the community where the outcome measurements may be changes in immune responses. It is hoped this book will provide sufficient knowledge to the uninitiated in this area to enable their appreciation of the significance of: (i) what is being supplemented and why? (ii) what is being assessed and evaluated as an outcome in response? (iii) how and why is it being reflected in an indicator of immune function and what is the scientific basis for expecting this change?

A student of nutrition on the other hand may benefit from understanding why a particular indicator of immune function has been chosen, while someone familiar with immunology might recognize the importance of a nutrient and the role it plays in maintaining this important immune function. The modular structure of this book caters to the needs of its intended wide audience by providing some information in boxes that can be studied or ignored depending on the individual needs of the reader. The boxes with case studies and other material culled from the literature emphasize and illustrate the significant points that are being made and provide some evidence base for the material in the text in the various chapters.

1.5   Structure of the Book

The book begins after this introduction with a general outline of the immune systems of the human body (Chapter 2). It describes first the defence mechanisms of the body including the physical barriers that prevent entry of infectious agents. It then provides a basic description of both innate and adaptive immunity. Innate immunity is mediated by cells that recognize, attack and deal with pathogens, aided by molecules such as complement. Adaptive

or acquired immunity occurs either by cell-mediated mechanisms or by humoral mechanisms characterized by the production of antibodies. Next, the specific role of nutrients, both macro and micro, that influence the immune system is described, along with the likely mechanisms that are affected in a deficiency of that nutrient (Chapter 3).

The next two chapters describe the consequences of moderate to severe undernutrition on immune function (Chapter 4) and the important role that episodes of infection have in inducing and perpetuating undernutrition, as well outlining the various ways in which they contribute to cause undernutrition (Chapter 5). The next three chapters address specifically the association between deficiency of vitamin A (Chapter 6), iron status (i.e. both deficiency and excess; Chapter 7) and zinc deficiency (Chapter 8) and the risk of infection.

The next set of chapters discusses the importance of nutrition and its interaction with the immune system in major public health problems such as diarrhoeal diseases and respiratory illness as well as killer diseases like HIV/AIDS and TB (the latter in Chapter 9). The following three chapters then address this important interaction and how it affects the nutrition and health of the most vulnerable groups, i.e. infants and children (Chapter 10), maternal nutrition and its impact on birth outcomes (Chapter 11) and the elderly (Chapter 12).

The last three chapters address important recent developments in the field of nutrition and immune function interactions such as those that affect cancer and autoimmune diseases (Chapter 13), the role played by probiotics and prebiotics which are food- and nutrient-based approaches to modify immune function (Chapter 14), and food allergy and food intolerance (Chapter 15).

Further Reading

Mata, L.J. (1978) *The Children of Santa Maria Cauque: A Prospective Field Study of Health and Growth.* MIT Press, Cambridge, Massachusetts. *An extraordinary account of a 9-year prospective incidence observation study of infection and nutrition in a community living in a Guatemalan highland village.*

Scrimshaw, N.S., Gordon, C.E. and Taylor, J.E. (1968) *Interactions of Nutrition and Infection.* World Health Organization, Geneva, Switzerland. *A comprehensive review of the then literature on the interrelationships of infectious disease and malnutrition, drawing attention to its public health importance.*

2 Immune Systems: The Defence Mechanisms of the Body

- The human body's defence mechanisms against infectious organisms consist of physical barriers that prevent entry of these agents and the immune system which fights them; the latter is composed of both innate and adaptive components.
- Physical barriers such as the integrity of the skin, the secretions of mucous membranes, the high acidity of the stomach and the normal bacterial flora of the gut act as a first line of defence for the body.
- The inflammatory process is characterized by redness, warmth, swelling, pain and loss of function, and is a manifestation of the tissue's response to the entry of a foreign body or agent.
- Innate immunity is mediated by cells that recognize, attack, engulf by phagocytosis and dispose of pathogens, aided by molecules such as complement.
- The adaptive or acquired immune response of the body occurs in two forms: by cell-mediated immune mechanisms mediated largely by T lymphocytes and by humoral mechanisms characterized by the production of antibodies mediated largely by B lymphocytes.
- Cytokines are proteins secreted by the cells of the immune system; they modulate the activity of the immune mechanism.
- Several tests are available to assess the normal functioning of the immune system.

2.1 Introduction

The environment surrounding us is crowded with organisms; not all of them are visible but some enter our body and cause harm, resulting in infection and disease. There are numerous others that do not always cause disease even when they use the human body as a host, and instead establish beneficial relationships with the human host. The organisms that get into the human body and do harm of some kind vary in magnitude from those visible to the naked eye like worms or helminths, to ones largely visible only under microscopy including fungi, protozoa, bacteria and viruses, to others not seen like prions. Such organisms that are agents of disease are referred to as *pathogens*.

The human body has a range of defence mechanisms to tackle these pathogens. The first line of defence is the ability of the human host to prevent entry of the pathogen and the next response is that mediated by the host's natural or innate immunity. If the pathogen overcomes these obstacles, the host has the ability to resist infection and

disease by resorting to adaptive immunity. Failure at any of these stages of the battle between the pathogen and the human host can result in disease and even death of the host. The human immune system is complex and highly organized, and functions to protect the individual from a range of environmental agents or pathogens that can infect the body and cause disease. From the perspective of this book it is important to note from the start that poor nutrition can compromise the body's ability to mount effective defence and immune responses, while infections, in turn, can undermine the normal nutritional status of an individual.

2.2 The Defence Mechanisms of the Body

The principal defence mechanisms of the body are based on the body's ability to distinguish and identify cells and molecules that are a part of itself, i.e. 'self', and those that are 'non-self' or foreign. It thus has the ability to distinguish friend

Box 2.1. Tests of Immune Function.

The outline in this box on tests of immune function is specifically directed towards the principal aim of this book to show the close interrelationships between nutrition, immune functions and infections. Hence it does not provide an exhaustive account of the various immune tests. It deals only with tests used in clinical practice or those that are favoured by researchers interested in studying the interactions between immune function and nutrition.

Changes in immune function are consistently seen during generalized malnutrition and in deficiencies of specific nutrients such as vitamin A, iron and zinc. The evidence that these changes in immune responses can be reversed by nutritional repletion or following supplementation of the specific nutrients that are deficient, suggests that the observed changes are due to the impact of changes in nutritional status. As a result, tests of immunocompetence have been used as a measure of the functional index of nutritional status. It is important to note, however, that these tests are not specific enough to detect individual nutrient deficiencies. There are many other factors that affect immunological responses and these include emotional stress and physical stress associated with trauma, surgery, anaesthesia, burns, etc. The immune response is also involved in the pathophysiology of several diet-related diseases like type 2 diabetes mellitus, cardiovascular disease and some cancers. The immunological tests should, therefore, be used in conjunction with other tests assessing nutritional status and should be interpreted in the light of other findings.

Although humoral immunity is generally less affected than cell-mediated immunity by changes in nutritional status, nearly all aspects of the immune system can be impaired by general or specific nutritional deficiency. The following tests of immune function are often used to complement the assessment of nutritional status in individuals and in clinical practice:

- lymphocyte count;
- T-lymphocyte count;
- lymphocyte proliferation assay (lymphocyte mitogen assay);
- cytokine assays;
- complement assays and acute-phase proteins;
- delayed cutaneous hypersensitivity (DCH) tests, also referred to as delayed-type hypersensitivity (DTH) tests.

Lymphocyte count

Of the total leucocytes in the blood of healthy, well-nourished individuals, lymphocytes account for 20–40% of white blood cells. The average total lymphocyte count is about 2750 cells/mm^3 (range 1500–4000 cells/mm^3), but is reduced in malnourished subjects. Lymphocyte counts ranging from 900 to 1500 cells/mm^3 are indicative of moderate nutritional depletion, while in severe nutritional depletion the lymphocyte count is below 900 cells/mm^3. Factors such as stress, sepsis, concurrent infection and some drugs (e.g. steroids) may affect the total lymphocyte count.

T-lymphocyte count

T lymphocytes constitute 75–80% of the circulating lymphocytes. They are reduced in both absolute number and relative proportion in the peripheral blood during malnutrition. In most instances, these changes are reversed following nutritional repletion; this demonstrates their sensitivity to nutritional status. Sequential counts of T cells can thus be helpful in assessing the response to nutritional repletion and recovery in malnourished individuals. T-lymphocyte numbers can be assessed by suspending washed lymphocytes in saline, mixing the suspension with sheep red blood cells, and calculating the proportion of lymphocytes that form 'rosettes' with three or more sheep red blood cells. Alternatively, T cells can be measured using CD3$^+$ surface markers. Measurement of T lymphocytes is now done by flow cytometry.

Lymphocyte proliferation assay (lymphocyte mitogen assay)

These assays measure the functional capability of lymphocytes. Lymphocyte function can be assessed by exposing the cells to antigens or mitogens, which cause them to divide and proliferate. In cases of immune dysfunction, mitogen-induced proliferation is decreased. The mitogens commonly used are concavallin A (Con A) and phytohaemagglutinin (PHA). This is a sophisticated test that measures the rate of DNA synthesis by counting the amount of ^{3}H-labelled thymidine incorporated following 16–24 h of incubation with the mitogen. These assays are a more direct measure of immunocompetence and assess cell-mediated immune response. Lymphocyte proliferation assays are more sensitive than total lymphocyte counts as they can pick up age-related reduction in immune response even in the absence of changes in nutritional status in the elderly.

Cytokine assays

Immunoassays can be used to measure levels of specific cytokines. The most popular technique is the ELISA, many of them now available as commercial kits. Currently these assays are largely research tools.

Continued

Box 2.1. Continued.

Complement assays and acute-phase proteins

Measuring the levels of complement, more specifically complement C3, is now increasingly popular. Complement C3 is an acute-phase reactant (acute-phase protein) and its level increases in healthy individuals in response to an acute infection. In malnourished individuals the levels of complement C3 are low and decrease even further during an infection.

Other acute-phase proteins such as C-reactive protein are also measured in clinical practice, which provides further evidence of an acute-phase response during an active infection or reactivation of a chronic condition.

Delayed cutaneous hypersensitivity test

The DCH test is a direct functional measure of cell-mediated immunity *in vivo*. When healthy individuals are re-exposed to antigens intradermally, the result is an induration (hardened area) and erythema (redness) in the skin. The size of the induration at the end of 48 h is a measure of the cutaneous cell-mediated immune response to the antigen. These skin reactions are decreased in malnourished individuals

(whether the malnourishment is generalized or due to specific deficiencies) and are reversed after nutritional repletion.

To conduct this test, a battery of specific antigens is injected intradermally in the forearm and the cutaneous response noted at the end of 24 and 48 h. The antigens commonly used are purified protein derivative (PPD), some antigenic derivative of the infective agent causing mumps, *Trichophyton*, *Candida* and dinitrochlorobenzene (DNCB). Many non-nutritional factors can affect DCH responses and hence reduce the specificity and sensitivity of the test. Several technical problems associated with DCH test, mainly due to reader variability and other factors, have been eliminated by the use of delayed hypersensitivity skin test kits. These kits consist of a sterile, disposable, plastic multi-puncture application instrument consisting of eight test heads preloaded with standardized doses of seven antigens (tuberculin, tetanus toxoid, diphtheria toxoid, *Streptococcus*, *Candida*, *Trichophyton* and *Proteus*). This test kit reduces false negatives, has increased sensitivity and is standardized for the reading of the skin response.

from foe. This ability to discriminate between 'self' and 'non-self' is fundamental to the body's defence system, the immune mechanism. However, other barriers, largely physical, are initially involved in defending the body from foreign agents and preventing entry of the pathogen into the human host. The best and simplest approach to understanding the host defence mechanisms would be to consider them separately at the three levels or stages of their operation or as 'lines of defence' (Fig. 2.1), although it is likely that in real life they may operate all at the same time during an infective episode.

The three levels of host defence mechanisms are the following:

1. Physical barriers or external defences that prevent the entry of the pathogen.
2. The *innate immune system* that utilizes already available cells and molecules in the host, which are deployed to confront and dispose of the pathogen.
3. The *adaptive immune system*, which utilizes specialized cells that identify and target the pathogen and also retain a memory of the pathogen for rapid and early mobilization in the future,

should a similar pathogen gain entry to the host organism.

The immune system is complex and comes into play when the pathogen has gained entry into the human host. The immune system is comprised of organs, cells and molecules dispersed throughout the body; this complex network functions due to both: (i) its ability to recognize the pathogen or infectious agent; and (ii) its capability to confront, eliminate and dispose of the pathogen. It has another important component – its sophisticated communication system – which coordinates the activities of the various recognition and attack or disposal components of this complex network of defence mechanisms. Recognition components operate on the basis of the host's ability to distinguish 'self' from 'non-self' (or foreign), and range from non-specific to very specific recognition. The non-specific recognition component is characteristic of innate immune mechanisms, while the adaptive immune systems are based on specific recognition. The attack and disposal component comprises the phagocytic cells of the host, which attack and phagocytose (or 'eat') the pathogen. These phagocytic cells have recognition capabilities built into their surface but also take advantage

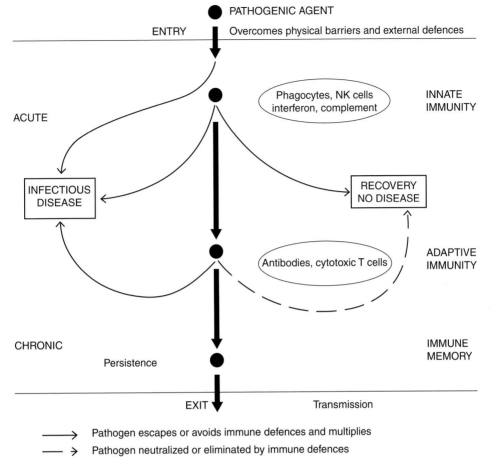

PATHOGENIC AGENT

ENTRY   Overcomes physical barriers and external defences

ACUTE

Phagocytes, NK cells
interferon, complement

INNATE
IMMUNITY

INFECTIOUS
DISEASE

RECOVERY
NO DISEASE

Antibodies, cytotoxic T cells

ADAPTIVE
IMMUNITY

CHRONIC

Persistence

IMMUNE
MEMORY

EXIT   Transmission

→ Pathogen escapes or avoids immune defences and multiplies

- → Pathogen neutralized or eliminated by immune defences

Fig. 2.1. Schematic illustration of the lines of defence against a pathogenic agent and the levels at which the two components of the immune system operate to deal with the pathogen after it breaks through the physical barriers of the body. (Adapted from Playfair and Bancroft, 2004.)

of circulating recognition molecules such as complement and antibodies. Phagocytes can attack, engulf and dispose of small pathogens like bacteria (intracellular killing), and they can attack other pathogens by attaching themselves from the outside and killing them (extracellular killing), some of which may need the assistance of antibodies. The cells of the immune system communicate with each other either by direct cell-to-cell contact or by a network of chemical molecules called cytokines. These chemicals have historically acquired different names based on the observation of their actions or functions (interferons, tumour necrosis factor, colony-stimulating factors, chemokines, etc.), but are now increasingly designated as they are discovered as interleukins, meaning 'between white cells' – obviously referring

to their principal function for communication between white blood cells.

The immune system demonstrates both a generalized response and processes directed at specific disease organisms or toxins. The former results in general processes which make the human body resistant to such diseases as paralytic virus disease of animals, hog cholera, cattle plague and distemper. This is called innate immunity. A comparison of the innate with the adaptive immune systems (Table 2.1) reveals the differences between these two components of the body's defence mechanisms. The innate system is old in evolutionary terms, being seen in the earliest animals both invertebrates and vertebrates, while adaptive immunity is a feature of vertebrates only and hence of relatively

Table 2.1. Comparison of the main features of the innate and adaptive immune systems. (Adapted from Playfair and Bancroft, 2004.)

	Innate immunity	Adaptive immunity
Origin	Early in evolution	More recent origins
Organisms	Invertebrates and vertebrates	Vertebrates
Specificity	Low	Very high
Response	Very rapid (minutes/hours)	Relatively slow (days)
Memory	No	Yes
Cells involved	Neutrophils	B lymphocytes
	Monocytes/macrophages	T lymphocytes
	Dendritic cells	CD4$^+$ cells
	Mast cells	CD8$^+$ cells
	Natural killer cells	
Chemical mediators	Complement	Antibodies
	Cytokines	Cytokines
	Interferons	
	Acute-phase proteins	
Mechanisms	Chemotaxis	Cell-mediated immunity
	Opsonization	Humoral immunity
	Phagocytosis	
	Intracellular killing	
Characteristic	First line of defence inside host	Flexible, vigorous but regulated

more recent origin. The emphasis of the innate system is on attack or disposal while that of the adaptive component is on very specific recognition, with disposal often left to the innate system.

The principal cells of innate immunity are phagocytes while lymphocytes are the main cells involved in adaptive immunity. Communication in both systems is by cytokines but the other principal circulating molecules aiding action are complement and antibodies in innate immunity and adaptive immunity, respectively. The specificity of recognition is broad and across the board in innate systems. On the other hand, the very highly specific recognition along with the development of memory constitutes the hallmark of adaptive immunity. There is no development of memory in innate systems but the speed of action is rapid, occurring within minutes to hours of the entry of the pathogen. The adaptive system is slow to respond, with the memory providing a relatively rapid response on subsequent exposure to the agent or pathogen. The adaptive response is flexible and vigorous and depends on regulatory mechanisms to prevent it from going on too long or causing damage to the host. The human body has both innate and adaptive components and both systems are required and act in concert to optimize actions during an infection.

2.3 Physical Barriers to Infectious Agents or Pathogens

The physical barriers that protect the body from invasion by infective agents or pathogens are:

- the integrity of the skin;
- the mucous membranes lining the hollow viscera such as the respiratory, intestinal and urogenital tracts, their cilia and secretions;
- antibacterial components in the skin and mucous secretions including sweat, sebaceous secretions and tears;
- the highly acidic pH of the stomach, which prevents passage of most organisms beyond the stomach;
- enzymes such as lysozymes in tears and other secretions;
- the normal bacterial flora of the skin and intestine.

Natural physical barriers to infectious agents are a simple yet effective means of defence. A major physical barrier is provided by the intact skin, which is generally impermeable to most infectious agents. Sweat glands and sebaceous glands in the skin seem ideal as potential points of entry for infectious agents. However, most bacteria fail to enter due to the low pH; the direct inhibitory effects of the various secretions of the glands in the skin and their potent antimicrobial proteins, such as lysozymes, lactoferrins, defensins and peroxidases; and the lactic acid and fatty acids in sweat and sebaceous secretions. The antimicrobial action may result from enzymatic digestion of the pathogen or by inflicting damage to the membrane of the pathogenic organism. If the continuity and the integrity of the skin is disrupted or broken it allows for easy entry of pathogenic organisms, resulting in the risk of infection.

The mucous membrane linings of hollow organs such as the respiratory, intestinal and urogenital tracts are more delicate and hence vulnerable to entry by pathogens. Mucus and other secretions of these tracts that connect the internal organs to the external body surfaces form an important form of defence. They trap and immobilize bacteria and thereby prevent adherence and colonization of epithelial surfaces. In addition, the outward or upward beating action of the cilia lining some of these tracts, e.g. the respiratory tract, helps move the trapped organisms in the mucus up to be coughed out or swallowed. Hairs at the external nares (the nostrils) of the respiratory tract prevent entry, while the cough reflex and the ciliated nature of the mucous membrane along with the mucus secretions, operating together and referred to as the 'muco-ciliary escalator', help drive entrapped organisms upwards and outwards to be expelled. Some organisms are capable of neutralizing the muco-ciliary escalator by forming firm attachments to the membrane of the respiratory tract and by inhibiting ciliary motion. The alveoli of the respiratory tract contain surfactant proteins which, in addition to helping reduce surface tension, contribute to aggregation and thus enhanced uptake of pathogens by phagocytic cells. Many antimicrobial proteins and peptides are present and function effectively from the thin layer of liquid between the mucus layer and the epithelium of the respiratory tract. Both the high acidity of the gastric secretions and the detergent actions of bile salts protect the digestive tract from pathogens, while protective antibodies and the normal bacterial flora of the gut also contribute to this defence function.

Other mechanical factors that help protect the body are the rinsing actions of tears, saliva and urine. Many bodily secretions contain bactericidal components, for example: hydrochloric acid in gastric juice; lactoperoxidase in breast milk; lysozymes in tears, nasal secretions and saliva; and the proteo-lytic enzymes in gastrointestinal digestive secretions. The normal bacterial flora of both the skin and the gastrointestinal tract also provide an important barrier of defence. They suppress the growth of potentially pathogenic bacteria and fungi by competing for essential nutrients or by producing substances that inhibit the growth of pathogens.

2.4 Inflammation and Innate Immunity

The human body has the ability to resist all types of organisms or infectious agents that are likely to attack and damage organ systems and tissues. The entry of infectious agents past the initial physical barriers leads to the initiation of processes that are aimed at dealing with and confining the spread of the infection. The special cellular systems for combating infectious agents after they have breached the physical barriers are the white blood cells or leucocytes. Leucocytes are immediately attracted to the point at which the infective agent has passed the barrier. This attraction of the white blood cells to the foreign agent is the result of a series of changes that occur in the tissues that are injured or breached by the infectious agent or pathogen.

Inflammatory response

The complex of characteristic changes that occur in tissues attacked by infective agents is called inflammation or the *inflammatory response*. The five features of tissue inflammation are redness, warmth, swelling, pain and loss of function. An inflammatory response is characterized by:

- dilation of local blood vessels with consequent excess local blood flow, resulting largely in redness and warmth;
- increased permeability of the capillaries with leakage of large quantities of fluid and proteins into the tissue spaces, causing swelling and pain;
- clotting of fluid in the tissue spaces, which may occur because of excessive amounts of proteins such as fibrinogen leaking from the blood vessels;
- migration of large numbers of leucocytes into the tissues – in particular, neutrophils and macrophages – along with other molecules in demand during an inflammatory response;
- swelling of the cells and tissue spaces contributing to the swelling and compounded by the pain, leading to loss of function.

Many tissue products are released in response to and as a result of the entry of infectious agents that are responsible for tissue inflammation. These products include histamine, bradykinin, serotonin, prostaglandins, reaction products of the complement system and the blood clotting system, along with a wide range of hormones and other chemicals such as cytokines and leucotrienes. Several of these substances not only increase blood flow to the region, they also attract the leucocytes to the region of tissue injury. This attraction is called *chemotaxis* and is aided by several of the reaction products listed above as well as by some bacterial toxins and by degenerative products of tissue injury (referred to as chemokines). Some of the chemicals released (e.g. histamine) are responsible for vasodilation, while others (e.g. bradykinin, histamine and leucotrienes) are responsible for an increase in permeability and the subsequent leakage of capillary blood leading to swelling and the pain associated with inflammation. So too are prostaglandins, since they generally induce vasodilation, increase sensitivity of nerves to pain stimuli, and may also induce fever in an individual with inflammation.

The earliest reaction to an infection is the inflammatory response, which is often accompanied by fever and other symptoms of an acute illness. This phase is characterized by the appearance of a range of proteins referred to as *acute-phase proteins*. These are produced by the liver, stimulated by the chemical mediators of innate immunity – the cytokines secreted by the phagocytes. While the levels of normal plasma proteins such as albumin, transferrin and lipoproteins are reduced, the level of acute-phase proteins rises in the circulation. These acute-phase proteins include protease inhibitors (antitrypsin and antichymotrypsin), components of complement, transport proteins like caeruloplasmin and haptoglobin, clotting factors like fibrinogen and more specific proteins like C-reactive protein (CRP) which appear to be antibacterial, as well as others like serum amyloid A protein and acid glycoprotein. The acute-phase response is caused by a wide range of stimulants. Raised CRP in the blood is often a useful sign of an acute infection, of the acute exacerbation of a chronic disease like rheumatoid arthritis, or of chronic infection.

Box 2.2. Acute-phase Response and Acute-phase Proteins.

Two important physiological responses associated with acute inflammation are fever and the acute-phase response. The first involves the alteration of the temperature set-point in the hypothalamus and the generation of the febrile response or onset of fever. The second involves alterations in metabolism and liver function. Three cytokines that are released from the site of tissue injury, i.e. interleukins IL-1, IL-6 and tumour necrosis factor (TNF-α), mediate fever and regulate the febrile response through the induction of prostaglandin E, possibly as a protective mechanism. The second important aspect of the acute-phase response is the alteration in the biosynthetic function of the liver. Under normal circumstances, the liver synthesizes a characteristic range of plasma proteins at steady-state concentrations. During acute inflammation, the plasma levels of several of these proteins increase (while some decrease), since many of these proteins have important functions and the higher plasma levels of these proteins are required during the acute-phase response following an inflammatory stimulus. Although most of these acute-phase proteins (APPs)

are synthesized by liver cells (hepatocytes), some are produced by other cell types, including monocytes, endothelial cells, fibroblasts and adipocytes.

Hence, APPs, also known as acute-phase reactants (APRs), are proteins whose concentrations in plasma or blood change and generally increase in response to inflammation resulting from infection, tissue injury or other forms of stress. Some proteins decrease in response to inflammation and are referred to as 'negative acute-phase proteins', as opposed to the majority of proteins whose levels increase and are called 'positive acute-phase proteins'. They include not only proteins but also cellular elements of blood clotting such as platelets. This response to inflammation is called the *acute-phase reaction* or acute-phase response.

During the inflammatory response to an injury or infection leucocytes such as neutrophil granulocytes and macrophages secrete a number of cytokines into the bloodstream, predominant among them the IL-1, IL-6 and IL-8, and TNF-α. The liver responds to these chemicals by producing a large number of APPs while the production of other proteins is reduced. Most APPs are specialized secretory products made by the liver and work outside the cell. Various APRs are induced to varying extents during inflammation. For instance, serum amyloid A protein increases over 1000-fold during an acute inflammation while α-antitrypsin increases only two- to three-fold. Some like haptoglobin (a haemoglobin-binding protein) are also antioxidants. Many are induced by cytokines, while others like CRP are not only released in response to cytokines but also affect the immune system themselves in turn, by regulating the secretion of cytokines.

Other APPs are not strictly immunological. Examples are iron-binding proteins such as transferrin, haptoglobin and haemopexin, which are released by the liver during an infection to mop up iron. This mopping-up role fulfils three important functions: (i) it keeps iron from being accessible to the invading organism; (ii) as cells die during an infection, these important nutrients are salvaged for reuse and prevented from inducing oxidative damage to the tissues; and (iii) the bound iron is taken up by host cells with appropriate receptors to allow host cells to survive protracted attack by the invading organism.

Thus APRs have a wide range of activities that contribute to host defence. They directly neutralize inflammatory agents and help to minimize the extent of local tissue damage, as well as participate in tissue repair and regeneration. There is a rapid increase in the plasma concentration of many complement cascade components, the activation of which ultimately results in the local accumulation of neutrophils, macrophages and plasma proteins. These participate in the killing of infectious agents, the clearance of foreign and host cellular debris, and the repair of damaged tissue. Coagulation components, such as fibrinogen, play an essential role in promoting wound healing. Proteinase inhibitors neutralize the lysosomal proteases released following the infiltration of activated neutrophils and macrophages, thus controlling the activity of the pro-inflammatory

enzyme cascades. The increased plasma levels of some metal-binding proteins help prevent iron loss during infection and injury, also minimizing the level of haem iron available for uptake by bacteria and acting as a scavenger for potentially damaging oxygen free radicals.

Positive APPs include C-reactive protein (CRP), D-dimer protein, mannose-binding protein, α_1-anti trypsin, α_1-antichymotrypsin, α_2-macroglobulin, complement factors, ferritin, serum amyloid, caeruloplasmin, haptoglobin and coagulation factors such as fibrinogen, prothrombin and factor VIII, von Willebrand factor and plasminogen. Positive APPs serve different physiological functions for the immune system. Some act to destroy or inhibit growth of microbes, e.g. CRP, mannose-binding protein, complement factors, ferritin, caeruloplasmin, serum amyloid A and haptoglobin. Others give negative feedback on the inflammatory response, e.g. serpins and α_2-macroglobulin, while coagulation factors affect the coagulation function. Serpins also act to down-regulate inflammation. Negative APPs are albumin, transferrin, transthyretin, transcortin and retinol-binding protein (RBP). Reduction in levels of transcortin for instance decreases the binding of cortisol during an inflammatory response. Most APRs are inducible by IL-1, IL-6 or TNF-α, while others like albumin, prealbumin, fibronectin, and caeruloplasmin are regulated only by IL-6.

The clinical significance of APPs is that they are useful markers of inflammation in a patient and correlate well with erythrocyte sedimentation rate. They are thus of value in following up response to treatment and in assessing prognosis. They may also indicate liver failure. The responsiveness of CRP to acute-phase stimuli, along with its wide concentration range and ease of measurement, has led to plasma CRP levels being used to monitor accurately the severity of inflammation and the efficacy of disease management during an infection.

Phagocytosis

In addition to the physical barriers that operate to help provide a major defence mechanism of the body, the two most important mechanisms involved in innate immunity are: (i) phagocytosis by neutrophils, macrophages and other cells; and (ii) the presence in circulating blood of certain humoral or chemical compounds that assist this process. These chemicals attach to foreign organisms or particles and toxins and help fight and contain the infection.

Phagocytosis is the ability of some circulating cells that migrate during an inflammatory response to ingest foreign agents or pathogens such as bacteria. It is a complex process resulting in the ingestion and subsequent killing or digestion of these pathogens (Fig. 2.2). The two principal phagocytes in the human body are the polymorphonuclear leucocytes or neutrophils and macrophages. There are others such as dendritic cells, mast cells and natural killer cells which also fulfil this function.

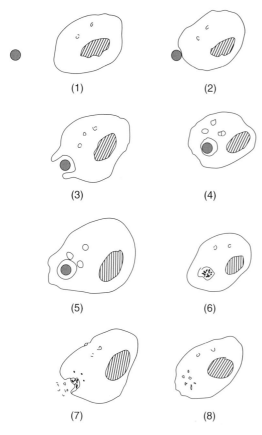

(1)　　　　(2)

(3)　　　　(4)

(5)　　　　(6)

(7)　　　　(8)

Fig. 2.2. Stages in the process of phagocytosis and the subsequent intracellular killing of pathogens by phagocytic cells such as polymorphonuclear leucocytes and macrophages. (1) Chemotactic attraction and movement towards the pathogen; (2) attachment to the cell wall, possibly assisted by complement or antibody; (3) phagocytosis and ingestion of the pathogen; (4) lysosomes coming into contact and (5) forming 'phagolysosomes'; (6) killing and digestion; (7) release of degradation products; (8) remains digested by enzymes inside the cell.

There are three essential prerequisites for *neutrophils* and *macrophages* to phagocytose specifically the infectious agents and not attack normal cells.

1. A rough surface increases the likelihood of phagocytosis.
2. Whereas the protective protein coat of most living cells prevents phagocytosis, dead tissue and foreign particles frequently have no protective coat. Many of these cells carry a negative charge, some because the lack of a cell membrane coat exposes the interior of the cell which is negatively charged. A strong negative charge makes them subject to phagocytosis.

3. The neutrophils and macrophages and other cells involved in innate immunity have a specific means of recognizing certain foreign materials and pathogens. This is mediated by the immune system through the interaction of two sets of complementary molecules, i.e. 'pathogen-associated molecular patterns' on the surface of the pathogen and 'pattern recognition molecules' on host cells. The pattern recognition molecules include immune mediators such as *complement* or Toll receptors and may be either humoral (soluble) or bound to the membranes of the phagocytes. They were historically termed 'complement' when it was initially recognized that antibodies needed another factor in some of their functions, although it is now known that complement activation does not always need an antibody. These recognition systems trigger the attack against infectious agents. The variable portions of complements or antibodies adhere to the bacterial membrane and make them susceptible to phagocytosis. Thus the presence of the complement or antibody on the pathogen makes the process of recognition and attachment by the phagocytic cell more effective since the phagocytes also have receptors for these molecules on their surface. This process that aids phagocytosis is called *opsonization*.

The process of phagocytosis (Fig. 2.2) begins with the attraction of the phagocyte towards the pathogen along a chemotactic gradient, and its attachment to the cell wall assisted by the complement or antibody. Neutrophils or macrophages attached to the infectious agents then put out pseudopodia ('fake feet') around the agents and engulf them. The agents are then localized within phagocytic vesicles (or *phagosomes*) inside the cytoplasm of the neutrophil and can be enzymatically digested or acted on by powerful oxidizing agents present in lysosomes. When a phagosome fuses with a lysosome it is often referred to as a *phagolysosome*. A neutrophil can usually phagocytose between five and 20 bacteria before it becomes exhausted and dies. Macrophages, on the other hand, are much more powerful phagocytes than neutrophils and are often capable of engulfing over 100 bacteria. They also have the ability to engulf much larger particles, for example whole red blood cells or malarial parasites. Unlike neutrophils, macrophages extrude residual products after digestion of ingested foreign particles and often survive for much longer. It is important to note that not all phagocytosis results in the killing of the pathogenic agent inside the cell. Sometimes pathogens use this mechanism as a survival strategy as some pathogens allow themselves to be engulfed but are not killed inside host cells.

Apart from neutrophils and macrophages which constitute the principal phagocytic cells, the other cells associated with innate immunity are dendritic cells, mast cells and natural killer cells.

Dendritic cells are characterized by processes projecting in many directions, which increases their surface area enormously and enables interaction with foreign organisms and immunological cells. Their main function is to present foreign organisms to lymphocytes and thus they specialize in recognition more than phagocytosis. They also secrete a wide range of cytokines.

Mast cells on the other hand participate in the acute inflammatory response by releasing a range of chemicals (such as histamine, leucotrienes and other similar molecules) that increase vascular supply and permeability of blood vessels in the region of an acute infection to mobilize leucocytes. They increase the delivery of complement and antibodies to initiate and promote the inflammatory response and the subsequent phagocytosis by other cells.

Natural killer (NK) cells are large granular lymphocytes, which were identified as having the ability to kill tumour cells. Unlike lymphocytes, which are associated with adaptive immunity, these cells with natural or innate type of killing function respond rapidly and have less specific or restricted recognition abilities. Hence they are more like innate immunity cells, in contrast to conventional cytotoxic T lymphocytes. NK cells are able to bind to cell surfaces, they are poor as phagocytes, they act to lyse cells infected with intracellular pathogens, and are also stimulated by cytokines. The important feature is that they act rapidly, unlike lymphocytes of the adaptive immune response.

Complement

Complement is the principal humoral mediator of innate immunity during the host's attack on the pathogen. The complement system consists of a cascade of chemically and immunologically distinct proteins, capable of interacting with each other, with antibodies and with cell membranes. The activation of this system results in a wide range of biological activity, from lysis of different pathogens to direct mediation of the inflammatory process. Complement is able to recruit and enlist the participation of other cellular effector systems, to induce

histamine release from mast cells, migration of leucocytes, phagocytosis and release of lysosomes from phagocytes.

There are two parallel but entirely independent pathways leading to the final active part of the complement system. The two pathways are called the classical and the alternative or lectin-mediated pathways. Each pathway is triggered differently but the end result is cytolysis or cytotoxicity. Thus the response of the integrated complement system is to produce inflammation and facilitate the localization of the pathogenic agent. Phagocytes bear receptors on their surface for antibody and for complement. The pathogen gets coated with *opsonins*, which are antibody and complement components or complement alone. This coating attracts the phagocyte bearing receptors for both antibody and complement and facilitates the process of phagocytosis. Complement also demonstrates other properties such as smooth muscle contraction, vascular permeability and chemotaxis of leucocytes, which promote the acute inflammatory response to the entry of the pathogen.

2.5 Adaptive or Acquired Immunity

In addition to innate immunity, the human body can develop extremely powerful and highly specific immunity against particular invading or infectious agents and against foreign cells or tissues from other individuals or species. This is called acquired immunity or adaptive immunity. It is referred to as adaptive because it allows the body to 'tailor-make' recognition molecules adapted to the pathogens it encounters rather than relying on the available systems and hoping that they will be able to tackle every infectious agent the body is exposed to. The characteristics or hallmarks of this form of acquired immunity are high specificity and immunological memory. While innate immune systems depend on phagocytic cells, adaptive immunity relies on lymphocytes which have the ability to circulate throughout the body and can proliferate and differentiate in response to demand.

Two different, but closely allied, types of adaptive immunity occur in the body. In one, the lymphocytes produce circulating antibodies, which are globulin molecules that are capable of attacking the invading agent. This is called *humoral immunity*. The second type of acquired immunity is mediated by the formation of a large number of activated lymphocytes that are specifically designed to destroy foreign agents. This is called *cell-mediated immunity*. Adaptive immunity of both types, i.e. humoral and cell-mediated, is mediated by lymphocytes. Lymphocytes circulate throughout the body policing and detecting the presence of foreign agents or molecules (termed *antigens*). Due to the possession of antigen-specific surface receptors, each lymphocyte is individually specific for the antigens it recognizes. On recognition of their specific antigen, they respond by proliferation of their numbers and by switching on a designated function such as cytotoxicity, secretion of an antibody or cytokines. On fulfilling their role, many functioning lymphocytes retain their immunological memory and remain in the body for years as memory cells which have the capacity to proliferate once more and produce a fast response should the same antigen enter the body again.

The two principal types of lymphocyte are *T lymphocytes* and *B lymphocytes*. Both T and B lymphocytes arise from bone marrow stem cells. B lymphocytes complete their maturation within the bone marrow while T lymphocytes undergo differentiation and selection within the thymus. Humoral immunity is mediated by B lymphocytes and is therefore often referred to as B-cell immunity. On the other hand, cell-mediated immunity is largely the function of T lymphocytes and hence is referred to as T-cell immunity. B lymphocytes operate largely in the extracellular fluid spaces of the body while T lymphocytes cater to the intracellular compartment. They interact with each other and depend on the innate immune systems (phagocytes, complement, etc.) to dispose of the foreign agent. Table 2.2 summarizes the differences between T and B lymphocytes.

The *lymphoid system* is the term used to describe the total mass of lymphocytes in the body, some of which are circulating while others are located in organs such as the lymph nodes, spleen, tonsils and in the fetus in organs such as the liver and thymus. Lymphoid system is classified as primary, i.e. the site where the lymphocytes are formed, and secondary, i.e. sites where they settle to police, recognize and deal with antigens. Secondary lymphoid organs are located in strategic parts of the body where the likelihood of encounter with a foreign antigen is highest, such as the tonsils in the throat, Peyer's patches in the intestine, lymph nodes and the spleen. Lymphocytes constantly circulate around the body, but during an infection or entry of a pathogen, lymphocytes are attracted to the site by chemicals called chemokines, which are special types of cytokine.

Both T and B lymphocytes excel in their recognition function although the surface molecules responsible are not the same. A combination of several genes is responsible for designing this surface recognition molecule, such that each lymphocyte carries a different combination and thus recognizes a different but specific antigen and hence demonstrates a different but high specificity for a specific antigen. When a lymphocyte recognizes its specific antigen it responds by proliferating into a population of similar lymphocytes with identical specificity. This population of similar lymphocytes is called a *clone* and the sequence from recognition to proliferation and formation of a clone of lymphocytes is referred to as *clonal selection*. When the lymph nodes in the groin enlarge as a result of an infection in the foot, it reflects the clonal expansion of the specific clone of lymphocytes, many of which will differentiate and fulfil their functions (as effector cells), while a few will remain behind as memory cells. During any subsequent entry by the same antigen these few lymphocytes with immunological memory will be

Table 2.2. Comparison of the characteristics of B lymphocytes and T lymphocytes of the adaptive immune system. (Adapted from Playfair and Bancroft, 2004.)

	B lymphocytes	T lymphocytes
Origin	Bone marrow Liver in fetal life	Bone marrow and maturing in thymus
Location	In circulation and in lymphoid organs	In circulation and in lymphoid organs
Specificity	Antigen specific	Antigen specific
Memory	Yes	Yes
Recognition	Specific antibody	T-cell surface receptor
Secreted product	Antibodies	Cytokines
Function	Assist phagocytosis	Cytotoxic T cells T helper cells

able to mount a faster and bigger response. Figure 2.3 demonstrates an example of this phenomenon when measured by levels of antibodies produced by lymphocytes during the first (primary) and subsequent (secondary) exposure to the specific antigen.

Other cell types are also essential in the acquired or adaptive immune response, specifically for the activation of T and B cells; they are termed accessory cells. Accessory cells include *antigen-presenting cells* (APCs). These features will be discussed in subsequent sections under humoral and cell-mediated immunity.

Humoral immunity and B lymphocytes

Humoral immunity is mediated through the production of specific antibody molecules which can bind to the antigen responsible for its production by the B lymphocytes. When a B lymphocyte recognizes its specific antigen, the cell undergoes a dramatic change and enlarges to form a plasma cell which is large relative to the size of a lymphocyte. These cells expand, divide rapidly and, when mature, produce antibodies at an extremely rapid rate. The antibodies are secreted into the lymph and carried into the bloodstream. However, some of the activated B cells do not become plasma cells, but form a moderate number of new B lymphocytes that are similar to the original clone. These cells reside throughout the body, inhabiting all the lymphoid tissue but remaining dormant until activated by the next fresh exposure to the same antigen. These B lymphocytes are called *memory cells* and are responsible for the rapid secondary response that occurs to a subsequent exposure to the same antigen (Fig. 2.3).

The coordinated recognition and response of the activated B lymphocyte on exposure to the specific antigen results in the production of the antibody; this is the same molecule as the surface antigen receptor since this molecule can bind to the specific antigen and thus help in its disposal. The process of antigen activation of the B lymphocyte, which occurs mainly in the lymphoid organs, may occur in three different ways depending on the antigen. Some antigen activation of B lymphocytes is dependent on T cells. Others are independent of T cells and the latter antigens are referred to as *T-independent* (or Ti antigens). Some Ti antigens have mitogenic activity, i.e. they can induce cell division, and can activate B cells directly to induce antibody production and secretion. Other Ti antigens have repeated identical antigenic determinants and can cross-link on the surface of the B cells which then recognize the antigen and can respond by division and secretion of antibodies. Both these T-independent activation processes are restricted to IgM (one type of immunoglobulin) production and do not show memory effects. However, most pathogenic antigens do not have these abilities and need several molecules to be

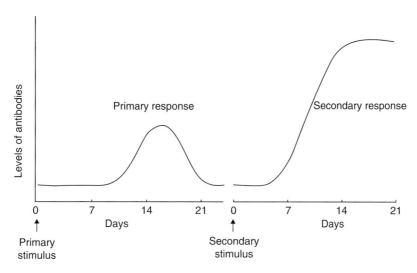

Fig. 2.3. Primary and secondary antibody responses to the same antigenic stimulus showing the slow appearance of antibodies and the weak response with a short life in the primary response, and the faster and greater response in the secondary response.

presented to the B lymphocyte simultaneously to activate them. This simultaneous presentation of the necessary molecules is carried out by special APCs found mainly in lymphoid organs and requires help from T lymphocytes, hence is referred to as *T-dependent* (TD).

The T-cell-dependent B-lymphocyte activation process occurs in the following manner. When the B lymphocyte is activated by the antigen on its surface receptor molecules, it then forms the B-cell receptor (BCR) complex. Without the BCR complex formation the B cell does not respond and inhibition of the BCR complex is one of the ways in which some pathogens evade recognition. The complex of the antigen and the BCR is taken into the cell by endocytosis and the antigen processed and digested. The antigen peptides resulting from this digestion are picked up by newly synthesized molecules called *major histocompatibility complex* (MHC) molecules, which are then transported to the B-cell surface. T lymphocytes are called T helper (Th) cells because they help with cytokine release and demonstrate other favourable actions. Th cells recognize the combinations of MHC–peptide complex on B cells (or even on APCs), which in turn results in the activation of Th cells and their consequent proliferation into a clone, thereby increasing the number of Th cells available to help any B cell carrying the same MHC–peptide complex. At the same time, the activation of the B cell by the pathogen as well as through the release of a range of cytokines (IL-2, -4, -5, -6) by T cells results in the simultaneous proliferation of B-cell clones, thus increasing both B cells and T cells.

Antibodies

Humoral immunity is mediated by the production of antibodies by activated B lymphocytes. Antibodies are globular proteins and, because of their immune function, are often referred to as *immunoglobulins*. Antibodies are made up of four polypeptide chains – two identical long or heavy chains and two short or light chains which are also identical, attached to form a Y-shaped molecule (Fig. 2.4). The stem of the Y is contributed only by the heavy chains (the constant region), while the two tips of the Y, made up of both light and heavy chains, comprise the variable region. The variable tips of the Y have the specific antigen-binding site while the constant region mediates different biological actions such as activation of the innate immune system to dispose

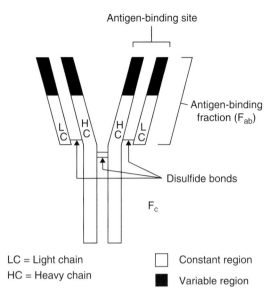

LC = Light chain   □ Constant region
HC = Heavy chain   ■ Variable region

Fig. 2.4. Diagrammatic representation of the structure of the antibody molecule. F_{ab} (fragment, antigen binding) is the site that binds antigens and recognizes specific antigens; F_c (fragment, crystalline) plays a role in modulating immune cell activity, binding to cell receptors and complement protein.

of the antigen bound to the other end. The antibody molecule is thus not only neutralizing the antigen, but also marking it for disposal by the innate immune systems.

Immunoglobulins are gamma globulins, constitute about 20% of the circulating plasma proteins and have molecular weights varying from about 150,000 to over 900,000. Irrespective of their antigen specificity, antibody molecules having a constant heavy chain region are termed as belonging to the same class. There are five principal classes of antibodies (or isotypes of immunoglobulin) (see Table 2.3). The five classes M, D, G, E and A (isotypes of immunoglobulins (Ig) designated as IgM, IgD, IgG, IgE and IgM, respectively) differ in their biological actions.

IgG is the most important, constituting 75% of serum immunoglobulins. It is active both in the blood and in tissue spaces and even crosses the placental barrier, thus conferring immunity to the fetus and newborn. However, it has a short half-life of only a few weeks and hence provides protection to the newborn until about 6 months of age, after which the infant has to produce its own antibodies. IgG functions in activating both complement and

Table 2.3. Classification of antibodies (immunoglobulins). (Adapted from Playfair and Bancroft, 2004.)

Class	Molecular weight	Biological function
IgM	970,000	Agglutination Activation of complement
IgD	184,000	Triggers B lymphocytes
IgG (subclass 1,2, 3 & 4)	146,000 to 170,000	Activation of complement Opsonization to aid phagocytosis Crosses placental barrier Enters tissue spaces
IgE	188,000	Binds mast cells Mediates allergic response
IgA (serum and secretory)	160,000 to 380,000	Secretory IgA appears in secretions such as breast milk

phagocytosis. IgM is the largest molecule (molecular weight 970,000) with ten antigen-binding sites in its pentameric structure and can thus immobilize and agglutinate (stick together) bacteria. Its large size does not allow it to get out of the bloodstream or cross the placenta. IgM can also activate complement. IgA is adapted to function at the mucosal surfaces of hollow organs such as the gut, lungs and urogenital tract, while IgE present in trace amounts is prominent during allergies. IgD is mainly found on B lymphocytes and is involved in their activation pathway.

Antibodies act in many different ways to protect the body against invading foreign agents and pathogens. They neutralize bacterial toxins by the ability of IgG molecules to block the binding of the toxin to the cell receptor, thus preventing its entry and consequent damage to the cell. This forms the basis of immunization (discussed below) – both of 'active immunization', when the injected antigen enables the body to stimulate the production of antibodies to the bacterial toxin and to retain that memory for a later occasion, and of 'passive immunization', when the specific antibody is injected to save life during an acute invasion and infection by a pathogen. Antibodies by binding to the specific antigen through pattern recognition can then bind to phagocytic cells like neutrophils and macrophages

for their eventual disposal. Antibody binding to the specific antigen also activates the complement pathway to enhance phagocytosis (opsonization). Thus antibody, complement and phagocytes operate together to deal with the infective agent. While antibodies can aggregate antigens for eventual disposal through their ability to activate complement, they facilitate both complement-mediated lysis of the pathogen and the lysis of pathogen-infected cells. Thus antibodies can directly attack the invading agent, as well as attack by activation of the complement system that leads ultimately to the destruction of the invading agent.

Cell-mediated immunity and T lymphocytes

A cell-mediated immune response occurs when lymphocytes are attracted and migrate to the site of entry of the infectious agent or the area of inflammation due to the pathogen. The important difference with respect to humoral immunity is that while B lymphocytes produce antibodies that can travel throughout the body and can act for weeks, the cell-mediated immune defence is the direct result of T lymphocytes and their cytokines acting directly although transiently – thus explaining the need to locate as closely as possible to the pathogenic agent. Often dendritic cells take up the pathogen and migrate to the lymph nodes, where they expect to contact the T cell with the specific receptor. As with innate immunity, the targeted migration of T cells is aided by chemokines and other molecules.

Resting T lymphocytes are very similar to B lymphocytes. When activated however, unlike B cells which form large plasma cells, T cells enlarge slightly and begin to secrete cytokines and other toxic molecules which have effects on other target cells over a short range with no antigen specificity. While the effect of the activity of these T cells is non-specific, it is important to note that their activation is highly specific: in response to the antigen presented as the MHC–peptide complex by only those T cells that have the capability of detecting this specific complex by means of their receptor. On activation the T cell initiates production of cytokines, particularly IL-2 as well as receptors for IL-2, the latter for stimulating itself to proliferate into a clone. The many cytokines produced in turn may activate B cells and macrophages. Unlike the Th cells which are cytokine-secreting cells, the cytotoxic T cells function to kill cells harbouring intracellular pathogens.

T lymphocytes are thus activated by recognizing fragments of the foreign protein (the antigen), on an APC or on a B cell, as the MHC–peptide complex which is recognized. The antigen peptides presented by the APC or B lymphocytes are bound to MHC molecules, which are glycoproteins. There are two types of MHC molecules, which present different types of antigen to the T lymphocytes: class I MHC molecules and class II MHC molecules. Class I MHC molecules are expressed by all nucleated cells (and platelets) and present antigens that are expressed intracellularly (e.g. viral antigens). Class II MHC molecules occur only in APCs and present extracellular antigens (e.g. bacterial proteins). Since the two different T-cell types (T helper and T cytotoxic) both recognize MHC–peptide complexes but have different effects on the target cell, they need another set of surface molecules on the T cells which helps to distinguish them. These surface markers have been classified according to an internationally recognized system of 'CD' numbers where CD stands for 'cluster of differentiation'. Class I MHC molecules are recognized by CD8+ T cells. The CD8+ T cells proliferate to form a clone of cytotoxic T lymphocytes (CTLs) which can directly lyse cells infected with virus. Class II MHC molecules are recognized by CD4+ T cells, which proliferate and activate B lymphocytes.

Viruses, unlike bacteria, infect and replicate in cells. CTLs are designed to kill both the virus and the cell. They are mainly CD8+ cells that recognize the viral peptides bound to class I MHC molecules and will destroy all cells with this combination. CD8+ T cells may receive help from CD4+ Th cells which secrete cytokines. CTLs kill by apoptosis or cell suicide by the transfer of granule-derived enzymes via the actions of perforin, which results in activation of an enzyme cascade, and by triggering a surface molecule called Fas, which also leads to apoptosis. CTLs are serial killers since the release of cytotoxic mediators by the CTL occurs quickly and the CTL is now able to disengage and attack another similar infected cell. CTLs may play this crucial role not only in viral infections but also in other intracellular infections like TB and malaria. CTLs are also implicated in rejection of transplanted organs and of some tumours.

The adaptive immune mechanism is thus reliant on both B and T lymphocytes, and their response to a pathogen is powerful, flexible, antigen specific and demonstrates immunological memory. B cells on activation initiate clones which secrete antibodies that are effective largely against extracellular agents such as bacteria and help neutralize their toxins. Th cells or CD4+ Th cells interact with B cells and macrophages to direct an antigen-specific immune response mediated through antibodies and cytokines to help neutralize the invading pathogen. CD4+ Th differentiation can be biased towards a type 1 (Th1) or type 2 (Th2) response. The Th1-biased immune response is characterized by IgG production and activation of macrophages, while the Th2-biased immune response results in IgE secretion and eosinophilia and is seen in helminthic infections and allergic diseases. CD8+ T cells are cytotoxic or killer T cells and act on intracellular infected cells.

Cytokines

Cytokines are other humoral mediators of the innate immune system and are essentially molecules that play an important role in communication; they lack any direct pathogen recognition or attack or disposal role. They are soluble proteins secreted by the cells of the immune system and are mainly released in response to invasion by foreign agents. They act on cells of the immune system to modulate their activity. There is now evidence to suggest that the ability to secrete cytokines is not restricted to cells of the immune system. Non-immune cells and tissues such as fibroblasts, endothelial cells and even the ovary can produce cytokines under certain circumstances. A number of cytokines act as growth factors and lead to the proliferation and differentiation of a wide range of cells. Cytokines are involved in promoting inflammatory responses, cell differentiation and proliferation, as well as cell movement and inhibition. They also form a special group of antiviral particles called interferons.

Cytokines can be divided into interleukins (IL), tumour necrosis factors (TNF), interferons, colony-stimulating factors and transforming growth factors. Some cytokines have widespread metabolic effects on the body and are often called *pro-inflammatory cytokines*. They are IL-1, IL-6 and TNF-α. Cytokines have several beneficial effects. They initiate local inflammatory responses as well as activating and recruiting leucocytes to the site of infection. Cytokines can increase vascular permeability and thus allow movement of immunoglobulins, complements and leucocytes to the site of infection. Some cytokines, such as IL-12, generate beneficial T-cell responses to intracellular pathogens, such as mycobacteria and toxoplasma. However, cytokines are not always

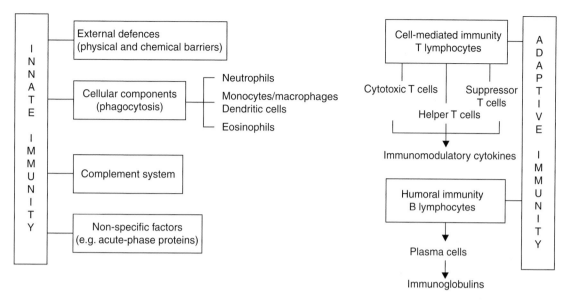

Fig. 2.5. Schematic representation of the innate and adaptive or acquired components of the human immune system. (Adapted from Wintergerst *et al.*, 2007.)

beneficial. The benefits depend on the secretion of cytokines in relatively low concentrations at the site of infection. If the infection disseminates and cytokines are released systemically, they may lead to detrimental effects. Systemic production can induce fever and can trigger septic shock, which may lead to death.

Figure 2.5 provides a schematic representation of the entire human immune system and Table 2.1 summarizes the major differences between the innate and adaptive immune systems with regard to the cells involved and the chemical molecules participating in the process.

2.6 Immunization

Immunization is the process of acquiring immunity against an illness due to an infective agent or pathogen. Immunization can be a passive or an active process. *Passive immunization* results from the passive transfer of antibodies, while *active immunity* is acquired by activation of the immune system within the body directed to a specific pathogen. Passive immunity is acquired by the newborn from the mother or by an individual who is administered preformed immunoglobulins.

In a newborn infant the maternal transfer of antibodies (IgG) that has occurred passively across the placenta before birth, provides a level of immu-

nity. Colostrum and breast milk also afford significant protection to the newborn infant. The major immunoglobulin in milk is the secretory IgA, which remains in the gut of the newborn, protecting the newborn's intestinal mucosal surfaces from enteric pathogens. It is believed that the antibodies are specific to the antigens in the maternal gut with IgA-producing cells migrating to the breast tissue and secreting specific antibodies which appear in milk, thus constituting an *'entero-mammary axis'*.

Gamma globulins administered as either whole serum or concentrated immune globulins are another means of acquiring passive immunity. Administration of such immune globulins, which is largely IgG, offers immediate protection to individuals who are at risk since active immunization may take 7–10 days for effective antibody production. Passive immunization is also useful over the short term, to immunize individuals who are unable to produce antibodies.

In addition to exposure and acquisition of the illness, vaccination is the other way of acquiring active immunity against an infectious agent. The advantages of active over passive immunization are the result of the host's immune system being stimulated to produce an immune response against a given antigen. This ensures the activation of both humoral and cellular immune mechanisms and provides an immunological memory which can be boosted on subsequent exposure to the antigen (Fig. 2.3). Antibodies so formed are longer lasting and continuously replenished as compared with passively acquired immunity. Active immunization can be achieved by injecting killed or live attenuated vaccines, toxoids and polysaccharide-conjugated vaccines.

Further Reading

Parham, P. (2005) *The Immune System*, 2nd edn. Garland Science, New York & London. *Aimed at students who are coming to immunology for the first time, emphasizing the functioning of the human immune system.*

Playfair, J.H.L. and Bancroft, G. (2004) *Infection and Immunity*, 2nd edn. Oxford University Press, Oxford, UK. *A compact textbook for any student who needs to know something about immunity and its basis in infectious diseases.*

Playfair, J.H.L. and Chain, B.M. (2005) *Immunology at a Glance*, 8th edn. Blackwell Publishing, Oxford, UK. *Concise introduction based on illustrations and sketches aimed at busy students whose work impinges on immunology.*

Roitt, I.M. and Rabson, A. (2000) *Really Essential Medical Immunology.* Blackwell Science, Oxford. UK. *Concise version of the original classic* Roitt's Essential Immunology, *now in its 11th edition, for busy students getting to grips with immunology.*

3 Role of Nutrients in Immune Functions

- The energy needs of the body may be increased during an infection to compensate for the increased energy demands due to fever and shivering associated with the infection.
- Protein requirements are increased during infections as more protein is required for the synthesis of cytokines and acute-phase proteins and the proliferation of immune cells.
- Some amino acids, like arginine, glutamine, methionine and cysteine, and free fatty acids have an important role in the normal functioning of the immune system.
- Vitamin A plays an important role in host defence mechanisms, including both cell-mediated immunity and humoral immune mechanisms.
- Both iron deficiency states and excess iron can exert adverse effects on the body's response to an infection.
- Zinc plays an important role in the body's immune function.
- Other nutrients that influence the immune system are trace minerals like selenium and copper and antioxidant vitamins like vitamin C and vitamin E.
- Several nutrients influence the cytokine functions of the body.

3.1 Introduction

This chapter on the role of nutrients in the immune response summarizes our current knowledge of the important role some specific nutrients play in maintaining the defence mechanisms and the integrity of the immune systems of the body discussed in Chapter 2. Nutrients present in the food that we consume in our daily diet are broadly categorized as *macronutrients*, i.e. those which constitute the bulk of the nutrients in the daily diet (see Box 3.1), and as *micronutrients*, i.e. nutrients present in small quantities and required by the body also in small quantities (see Box 3.2). Macronutrients, like protein and fat as well as many micronutrients such as vitamin A, iron and zinc play an important role in the body's defence to an infection and particularly in the immunological response it mounts. This chapter examines the exact role these nutrients play in enabling the optimal functioning of the immune systems, thus helping protect the human body against infectious agents and pathogens. This discussion is distinct from the broad interactions between poor nutritional status on the host's defence mechanisms and the increased risk of infection that

undernourished individuals are susceptible to, which will be discussed in Chapter 4.

3.2 Energy and Protein

Macronutrients (carbohydrates, protein and fats) are the main source of energy for the body. They also meet the body's needs for growth, for the repair and replacement of dead and dying cells, and for the day-to-day maintenance of the body. Infections have profound effects on the body's needs for energy and protein and on the subsequent metabolism of these nutrients. An important part of the body's response to an infection is the raising of body temperature, which may eventually manifest as a fever. For every degree Centigrade rise in temperature the basal metabolic rate increases by 13%, and in sick patients the increase in resting metabolism may be as much as 30–40% above normal. The energy requirements of the body are thus proportionally increased and a significant increase in food consumption is needed to supply the extra energy. Without an appropriate increase in food consumption, the energy has to be provided

Box 3.1. Macronutrients.

Food consumed as our daily diet consists mostly of macronutrients. Macronutrients (carbohydrates, protein and fats) are the main source of energy for the body. They also meet the body's needs for growth, for repair and replacement of dead and dying cells and for day-to-day maintenance of the body.

Carbohydrates

Carbohydrates generally provide the bulk of the diet and are a major source of energy. Carbohydrates contain atoms of carbon, hydrogen and oxygen in their molecules. The hydrogen and oxygen atoms are always present in the same proportion as in water (2H:O) and are attached to carbon atoms – hence the name carbohydrate. The carbohydrates in food are broadly classified as sugars and polysaccharides. Sugars are small, sweet-tasting molecules. They can be joined into long chains (when they no longer taste sweet); chains of ten or more sugar molecules are called polysaccharides. Carbohydrates are generally divided into three groups:

1. Monosaccharides, examples of which are glucose, fructose and galactose;
2. Disaccharides, examples of which are sucrose, lactose and maltose;
3. Polysaccharides, examples of which are starch, glycogen and cellulose.

The three commonest sugars in foods are sucrose (cane sugar), glucose (grape sugar) and fructose (fruit sugar). Other sugars that occur in smaller quantities in foods, and do not taste as sweet, are lactose (milk sugar) and maltose (malt sugar).

Carbohydrates are synthesized in green plants by photosynthesis. The primary products are sugars which are then polymerized to form polysaccharides. Plants contain two distinct types of polysaccharides, i.e. starch and non-starch polysaccharide (NSP). Animal tissues also contain carbohydrate polymers; for example glycogen, a storage polysaccharide with a similar structure to starch. However, cereals are the principal source of starch in the diets of most communities; they also provide a rich source of NSP. Potatoes and bananas are good sources of starch. Other sources of carbohydrate in the diet are vegetables including legumes, and fruit.

Proteins

Proteins differ from both carbohydrates and fats in that they contain nitrogen and sometimes sulfur in addition to carbon, hydrogen and oxygen. They also have complicated structures. Proteins are macromolecules built up of relatively simple units or building blocks called amino acids, which link together by peptide bonds to form long polypeptide chains. Proteins are the most complex of food chemicals, not only because there are 20 different amino acids that may be involved in their structure, but also because of their special three-dimensional configuration achieved by coiling and cross-linking.

Plants synthesize amino acids from inorganic chemicals while animals do not have this ability and hence need to derive the required amino acids from consuming plant- and animal-based foods. The human body is also limited in its ability to convert one amino acid into another. Of the 20 amino acids needed by the body, nine have been found to be essential and hence are termed 'essential' or 'indispensable' amino acids; the others are considered 'non-essential' or 'dispensable'. However, among the latter are several that become 'conditionally indispensable' depending on the limited availability of precursor amino acids or on the demands made by the body in some situations.

Proteins generally comprise between 10% and 15% of the energy content of a diet. However, they are the main functional and structural components of animal cells, not merely sources of dietary energy. Thus, adequate protein and amino acids in the diet is essential to maintain cellular integrity and function. Because the characteristic element of protein is nitrogen, which constitutes 16% of its weight, nitrogen metabolism is often considered to be synonymous with protein metabolism in the body. The principal source of animal protein in the diet is provided by meat, fish and related products. Plants such as cereals, legumes and pulses provide vegetable protein. There is no evidence that protein of animal origin is in any way superior to vegetable protein. Proteins are necessary for proper growth and development, for maintenance and repair of worn and damaged tissues, and for the synthesis of enzymes and hormones.

Fats

Fats, as a term, generally refer to those foods which are fatty in nature; they are greasy in texture and taste and not miscible with water. Fats are an important source of energy in the diet. Chemically they are composed of esters of glycerol with fatty acids. Fats and oils are chemically similar, although the former are solid and the latter are generally liquid at ambient room temperature. Edible fats, however, are triacylglycerols and are chemically distinct from the oils derived from petroleum products. The melting points of triacylglycerols and the degree of 'hardness' of fats increase with the chain lengths of the constituent fatty acids and their degree of saturation (fatty acids are said to be 'saturated' when each carbon atom in the chain carries all the hydrogen atoms possible). Thus, hard fats like lard contain a relatively high proportion of saturated long-chain fatty acids.

Two other terms related to fats need to be understood. Biochemists tend to use the term 'lipids' which include a far wider range of chemical substances than simply triacylglycerols. Lipids include phospholipids, glycolipids, sterols and fat-soluble vitamins. In nutrition and dietetics, a distinction is also made between visible and invisible fats. Visible fats are those that are apparent in the diet, and include the fat on meat and in spreads such as butter or margarine. Invisible fats are hidden in the food and include those that are incorporated during preparation or cooking, for example the fat in cakes and biscuits, as well as those that are present as constituents of cell membranes of plant or animal tissues.

Fats are generally categorized on the basis of their functions into structural fats, storage fats and metabolic fats. Structural fats contribute to the architecture of cells, mainly as constituents of biological cell membranes and of mitochondria and other organelles inside cells. Storage fats provide a long-term reserve of metabolic fuel for the organism, mostly in adipose tissue. Metabolic fats are those lipid molecules that undergo metabolic transformations to produce specific substances of physiological and nutritional importance. However, it is important to remember that there is a considerable overlap in the functions of the three types of fat, and sometimes all three roles are fulfilled by the same fat molecule.

Like amino acids are to proteins, fatty acids are the main components of fats. Fatty acids vary in length from one to more than 30 carbon atoms. Fatty acids are broadly divided into saturated fatty acids which contain no double bonds, e.g. palmitic acid, and unsaturated fatty acids which do have double bonds, e.g. oleic acid. Unsaturated fatty acids occupy more space structurally as the double bonds allow for a large amount of structural variety, and are further classified as monounsaturated (i.e. a single double bond) and polyunsaturated (i.e. more than one double bond). Fatty acids are also categorized according to their chain length, which is based on the number of carbon atoms in their structure. Those fatty acids with less than eight carbon atoms are referred to as short-chain fatty acids and are water soluble, being present mainly in dietary products containing milk fat. Medium-chain fatty acids have between eight and 14 carbon atoms; they are mostly intermediates in the synthesis of long-chain fatty acids (more than 14 carbon atoms) but are also present in milk fat. Long-chain fatty acids are the main constituents of dietary fat and may be long-chain saturated (SFA) (mainly as animal fats and butter), long-chain monounsaturated (MUFA) (fats in olive oil) or long-chain polyunsaturated (PUFA) (sunflower, safflower and flaxseed oil fats). Fats are esters of fatty acids with glycerol (mostly as triacyglycerols; also called triglycerides) which are primarily sources of energy in the diet. Other fats include phospholipids, which are important components of cell membranes, and cholesterol. Cholesterol has important functions as a precursor of steroid hormones and of bile salts which help in fat digestion.

The important dietary sources of fat include fats stored in the meat and organs of animals, eggs, milk and fish, and vegetable oils from seeds and plants and in nuts. Oils and fats are liable to spoilage which results in the production of unpleasant odours and flavours. Such spoilage is called rancidity. Different types of oils and fats show different degrees of resistance to rancidity: vegetable oils deteriorate slowly, animal fats deteriorate more rapidly, while marine or fish oils spoil very readily unless refined and hydrogenated. In general all fats consumed by man are a mixture of saturated and unsaturated fats. Dietary fats sourced from land animals contain more SFAs, while the fats from plant sources and from fish have more unsaturated fatty acids; in the case of the latter they are mostly PUFAs. PUFAs include two unsaturated fatty acids – linoleic and linolenic – which are termed 'essential fatty acids' as they are needed for good health. There are others like arachidonic acid and docosahexaenoic acid that have been termed as 'conditionally essential' fatty acids because of the benefits that accrue from their adequacy during growth and development in children.

from tissue stores, i.e. energy stored in the body, or from breakdown of body tissues.

To some extent, the severely restricted levels of physical activity and the sedentary or recumbent posture of a sick person reduce total energy expenditure. However, it is vital to remember that fevers are associated with quite severe anorexia (poor appetite) which drastically reduces the amount of energy-supplying food consumed by the individual. This reduction in intake may be compounded by the fact that some infective fevers are associated with bouts of shivering (involuntary muscle contractions), which increase the

Box 3.2. Micronutrients.

Micronutrients are essential constituents of the diet but are present in only small quantities, and are required by the body in small quantities. They are vitamins, minerals or trace elements and fulfil a range of crucial functions in the body; thus they are essential for the normal and optimal functioning of the body.

Vitamins

Vitamins are organic substances present in minute quantities in the food we ingest daily and are essential for normal cellular metabolism. Vitamins probably function like catalysts (compare enzymes) or as cofactors in enzymatic reactions in the body. Most vitamins are derived from the diet but some vitamins can be made available to the body following synthesis by microorganisms in the gastrointestinal tract.

Vitamins are grouped together as an entity, but not because of their related chemical structure or their similar function in the body. The term 'vitamin' was derived from the discovery of vital factors other than macronutrients in the diet, the lack of which resulted in manifest deficiency diseases. Vitamins are broadly classified on the basis of their solubility in water as those that are water soluble (B group vitamins and vitamin C) and those that are fat soluble (vitamins A, D, E and K). Each vitamin has a unique role in the human body. A broad outline of their sources in the diet and their functions in the body, along with important manifestations resulting from their deficiency in the diet, are summarized in Table 3.1.

Table 3.1. Dietary sources of vitamins and minerals, their functions and manifestations of deficiency states.

Vitamin/ mineral	Dietary sources	Functions	Effects of deficiency
Vitamin A	Milk and dairy products, eggs, meat, liver, margarine, fish and fish-liver oil. Its precursor carotene is present in green leafy vegetables and pigmented fruits (papaya) and vegetables (carrots). Present in yellow maize	Necessary for healthy skin and mucus surfaces, for normal growth, development and cellular differentiation. Essential for normal visual function. Also required for the normal production of red blood cells	Affects normal growth. May lead to disorders of the skin and mucous membranes resulting in *follicular hyperkeratosis* and *xerophthalmia* and corneal ulcers. Lowered resistance to infections (anti-infective function) and disturbances of vision such as night blindness. Nutritional anaemia
Vitamin B complex	Cereal grains, pulses and legumes, bread and flour, meat, milk, eggs, potatoes, green vegetables, yeast extract	Functions as a coenzyme in many reactions in the body; in tissue oxidation and amino acid metabolism. Essential for red blood cell production	Loss of appetite, impaired general health. Severe deficiency includes *beriberi* and *Wernicke's encephalopathy* (thiamin), *pellagra* (niacin), angular stomatitis (riboflavin), peripheral neuropathy (pyridoxine) and anaemia (folate and B_{12})
Vitamin C	Fruits, green vegetables, potatoes, sprouted cereals and pulses	Necessary for the proper formation of collagen, bones and blood vessels. Involved in several metabolic pathways and has antioxidant function	Affects growth of children and causes bleeding from gums. Prolonged severe deficiency may lead to *scurvy*
Vitamin D	Eggs, milk and dairy products, margarine, fish-liver oils and fatty fish. Synthesized in skin on exposure to sunlight	Necessary for the proper absorption of calcium and formation of strong bones and teeth	Deficiency may result in rickets and osteomalacia
Vitamin E	Vegetable oils, wholegrain cereals, egg yolk, nuts and leafy vegetables	Powerful antioxidant and protects cell membranes from free radical damage	Effects of deficiency not known and probably rare

Table 3.1. Continued.

Vitamin/ mineral	Dietary sources	Functions	Effects of deficiency
Vitamin K	Liver and green vegetables; also synthesized in the body	Necessary for normal blood clotting or coagulation	A blood clotting disorder similar to haemophilia
Calcium	Milk and dairy products, soya milk	Most of the body calcium (99%) is in bones. Ionic calcium essential for muscle contraction, nerve conduction, blood clotting, secretion of hormones and activation of enzymes	Low blood calcium (hypocalcaemia) causes seizures and tetany due to increased neuromuscular activity. Deficiency may be associated with osteoporosis
Iron	Meat, liver, eggs, fish, legumes, fruits and green leafy vegetables; also all cereals. Milk is a poor source of iron	Required for the synthesis of haemoglobin present in red blood cells which transports oxygen. Also in myoglobin in muscle and in some enzymes	Iron deficiency disorders including anaemia
Zinc	Meat, liver, seafood and eggs	Component of several important enzymes essential for metabolism and for synthesis and action of hormones like insulin	Stunted growth in children, alteration of taste and impaired immune function. Severe deficiency associated with dwarfism and hypogonadism
Iodine	Sea fish, seaweeds, soil	Essential for the synthesis of thyroid hormones	Iodine deficiency disorders include abortion, stillbirths, cretinism, mental retardation and goitre

Minerals and trace elements

These micronutrients – essential minerals and trace elements – are largely inorganic and account for 4% of total body weight. Minerals include sodium, potassium, phosphorus, calcium, sulfur, iron and chloride. Minerals fulfil a wide range of functions in the body. In addition to the elements classified as minerals, the body needs some other elements in even smaller quantities. These are known as trace elements. They include cobalt, copper, magnesium, zinc, selenium, fluoride, iodine and chromium. Water, as well as food, is an important source of trace elements.

The physiological functions, dietary sources and deficiencies of some important minerals and trace elements of nutritional significance are provided in Table 3.1.

Deficiencies of only four of these inorganic elements or minerals are known to occur in human populations. They are:

1. Iodine deficiency, which compromises thyroid hormone function and can lead to mental retardation and cretinism in newborn infants and children;
2. Iron deficiency, which affects the ability of the body to produce haemoglobin by the red blood cells and thus impairs work performance, and may cause anaemia;
3. Zinc deficiency, which if severe manifests with signs of growth retardation, sexual and skeletal immaturity, skin disorders and mental disturbances;
4. Selenium deficiency, which may present as *Keshan's* disease (a cardiomyopathy) or as *Keshin–Beck* disease (a chronic osteoarthropathy).

Deficiencies of iodine and iron are widespread globally and affect large segments of the population, while severe deficiencies of zinc and selenium are rare and confined to specific population groups in the world. However, suboptimal deficiencies of all four are common and compromise normal health; particularly in the case of iodine, iron and zinc.

energy expenditure of the infected individual. Thus, contributions of endogenous tissue sources to meet the energy needs are inevitable. The weight loss or evident wasting seen during infections is due to both loss of fat and muscle (hence the term 'consumption' for the chronic wasting of infectious diseases like TB). The reduction in muscle mass is due to breakdown of muscle protein far in excess of the protein synthesized.

It is now well known that these changes in body tissues, including the fever, are due to a pyrogen – a cytokine peptide identified as IL-1.

It is also now well recognized that the increase in the need for synthesis of the entire range of cytokines and acute-phase proteins, along with the proliferation of immunologically competent cells (B and T lymphocytes), macrophages and other leucocytes and their various products (such as immunoglobulins and cytokines), generates an enhanced demand for both energy and protein. Increasing levels of amino acids are required for the increase in synthesis of these various proteins and cellular elements. Increased protein synthesis in turn requires increased energy demand in the face of the lowered food intake due to the anorexia common to most infections. Since the body reserves of carbohydrate (glycogen) do not last for more than a day, stored fat must be mobilized. However, the cytokine and other hormonal responses seen during an infection often tend to inhibit the efficient use of lipids. Hence, the body increasingly depends on tissue protein breakdown (such as that of muscle) to provide amino acids – both to meet the protein synthetic need and to generate an energy source like glucose (by gluconeogenic pathways) to provide the energy needs. Protein and energy provided by macronutrient intake and from the mobilization of body tissue are therefore essential during infection, and influence the immune response.

The role of macronutrients during an infection or inflammatory response is best seen in clinical situations when patients lose weight and the lean body mass (i.e. non-fat tissues) and muscle mass progressively decrease – a phenomenon that surgeons sometimes refer to as 'auto-cannibalism'. Along with the general increase in demand for nutrients, this condition is associated with a restriction in the utilization capacities of macronutrients like glucose and fatty acids and an increase in the demand for amino acids. There is increased gluconeogenesis and lipolysis; both metabolic processes not influenced very much by providing exogenous glucose to the patient. Macronutrient metabolic products – glucose (carbohydrate), amino acids (protein) and fatty acids (fat) – are all sources of energy at the same time, thus manifesting the utilization of mixed carbon sources for energy. The breakdown or catabolism of body tissue protein increases the urinary excretion of the end products of their metabolism like urea. The mobilized amino acids are prioritized for the synthesis of proteins related to and needed for the inflammatory response such acute-phase proteins

and white blood cells. As with carbohydrate and fat metabolism, even protein catabolism is influenced little by the provision of exogenous amino acids to the patient. Although protein synthesis responds to the administration of amino acids, excess of amino acids contributes only to synthesis and excretion of more nitrogenous end products. An understanding of these alterations in the metabolism of macronutrients during severe infections and trauma enables better clinical management of surgical patients.

During an episode of infection, substantial increases are observed in protein synthesis rates. It has been estimated that approximately 45 g of protein are required daily to provide for the increased proliferation of leucocytes and the synthesis of acute-phase proteins during an infection. This demand for protein will impact on other physiological processes that need protein, such as growth in children, and pregnancy and lactation in women. Since protein in the diet is unlikely to meet this demand, breakdown of skeletal muscle protein takes place to provide for the amino acid needs for synthesis of other proteins. These changes contribute to the wasting of muscles evident in patients with chronic infections. The production of cytokines and acute-phase proteins is thus largely dependent on the adequacy of protein intake, in particular those proteins with sulfur-containing amino acids. It is also observed that antioxidant defences are compromised on low protein intakes.

Amino acids

This section discusses the amino acids arginine, glutamine, and the sulfur amino acids methionine and cysteine, and their role in the functioning of the immune system.

Arginine

One of the amino acids needed by the body, arginine is considered conditionally essential or conditionally indispensable since it becomes essential or indispensable only during times of growth and during situations of metabolic stress such as following trauma, burns and infections or sepsis. Arginine is required for the normal functioning of the immune system in several instances. Nitric oxide is synthesized from arginine and is important in immune systems since the inhibition of nitric oxide production increases the host's susceptibility to infectious agents. Nitric oxide production is induced in macrophages in response to several stimuli, which include cytokines produced by

Th cells such as interferon (IFN-γ) and tumour necrosis factor (TNF-α). Nitric oxide plays an important role in cytotoxicity and in cell death (apoptosis) seen in infected and tumour cells. Nitric oxide is also involved in regulating the expression of the class II MHC–peptide complex in APCs. Arginine by its ability to increase secretion of various hormones such as prolactin, growth hormone and insulin-like growth factor (IGF-1) can influence indirectly immune mechanisms. Prolactin increases class II MHC molecules, increases T-cell activation and stimulates the release of cytokines. Growth hormone potentiates the cytokine responses of T cells while IGF-1 plays an important role in the maturation of lymphocytes. Supplementation of arginine benefits the innate immune response by increasing macrophage activity and NK-cell cytotoxicity, and beneficial effects are also observed in wound healing largely the result of increased collagen synthesis. In summary, arginine supplementation is beneficial in reducing trauma-induced immunosuppression manifested as reductions in T-lymphocyte mitogenesis, macrophage and NK cytotoxicity, and in delayed hypersensitivity test responses; at the same time improving wound healing. These are effects that manifest as being beneficial in clinical situations such as surgery and in patients with trauma or burns.

Glutamine

Glutamine is another conditionally essential (conditionally indispensable) amino acid that has immunomodulation effects and has demonstrated benefit in clinical situations. The enzyme glutaminase which converts glutamine to glutamate is present in high concentrations in all lymphoid organs and in lymphocytes, macrophages and neutrophils. Mitogenic stimulation of lymphocytes increases their glutaminase activity as well as glutamine uptake and utilization, indicating the importance of this amino acid in the optimal functioning of these cells. Glutamine is essential for mitogen-stimulated proliferation of lymphocytes and the extent of proliferation of these cells is related to the concentration of the amino acid. The activation of B lymphocytes to synthesize antibodies is dependent on glutamine and so too are related activities involved in antigen presentation using MHC molecules and in phagocytosis. Glutamine availability increases phagocytic activity and the bactericidal activity of neutrophils. Glutamine also increases secretion of cytokines and increases are seen in IL-1, interleukin receptors and interferons

(INF-γ) with increasing availability of glutamine. Clinical benefits were seen following the administration of glutamine in patients, with reduced infection rates and shortened hospital stays. Glutamine treatment of patients resulted in greater numbers of total lymphocytes, T lymphocytes and CD4+ lymphocytes but not in B lymphocytes. One can safely conclude that the amino acid glutamine is needed by the cells of the immune system and influences key functions of these cells, reducing the risk of infections in stress situations such as surgery, trauma and burns.

Methionine and cysteine

Of the sulfur amino acids, methionine is considered essential (indispensable) while cysteine is only conditionally essential (conditionally indispensable). Their metabolism is linked; they exert their effects on the immune system through their end products such as glutathione and taurine by providing the sulfur moiety that is incorporated into these end products. Immune cell function is sensitive to glutathione, which is an important antioxidant. Oxidative stress occurs as a result of generation of reactive oxygen species which can damage tissues. Antioxidant systems can either prevent or quench the harmful effects due to reactive oxygen species. Glutathione levels go down during infection, injury or surgery, thus weakening antioxidant defences of the body. The immune system is vulnerable to oxidative stress since many of the cells of the immune system produce these reactive compounds during their normal function. Hence glutathione and other antioxidants have an important role in the optimal functioning of the immune system. Direct effect of glutathione on the immune system is manifested as increased numbers of helper (CD4+) and killer or cytotoxic (CD8+) T cells with increasing cellular glutathione concentrations and administration of cysteine results in immune-enhancing effects manifested as an increase in lymphocyte numbers. Recent evidence indicates that glutathione promotes interleukin production by APCs, and that raising blood glutathione levels increases NK-cell activity and T-cell activation by mitogens. Taurine also has antioxidant and immunomodulatory properties, and regulates the release of cytokines.

3.3 Fats and Fatty Acids

Dietary fat, depending on the source, contributes varying amounts of fatty acids. Vegetable oils (corn, sunflower, safflower) are rich in *n*-6 polyunsaturated fatty acids (PUFAs) while fats from marine or sea foods are rich in *n*-3 PUFAs. Olive oil and butter are rich in monounsaturated fatty acids (MUFAs), while fats from animal sources have high concentrations of saturated fatty acids (SFAs) and low levels of PUFAs. Unsaturated fatty acids compete for insertion into cell membranes and hence the fatty acid composition of the membrane phospholipids reflects to some extent the profile of unsaturated fats in the daily diet.

High-fat diets appear to diminish innate immune responses. Reducing total fat intake to less than 30% of the total energy in the diet significantly increases NK-cell activity in human subjects. Animals on diets deficient in *n*-6 and *n*-3 fatty acids exhibit decreased neutrophil chemotaxis and macrophage-mediated phagocytic and cytotoxic activity. Animal experiments demonstrate that both deficiency and excess of essential fatty acids impairs innate immune response; high intakes of linoleic and α-linolenic acids suppress NK-cell activity. However, the amount of these essential fatty acids that people habitually consume does not influence adversely their innate immune systems and does not affect either NK-cell activity or cytokine production. Studies in experimental animals and man demonstrate that increasing intakes of fish oils or their component fatty acids, i.e. *n*-3 PUFAs, exert potent anti-inflammatory effects. They result in decreased neutrophil and macrophage chemotaxis and cytokine production; indicating that while these fatty acids compromise immune function in healthy and immunocompromised individuals, they may be of benefit to those who suffer the consequences of excess production of these molecules such as those with chronic inflammatory conditions like rheumatoid arthritis, ulcerative colitis and psoriasis. Clinical trials in patients with these conditions have demonstrated definite benefits of *n*-3 PUFA supplementation in terms of suppression of symptoms and reduction in episodes or relapse rates.

High-fat diets also affect adaptive immune response by suppressing T-lymphocyte proliferation. Essential fatty acid (linoleic and α-linolenic) deficiencies in animals suppress cell-mediated immunity and antibody production, while high intakes of linoleic and linolenic acids also suppress adaptive immune responses. Thus, with both linoleic acid and α-linolenic acid, increased and deficient intakes can suppress immune function. However, as with innate immunity, even adaptive immune function is not affected by reasonable changes in the intakes of these essential fatty acids.

While animal studies show that long-chain *n*-3 PUFAs inhibit lymphocyte proliferation, IL-2 and INF-γ production and delayed hypersensitivity responses, feeding moderate amounts of these *n*-3 PUFAs does not unequivocally exhibit immunosuppressive effects in man.

Experimental studies have shown that fats rich in *n*-3 PUFAs and MUFAs suppress inflammatory response and responsiveness to cytokines, while fats rich in *n*-6 PUFAs exert the opposite effect. Fats modify cytokine functions at several levels. Changes in fat intake change the fatty acid composition of membrane phospholipids and thus influence the type and amount of prostaglandins and leucotrienes produced when cytokines act on target tissues. The beneficial effects of *n*-3 PUFAs on cytokine production is exemplified by trials with fish oil which show improvements in symptoms of inflammation in rheumatoid arthritis, psoriasis, Crohn's disease and ulcerative colitis.

Fats and fatty acids thus demonstrate the potential to influence the immune systems with both the innate and adaptive components affected. The important link between fatty acids and immune function is by the mediation of compounds called eicosanoids (prostaglandins, leucotrienes, thromboxanes) synthesized from PUFAs. They also modulate the intensity and duration of the inflammatory response. Arachidonic acid is required for the synthesis of this group of inflammatory compounds. Dietary fatty acids influence the synthesis of eicosanoids by altering the amounts of arachidonic acid in the membranes of immune cells and thus reducing the availability of arachidonic acid for the synthesis of eicosanoids. *n*-3 PUFAs can hence be considered as arachidonic acid antagonists with important immunomodulating actions. Of these PUFAs, ones of marine origin – i.e. fish oils rich in eicosapentaenoic acid (EPA) and docosahexaenoic acid (DHA) – are the most biologically potent. Clearly fatty acids play an important role in both health and disease, and a central role in immune cell function and regulation, largely the result of their location and organization within cell lipids and as part of the structure of cell membranes and their contribution to fatty acid-derived inflammatory mediators.

3.4 Vitamin A and the Immune Response

Vitamin A (retinol) is important in normal visual function, in the differentiation of epithelial cells and in the immune system. The role of vitamin A in the immune system is not confined to the actions of retinol alone, but also includes the actions of carotenoids, which are the precursors of vitamin A and constitute much of the vitamin A in the diet. In the light of our current understanding of the role of vitamin A in the body, it is not surprising that when it was first discovered, early in the 20th century, it was called the 'anti-infection vitamin' because of its ability to prevent death due to infections in laboratory animals. However, the role of vitamin A in the prevention of blindness took centre stage for a long time, and it is only over the last few decades or so that its role in reducing infective morbidity and mortality has been highlighted once again.

Vitamin A in host defence mechanisms

Among micronutrients, vitamin A plays an important part in host defence mechanisms. It is essential for the maintenance of integrity of epithelial surfaces; vitamin A deficiency states manifest with stratification of cells, followed by squamous metaplasia (change of one kind of tissue into another) and eventually by keratinization. These changes, along with desquamation (scaling-off of the superficial layer) of cells and reduced mucus production, are widespread and compromise the physical barriers in the host defence systems. This allows invasion of the body by microorganisms that colonize the mucosal surfaces. Deficiency of vitamin A impairs DNA synthesis and reduces the turnover of the epithelial cells, and while bacterial cell adhesion in the respiratory tract is increased, these changes along with the desquamation and loss of muco-ciliary function, particularly in the small airways of the respiratory tract, predispose the individual to respiratory infection.

Vitamin A plays an important role in ensuring the normal and optimal functioning of the mucosal surfaces and its deficiency impairs mucosal function in the respiratory, gastrointestinal and genito-urinary tracts. Vitamin A deficiency results in loss of cilia from the respiratory mucosal lining, loss of microvilli in the gut mucosa and loss of mucin and goblet cells in the mucosal lining of all these organs. There is a tendency for squamous metaplasia (abnormal change) and keratinization in the respiratory and genito-urinary tracts. There is also impairment of the mucosal immune cell function and alterations in the antigen specificity of secretory immunoglobulins produced by these mucosae.

The mucosal lining of the eye, i.e. the ocular surface, also undergoes similar changes with loss of mucin and goblet cells, and the occurrence of squamous metaplasia. The loss of mucin secretion in all these mucosal linings seriously impairs their mucosal immunity. The gut mucosa not only shows poor antibody response to pathogens but also demonstrates a marked reduction in its integrity, with evidence of increased permeability.

Vitamin A deficiency affects the production of immune cells as it impairs the development of primary lymphoid organs and their cellular proliferation. Neutrophil function is markedly impaired and manifests as impaired chemotaxis and adhesion. The phagocytic activity of neutrophils is also markedly depressed in states of vitamin A deficiency as well as their ability to generate oxidative molecules to dispose of the phagocytosed pathogens, along with reduced complement-mediated lysis. However, in the absence of secondary infections, neutrophil numbers are not usually altered. Vitamin A deficiency reduces the numbers of circulating NK cells and impairs the cytolytic activity of these NK cells. Children with AIDS show dramatic increases in circulating NK cells when administered two doses of vitamin A, compared with children with AIDS who receive a placebo. Vitamin A deficiency also impairs the production of other blood cells such as red cells (erythrocytes) and lymphocytes. Deficiency states are characterized by decreased total lymphocyte and CD4[+] lymphocyte counts.

Vitamin A and cell-mediated immunity

In vitro studies of cell-mediated immunity show that responses to mitogenic stimuli such as concavallin A (Con A) and phytohaemagglutinin (PHA) are significantly reduced in vitamin A deficiency; and supplementation with vitamin A for a mere 3 days restores this function. Retinoic acid, a derivative of retinol, enhances NK-lymphocyte activity; this effect has been attributed to the alteration in cell surface structure and an increase in cell-surface receptor expression. Retinoids have also been shown to improve the phagocytic activity of both alveolar and peritoneal macrophages. The normal expression of phagocytic cells associated with the immune response, e.g. the production and normal differentiation of B cells and T cells, is also responsive to vitamin A status. It appears that vitamin A modulates the balance between Th1 and Th2 responses. Impaired responses to delayed cutaneous hypersensitivity (DCH) tests have been noted in vitamin A-deficient states. Specifically, the DCH response to the skin antigen dinitrochlorobenzene (DNCB) was examined and found to be impaired. Recent studies have shown that oral vitamin A administration increases DCH response in infants.

Vitamin A and humoral immunity

Vitamin A deficiency impairs the growth, activation and normal functioning of B lymphocytes, and a characteristic feature of vitamin A deficiency is an impaired capacity to generate an antibody response to both Ti and TD antigens. Retinoic acid, a metabolite of retinol, has been shown to favour the differentiation of activated B lymphocytes to antibody-producing cells which then increase the synthesis and secretion of immunoglobulins, IgM and IgG. Other studies have shown that animals deficient in vitamin A had lower levels of the secretory component of immunoglobulins (secretory IgA) but no alterations were seen in serum IgA and IgG levels. There was, however, a slight decrease in antibody affinity. Young mice that are deficient in vitamin A demonstrate decreased antibody responses to protein antigens, and the effect is more pronounced the longer and more severe the deficiency. This is not the case with older mice. There is evidence that mucosal immune systems are more affected thereby allowing easier access to the pathogen. Once invasion occurs, there is evidently a satisfactory antibody response suggesting that humoral immunity is relatively unaffected. There is some experimental evidence that disputes the latter finding and suggests that humoral antibody responses to diphtheria toxin, for instance, are also compromised.

Vitamin A-deficient children show a depressed antibody response to tetanus toxoid used as an antigen. Repeating these studies in animals using tetanus toxoid also shows an impaired antibody response during a primary exposure. However, if the same antigen is given to evoke a secondary response in these animals, after correction of the vitamin A deficiency the secondary immune response is comparable to that of normal animals, indicating that vitamin A deficiency – while lowering the ability to produce antibodies – does not affect the immunological memory of the immune cells. Studies on healthy children also show that vitamin A administration does not enhance antibody responses to tetanus toxoid

and that this effect of an enhanced antibody response is only seen in vitamin A-deficient children who are supplemented with the vitamin. Vitamin A supplementation has also been shown to improve antibody titre response to various vaccines.

Summary of the role of vitamin A in immune response

Vitamin A deficiency results in impaired humoral and cellular immunity and, with decreased activity of complement in serum, decreased activity of lysozymes in leucocytes. There are profound changes in the mucous membranes, which become keratinized; the production of secretory IgA is reduced along with a decrease in mucus production as a result of a reduction in glycoprotein synthesis. These changes impair the integrity of membranes and their resistance to bacterial invasion. At the same time, vitamin A deficiency increases bacterial cell adhesion and increased binding of bacteria to respiratory epithelial cells has been demonstrated in children with low vitamin A status. Table 3.2 summarizes the main features of the vitamin A-deficient immune system.

Table 3.2. Effects of vitamin A deficiency on the immune systems of the host. (Adapted from Semba, 2002.)

On protective barrier	Loss of cilia in respiratory tract mucosa
	Loss of microvilli from gastrointestinal tract mucosa
	Keratinization of respiratory, gut and ocular epithelial lining
	Decrease in goblet cells and mucin production of mucosal epithelium
On innate immune response	Impaired neutrophil function – impaired chemotaxis, adhesion and phagocytosis
	Decrease in NK cells and their impaired functioning
On adaptive immune response	Decrease in number and function of B lymphocytes
	Impaired antibody responses to Ti and TD antigens

There is increasing evidence that the role of vitamin A in immune response is not necessarily mediated by the conversion of pro-vitamin carotenoids in the diet and that carotenoids themselves may contribute to this important role in immunity. The support for this view emerges from non pro-vitamin A precursor carotenoids like lutein and lycopene being as active, and at times more active, than the vitamin A precursor β-carotene in enhancing cell-mediated and humoral immunity. The specific role for carotenoids directly on the immune system can be demonstrated in animals such as the domestic cat, which is an inefficient converter of carotenoids to active vitamin A. The direct effects of β-carotene in enhancing immune cell function are supported by other animal studies showing that addition of carotenoids to the diet improves resistance to infective agents and prevents stress-related involution of the thymus. These animals also show increased numbers of circulating lymphocytes and enhanced lymphocyte proliferation and cytotoxic T-cell activity. Several studies in human subjects have shown administration of carotenoids to increase CD4+ lymphocytes and NK-cell activity, particularly among elderly individuals. Other studies however have been unable to reproduce some of these beneficial effects of β-carotene, although the effects of carotenoids on NK-cell activity were observed, particularly in the elderly subjects. Exposure to ultraviolet light suppresses immune function. β-Carotene treatment prevents the immune-suppression effects of ultraviolet light, estimated as suppression of delayed hypersensitivity responses.

APCs initiate the adaptive immune response by presenting the antigenic peptide with the class II MHC molecules to Th lymphocytes, which then secrete cytokines. Carotenoids probably influence this mechanism by enhancing cell surface expression of the MHC and other related molecules that promote adhesion. This conclusion is supported by studies of β-carotene administration which are suggestive of a moderate enhancement of cell-mediated immunity even over a short period of time. It has also been suggested that, due to their antioxidant actions, carotenoids can modulate to influence the production of eicasonoids like prostaglandins, since β-carotene has been shown to alter the activation of the arachidonic cascade and thus suppress the production of these inflammatory compounds. There is little doubt that the range of carotenoids in our daily diet, provided largely by the fruits and vegetables we consume, have beneficial effects on the immune system independent of their role as precursors of vitamin A.

3.5   Iron and the Immune Response

At the onset of an infectious episode, dramatic changes are seen in the distribution of iron in the body, particularly a striking shift of extracellular iron to the intracellular compartment. These changes probably have an important survival value since iron is an essential element for the growth and replication of microorganisms. It has been hypothesized that the acute response of the body to shift nutrients such as iron from the circulation to the intracellular compartment represents a strategy by the body to deprive invading pathogens of an essential nutrient. This mechanism has been termed 'nutritional immunity' by some workers, and may have more than academic interest since it has enormous implications for public health interventions.

Two crucial observations highlight the role of iron in nutritional immunity:

1. The decrease in circulating iron levels with iron rapidly taken up by tissue stores during acute infections;
2. The apparent increase in susceptibility to infections of individuals with iron overload and the resurgence of infections following nutritional supplementation or repletion of undernourished or nutritionally depleted individuals.

The latter observation also implies that excess iron promotes infection or that low iron states reduce some infections.

Iron and the pathogen

Iron exists in two main forms: ferric (Fe^{3+}) and ferrous (Fe^{2+}). It is required by all living cells for many important cellular biochemical reactions. The ease with which iron undergoes reduction and oxidation in the body enables its easy participation in cellular redox reactions. Iron in the free state is highly reactive and readily catalyses oxidative and peroxidative reactions, resulting in unstable, toxic and reactive oxygen intermediates that can damage cell membranes and DNA. To limit this oxidative tissue damage, iron in the human body is strongly bound to metalloproteins, enzymes, and transport and storage proteins. Since the body is a poor source of free iron, pathogens that need free iron have developed mechanisms to obtain it within their host. They produce high-affinity iron chelators (siderophores) that are able to strip iron from the host's iron-binding proteins (e.g. transferrin) even when they are bound with high affinity. The microorganism genes responsible for this function have been identified and are part of the complex of iron regulatory genes that are turned on by the low free iron concentration within the mammalian host. The pathogens thus have the ability to acquire free iron under adverse conditions within the host. The low free iron levels also act as a signal to make microbial virulence factors since the iron-regulating genes act as a master switch to turn on a number of genes, many of which are virulence genes.

Iron and the host

Iron is required for DNA synthesis and is hence required for the proliferation of lymphocytes involved in the immune response. Ribonucleotide reductase, a rate-limiting enzyme for DNA synthesis, is an iron metalloenzyme and must be continuously synthesized; hence the need for a continuous supply of iron. This important role of iron in lymphocyte proliferation may explain the defects in immune response in iron deficiency states. Other iron-dependent host defence mechanisms are also known and these are likely to be affected by iron deficiency states in the host.

The neutrophil iron metalloenzyme, myeloperoxidase, catalyses the generation of bactericidal reactive halide radicals during the oxidative burst initiated during phagocytosis by neutrophils. This enzyme activity is inhibited in iron deficiency states. Iron also catalyses the production of bactericidal oxygen radicals by neutrophils. A defect in this defence mechanism is observed in iron-deficient states with a corresponding decrease in bacterial killing capacity, but iron-independent functions such as phagocytosis are not affected.

Clinical studies support a role for iron in the increase of susceptibility to infections. Clinical states with iron overload are generally characterized by saturation of the iron transport protein, transferrin, and excess iron circulating as low-molecular-weight, loose protein complexes that are readily available to pathogens. Clinical iron overload states are not only associated with increased susceptibility to infections; the infections to which iron overload states are predominantly susceptible are those caused by organisms that lack an effective iron-acquisition system (e.g. *Yersinia enterocolitica*).

Iron overload states also show impaired immune function, as exemplified by diminished neutrophil superoxide and hydrogen peroxide production, diminished nitroblue tetrazolium reduction, and reduced bactericidal activity.

It thus appears that both iron deficiency and iron excess exert adverse effects on immune responses and influence the metabolism and growth of pathogens in the host. The relationship between iron and infection depends on both the causative organism and the state of iron nutrition of the host. The effects of iron deficiency and iron overload on the immune response of the body are now discussed separately.

Effects of iron deficiency on immune function

Iron deficiency affects the innate immune function. Although neutrophil numbers are not altered, and phagocytosis appears to be normal, intracellular killing of pathogens is markedly impaired in iron deficiency. Macrophages also show slight reduction in their cytotoxicity. However, both humoral and cell-mediated mechanisms of adaptive immunity are affected by iron deficiency in human subjects and experimental animals. T lymphocytes in their resting or dormant state do not express transferrin receptors on their cell surface and hence do not demonstrate uptake of iron from their immediate environment. When T cells are activated they show an increase in surface transferrin receptors, which ensures adequate uptake of iron for the biosynthesis of DNA by the cell. Iron deficiency often manifests with a decrease in total T-lymphocyte count and a reduction in the proportion of CD4$^+$ and CD8$^+$ cells, and also a decrease in both helper and cytotoxic T lymphocytes. Iron deficiency states in human subjects consistently show anergy (absence of normal immune response to a particular antigen or allergen), depressed delayed-type hypersensitivity (DTH) reactions, decreased secretion of IL-2 and IFN-γ, poor lymphocyte proliferation responses to an antigen, and a decrease in antibody-dependent cytotoxicity. Increase in surface transferrin receptors occurs in B lymphocytes too, indicating uptake of iron on activation. However, other functions associated with humoral immunity are not evident in iron-deficient states in man. Total B-cell numbers, immunoglobulin levels and antibody response to tetanus toxoid do not seem to show any impairment.

Effects of iron overload on immune function

Iron overload, for instance following multiple blood transfusions, is associated with reduced phagocytosis by neutrophils, along with reduced opsonization and bactericidal activity. Iron overload does not seem to affect phagocytosis by macrophages or their killing ability, but it reduces their secretion of TNF-α and IL-1. Iron overload states are characterized by reduced T lymphocytes, CD4$^+$ cells and a reduced ratio of CD4$^+$/CD8$^+$ cells. T-lymphocyte proliferative responses to antigens are reduced and so are delayed hypersensitivity skin responses. Although iron overload has significant effects on cell-mediated immune responses, it seems to have no effect on humoral immunity and B-cell function.

In summary, the two extremes of iron nutritional status, i.e. iron deficiency and iron overload, both have detrimental effects on the immune mechanisms of the body and hence increased susceptibility to infections is seen in both conditions. Table 3.3 summarizes some the effects of iron deficiency states and iron overload in man.

3.6 Zinc and the Immune Response

Zinc, like iron, shows a shift from the circulation into the intracellular compartment during an infection. However, in the case of zinc this acute transfer into the intracellular compartment may be related to the role of zinc metalloenzymes in DNA transcription and RNA translation in lymphocytes, since zinc influences the activities of numerous enzymes involved in replication and transcription. The activation and proliferation of lymphocytes is promoted by zinc and host defence is thus enhanced, since zinc participates in multiple aspects of the T-lymphocyte activation process. Zinc deficiency can therefore result in diminished lymphocyte proliferation and impaired host defence. Defects in cell-mediated immunity and increased susceptibility to infections have been seen in patients with zinc deficiency such as *acrodermatitis enteropathica*. Zinc deficiency also manifests with a depression in delayed hypersensitivity responses since they are largely manifestations of cell-mediated immunity. Zinc also plays an important part in apoptosis or cell

Table 3.3. Effects of iron deficiency and iron overload on the immune systems of the host. (Adapted from Kuvibidila and Baliga, 2002.)

		Iron deficiency	Iron overload
On innate immune response	Neutrophil migration – chemotaxis	↓	ND
	Neutrophil phagocytosis	↔	↓
	Neutrophil killing capacity	↓	↓
	Macrophage phagocytosis	↓	↓ or ↔
	Macrophage killing capacity	↓	↓ or ↔
	NK-cell activity	↓	↓
	Interleukin (IL-1) secretion	↔	
	INF-γ secretion	↓	ND
	TNF-α secretion	↓	↔
	Complement	↓	ND
On adaptive immunity (T-cell function)	Total T lymphocytes	↓ or ↔	↔
	CD4$^+$ cells	↓ or ↔	↓
	CD8$^+$ cells	↓ or ↔	↔
	CD4$^+$/CD8$^+$ ratio	↓ or ↔	↓
	Lymphocyte proliferation	↓	↓, ↑ or ↔
	Antibody-dependent cytotoxicity	↓	
	Interleukin (IL-2) secretion	↓ or ↔	↓
	DTH response	↓	↓
On adaptive immunity (B-cell function)	Total B lymphocytes	↓, ↑ or ↔	↑
	Immunoglobulin levels	↑ or ↔	↑
	B-cell proliferation	↓	↓ or ↔
	Antibody production (tetanus toxoid)	↔	

↑, increased; ↔, no significant change; ↓, decreased; ND, not determined.

death. Zinc-deficient animals exhibit enhanced spontaneous and toxin-induced apoptosis, while zinc supplementation decreases induced apoptosis of macrophages and T cells. Thus it appears that zinc functions as a major intracellular regulator of apoptosis and a dose–response relationship can be shown between intracellular levels of zinc in the immune cells and their degree of susceptibility to apoptosis. Zinc plays a role in regulating activation of the acute-phase reaction which is part of the acute-phase response mediated by cytokines (discussed below). Another essential role of zinc in the host's immune response is its binding to certain thymus-derived peptides that are responsible for the differentiation of T cells. Zinc deficiency results in a decrease in numbers of mature T cells and an increase in immature ones, thus increasing susceptibility to infections. Overall, the consistent finding of an important role for zinc in the host's immune response would explain the association between zinc-deficient states and increased morbidity due to infections.

Zinc affects immune function at many levels. Zinc deficiency damages the protective barrier to entry of pathogens, with the skin, respiratory and gut linings damaged by zinc deficiency. Chemotaxis and other functions of neutrophils are impaired and so is the chemotactic activity of macrophages, suggesting that the deficiency of zinc impairs innate immunity. However, the situation is a little complex since high levels of zinc also inhibit macrophage activation, possibly because high zinc levels inhibit complement-mediated phagocytosis by macrophages. NK-cell activity is also reduced in zinc deficiency. Zinc also shows profound effects on adaptive immunity. Lymphopaenia is a common feature of zinc deficiency in man; numbers of B lymphocytes are reduced and so are T lymphocytes along with decreased CD4+/CD8+ cell ratios. This is characteristic even of marginal zinc deficiency and is reversed by zinc supplementation. T-cell activation to an antigen and the consequent proliferative response, as well as T-cell cytotoxicity and DTH test responses, are suppressed in zinc deficiency states and are reversed when zinc is supplemented. DTH test responses are also suppressed in malnourished children and restored following zinc supplementation. The production of IL-2 and IFN-γ is decreased and it appears that there is an imbalance between Th1 and Th2 function in zinc deficiency. B-lymphocyte function is also compromised in zinc deficiency as B-cell proliferation and antibody responses both to Ti and TD antigens are suppressed. In summary, zinc has numerous key functions in the immune system at all levels and zinc deficiency manifests with increased susceptibility to infectious agents. Table 3.4 summarizes some of the main features of zinc deficiency on immune function.

Table 3.4. Effects of zinc deficiency on immune functions.

Thymus size	↓
T lymphocyte proliferation	↓
Cytokine production (IL-2, IFN-γ, TNF-α)	↓
CD4+/CD8+ ratio	↓
Th-cell function	↓
NK-cell activity	↓
DTH response	↓

↓, decreased.

3.7 Other Micronutrients and Immune Function

In addition to the micronutrients discussed in some detail above, several other vitamins and minerals influence the normal functioning of the body's immune system. Antioxidant vitamins like carotenoids were discussed earlier, while other antioxidant vitamins like vitamin C and vitamin E are discussed below.

Vitamin B$_6$

Vitamin B$_6$ per se has no antioxidant properties, but exerts important antioxidant actions because of its crucial role in the metabolic pathways involved in the formation of cysteine which is a precursor for glutathione, an important antioxidant with effects on the immune system. In experimental animals B$_6$ deficiency manifests with thymic atrophy and lymphocyte depletion from lymphoid tissues. Production of antibodies is also affected. In elderly subjects experimental deficiency reduces total lymphocyte numbers and decreases the proliferative response of mitogen-exposed lymphocytes and IL-2 production.

Folate

Folate, along with vitamins B$_6$ and B$_{12}$, plays an important role in nucleic acid and protein synthesis.

Folate deficiency alters the immune response, which affects mainly cell-mediated immunity by reducing the proportion of circulating T lymphocytes and their proliferation following exposure to a mitogen. Folate deficiency reduces the capacity of CD8+ cells to proliferate in response to mitogen activation. Folate supplementation in the elderly improves immune function by altering the age-associated decrease in NK-cell activity and there is evidence that folate supplementation also improves NK-cell cytotoxicity.

Vitamin B$_{12}$

Vitamin B$_{12}$ interacts with folate since they both act together with vitamin B$_6$ in DNA and RNA synthesis. Vitamin B$_{12}$-deficient individuals show a decrease in total numbers of lymphocytes and CD8+ cells and in the proportion of CD4+ cells. Deficient states show an abnormally low CD4+/CD8+ ratio and suppressed NK-cell activity. All these changes in immune response are reversed following the administration of vitamin B$_{12}$. Elderly individuals with low B$_{12}$ levels also show impaired antibody response to antigens.

Other B-complex vitamins

Other B-group vitamins also influence the immune system. They include *biotin*, whose deficiency manifests with reduction in the weight of the thymus and a decrease in lymphocyte proliferation and antibody production. *Pantothenic acid* deficiency also reduces antibody responses. Deficiency of *thiamin* (vitamin B$_1$) reduces thymic weight and manifests with reduced neutrophil motility and decreased antibody secretion, while *riboflavin* (vitamin B$_2$) deficiency decreases antibody responses and the numbers of circulating lymphocytes.

Vitamin C

The high concentrations of vitamin C in leucocytes which is rapidly utilized during infections, and the reduced immune function seen when plasma vitamin C levels are lowered, highlight the role this antioxidant vitamin plays in immune function. Vitamin C deficiency in man does not seem to impair lymphocyte proliferation or alter the numbers of CD4+ and CD8+ cells, although vitamin C administration increases T-cell proliferation as well as neutrophil motility. It also seems to increase circulating immunoglobulin levels. Vitamin C-deficient diets result in decreased DTH response which recovers following supplementation of vitamin C. Vitamin C also provides useful antioxidant protection in inflammatory sites and prevents oxidant-mediated tissue damage.

Vitamin D and 1,25-dihydroxycholecalciferol

Vitamin D and its biologically active metabolite, 1,25-dihydroxycholecalciferol, are potent immunomodulators. Significant quantities of vitamin D receptors are located in most tissues and cells of the immune system such as thymus, monocytes and macrophages; most cells of the immune complex apart from B cells express vitamin D receptors. 1,25-dihydrocholecalciferol down-regulates the production of IL-12 and protects from the occurrence of Th1-mediated autoimmunity. It also prevents excessive expression of inflammatory cytokines while promoting the oxidative burst potential of macrophages, thus assisting intracellular killing. It stimulates the expression of potent antimicrobial peptides in neutrophils, macrophages, NK cells and epithelial cells of the respiratory tract.

Vitamin E

Vitamin E is also involved in maintaining normal immune cell function. Low vitamin E levels are associated with lowered lymphocyte proliferation responses and serum IgM concentrations. DTH responses reflect vitamin E status, with reduced levels leading to poor responses. Vitamin E administration to infants increases neutrophils' phagocytosis but lowers their ability to kill pathogens, possibly due to its potent antioxidant action in reducing the free radicals that mediate this role. Supplementation of the diet of elderly with vitamin E increases lymphocyte proliferation, IL-2 production and DTH response, but does not influence CD4+ cell numbers or levels of circulating immunoglobulins. It also seems to prevent exercise-induced neutropaenia and interleukin production, thus reducing exercise-induced muscle damage.

Selenium

Selenium is another trace mineral that exerts antioxidant activity and manifests several functions in the body, many of which are mediated through the synthesis of a wide range of selenium-containing proteins (selenoproteins). Selenium modulates immune function and it is now well recognized that adequate intake of selenium is essential for both cell-mediated and humoral immunity as well as the innate immune response. Selenium deficiency compromises neutrophil chemotaxis and the subsequent killing of phagocytosed bacteria by intracellular mechanisms, which are often achieved through the generation of reactive oxygen species. This respiratory burst reaction, although very effective, is harmful to the host cell; selenium plays an important role in preventing this host cell damage and quenching the toxic radicals generated in the process. Selenium deficiency results in the cell's inability to remove these toxic peroxides and thus damages the enzyme systems that generate the respiratory burst which kills the bacteria. Similar changes to that evident in neutrophils are also seen in macrophage function with regard to chemotaxis and intracellular killing. Thus selenium deficiency compromises the body's defence by impairing the detoxification of peroxides, leading to increased damage to cells and tissues. In summary, selenium increases chemotaxis, phagocytosis and complement-mediated phagocytosis, as well as bacterial parasite killing by neutrophils and macrophages.

Selenium stimulates lymphocytes and NK cells. It increases the expression of IL-2 receptors on the cell surface of B and T lymphocytes, thus increasing the ability of these cells to be stimulated by cytokines such as IL-2. It increases the number of lymphocytes, potentiates the cytotoxicity of killer cells, and promotes antibody production by B lymphocytes. Thus selenium increases B-lymphocyte numbers and their antibody secretion, increases CD4+ cell numbers and their response to mitogens (a substance that induces and stimulates mitosis), increases Th cells and increases IL-2 receptor expression. It also improves DTH responses and CD8+ T cells show increased cytotoxic action against virus-infected cells when selenium is supplemented.

Copper

Copper functions primarily as a cofactor in cellular metabolic reactions and copper-dependent enzymes catalyse reactions that involve molecular oxygen species. Several copper enzymes play an important role in antioxidant defence of the body. Copper deficiency

in animals manifests among other features with specific impairments in immune function. These include reduced thymus weight, decreased responsiveness of lymphocytes to mitogens, decreased production of antibodies, decreased activity of NK cells, and decreased antimicrobial activity of phagocytes.

Magnesium

Magnesium is another mineral trace element which is a component of metalloenzymes and plays a role in the normal functioning of the immune mechanisms of the body. Magnesium deficiency increases thymus cell proliferation, and increases the levels of interleukins (IL-1 and IL-6) as well as of TNF-α, while reducing the levels of acute-phase proteins and complement. Magnesium also influences the cytotoxicity of T cells and the functioning of adhesion molecules.

Manganese

Manganese is yet another trace mineral which is part of several enzymes in the body and hence exerts some influence on immune function. Deficiency states (which are rare in man) show lowered lymphocyte antioxidant enzyme activity such as that of superoxide dismutase; in experimental animals deficiency states manifest with deficient antibody synthesis and secretion.

Table 3.5 summarizes the levels of defence that are influenced by the various micronutrients discussed above, while Table 3.6 summarizes the main effects of micronutrient deficiencies on immune function.

3.8 Nutrients and Cytokines

It is clear from the preceding sections that macronutrients and micronutrients play an important role in the body's response to infection. Micronutrients such as vitamin A, iron and zinc not only modulate immune cell function but are also incorporated into acute-phase proteins and into enzymes associated with antioxidant defence mechanisms. Several trace elements such as zinc, copper, selenium and magnesium are important elements of acute-phase proteins like metallothionein, caeruloplasmin, superoxide dismutase and glutathione peroxidase. Iron excess increases cytokine production while iron deficiency decreases the ability of cells to produce cytokines. Vitamins also exert a number of

Table 3.5. Summary of the role of micronutrients on immune function. (Adapted from Maggini *et al.*, 2007.)

	External barrier	Cell-mediated immunity	Humoral immunity
Vitamins	Vitamin A	Vitamin A	Vitamin A
	Vitamin C	Vitamin B (B_6, B_{12})	Vitamin B (B_6, B_{12})
	Vitamin E	Vitamin C	Vitamin D
		Vitamin D	Vitamin E
		Vitamin E	Folate (folic acid)
		Folate (folic acid)	
Minerals		Iron	Zinc
		Zinc	Selenium
		Selenium	Copper
		Copper	

Table 3.6. Summary of the main actions of micronutrient deficiencies on immune function.

	Cell-mediated immunity	Humoral immunity	Phagocytic response of leucocytes
Vitamin deficiency			
Vitamin A	↓	↓	↓
Vitamin B complex			
Riboflavin			↓
Folic acid			↓
Pyridoxine	↓	↓	↓
Pantothenic acid	normal	↓	
Vitamin B_{12}	?	?	↓
Vitamin C		?	↓
Minerals/trace element deficiency			
Iron	?	normal	↓
Zinc	↓	↓	↓
Magnesium		↓	
Copper		↓	↓

↓, decreased function; ?, data equivocal.

effects on cytokine production. Both vitamin A and vitamin E have been shown to have effects on cytokine production. More recent research supports a role for vitamin D in the production of TNF-α, while vitamin B_6 has been shown to increase the production of IL-2 in elderly subjects. Despite the unprecedented interest in vitamin C in preventing infections, no effects of the vitamin have been dem-onstrated on the production of pro-inflammatory cytokines.

Pro-inflammatory cytokines (IL-1, IL-6 and TNF-α) have widespread effects on body metabolism. At the cellular level, they activate a number of intracellular signalling pathways including prostaglandins, leucotrienes, cyclic AMP and protein kinase C. Thus, there are many levels at which nutrients can influence the body's inflammatory response to the entry of pathogenic agents. The earliest evidence of the role nutrition plays in influencing cytokines came from studies in undernourished patients. Leucocytes from undernourished patients have a reduced capacity to produce cytokines, and protein supplementation improved cytokine production. Experimental studies in animals and observations in human subjects have shown that fats, amino acids and micronutrients can alter the ability of mammals to produce and to respond to IL-1, IL-6 and TNF-α.

Further Reading

Calder, P.C., Field, C.J. and Gill, H.S. (eds) (2002) *Nutrition and Immune Function*. CAB International and The Nutrition Society, Wallingford, UK. *A book aimed at graduate students offering syntheses of knowledge in the form of state-of-the art reviews on the interaction between immunity and nutrition, with emphasis on the mechanisms of action of the nutrients and their impact on human health.*

4 Undernutrition, Host Defence Mechanisms and Risk of Infection

- Undernutrition is associated with increased morbidity and mortality that is directly related to compromise in the host's defence mechanisms.
- Undernutrition induces a wide range of effects on the host's defence mechanisms and on the immune system and the immunological response.
- In undernutrition, circulating levels of T lymphocytes are reduced but there is no alteration in B-lymphocyte numbers.
- Although the number of polymorphonuclear leucocytes is unaffected, compromise in their function often accompanies undernutrition.
- Other changes such as altered complement levels and lysozyme secretion also occur with poor nutrition.
- Undernutrition in infants and children is associated with an increase in morbidity and mortality due to an increase in the risk of infection from a variety of bacterial, viral, parasitic and other infectious agents.
- Adult undernutrition is probably the underlying cause of increased morbidity due to infectious diseases, and is often the cause of absenteeism, loss of employment and decreased productivity.
- Immunological tests are sensitive to changes in nutritional status and are valuable indicators of deterioration in nutritional status and recovery from undernutrition.

4.1 Introduction

Undernutrition is an important determinant of morbidity and mortality due to infections, especially in infants and young children. According to the WHO, more than 9 million children in developing countries die before they are 5 years old and many of these deaths are due to infections like acute respiratory infections, diarrhoeal disease, measles and malaria. More than half of these children are at increased risk of infections due to underlying undernutrition, which increases substantially their risk of developing infections (Fig. 4.1). Undernutrition and infection interact closely in a vicious negative cycle (see Chapter 5) – poor nutritional status weakening the body's defence mechanisms, with episodes of infection in turn predisposing to poor nutritional status.

Knowledge of the interactions of undernutrition and infection has progressed considerably, enabling us to understand how infections play a role in the aetiology and pathogenesis of undernutrition. This topic is discussed at length in Chapter 5. It is also now clear that undernutrition in turn has deleterious effects on the host's defence mechanisms against infective agents and more specifically on the immune functions of the host. Compromise of the host's defence mechanism may be causally linked to the increased incidence and severity of infectious diseases in undernourished individuals. In turn, infection may lead to loss of nutrients due to vomiting, diarrhoea and malabsorption, which then aggravates the poor nutritional status of the host and further compromises the host's defences.

Since the 1970s reports have appeared in the literature of impaired immune responses in malnourished or undernourished children. Both humoral and cell-mediated immune responses are impaired, as well as several other aspects of the range of responses the body mounts in defence against a pathogenic agent, such as complement activity and antibody responses. The impairment of immune function and the increased risk of infection in malnutrition indicate that the body's defence mechanisms are compromised. Malnutrition enhances the risk and severity of infections not merely in children, but in

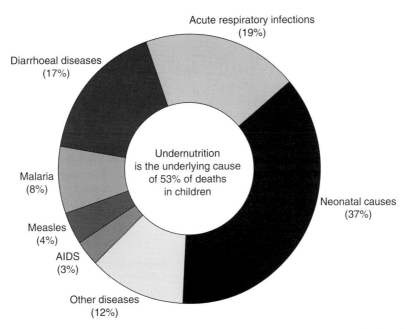

Fig. 4.1. Distribution of the causes of mortality in children under 5 years of age and the contribution of undernutrition as the underlying cause. (WHO estimates for 2000–2003 from Bryce *et al.*, 2005.)

all vulnerable groups such as hospitalized patients and the elderly as well as young adults who become undernourished secondary to conditions like anorexia nervosa. In these conditions, multiple nutrient deficiencies may exist alongside the major deficiency of energy and/or protein. Thus what is seen in an undernourished individual is the sum of the impaired

and compromised responses in the immune system that have been altered in a complex manner by more than one nutrient deficiency. This chapter, unlike the earlier one (Chapter 3), outlines the effects of the severe undernourished state in an individual on the host's defence mechanisms and the host's immune responses.

Box 4.1. Nutritional Anthropometric Assessments.

The objective of nutritional anthropometric assessment at the community level is to provide an estimate of the prevalence and the severity of malnutrition or under-nutrition. The incorporation of measures of nutritional anthropometry into the design of studies or surveys requires several important considerations. For meaningful information generation the sampling protocols must be well designed and strictly adhered to, in order to ensure that the sample is random and representative of the population being studied. One needs to distinguish between anthropometric measurements, indices and indicators used in assessing the nutritional status of children and adults. The basic anthropometric measurements made are weight and height, and age is often used as an additional measure particularly in children.

Anthropometric indices are a combination of measurements. For instance, the height of a child has no

meaning unless it is related to the child's age. Anthropometric indices have two functions – they are essential for the interpretation of measurements and for grouping them. An *anthropometric indicator*, on the other hand, relates to the application of the indices and is often constructed from the indices. Thus the proportion of children under 5 years old with weight-for-age below a certain level (considered as the cut-off) is widely used as an indicator of the nutrition of the whole community. Sometimes an index and an indicator may be the same. A good example is how infant mortality rate, which is an index of the number of infant deaths (under 1 year of age) per 1000 live births, is also used as an indicator of the state of public health or even development of a country. An index is thus generally a biological concept. Indices are continuous variables and their biological interpretation may change with

Continued

Box 4.1. Continued.

age. On the other hand, indicators represent a social concept. They are derivations of measures and indices used in social, medical or public health decision making at the population level. Indicators are used for population assessments and have little meaning for the individual. Indicators may provide a direct estimate of the underlying situation (e.g. loss of weight in children during a famine) or may serve as a proxy for some constraining factor in the environment (e.g. poor growth in children may be associated with inadequate diet and/or presence of infectious disease). The anthropometric indicators chosen should be the most appropriate and the following need to be considered carefully in their selection.

- *Validity* of a nutritional anthropometric index, i.e. the adequacy with which the index reflects the nutritional status being assessed. For example, 'weight-for-age' is a 'valid' reflection of acute malnutrition in children. The term 'valid' is more appropriate than 'accurate' since the latter is best used in a restricted statistical sense.
- *Reliability* of a nutritional anthropometric index, i.e. the degree to which repeated measurements of an anthropometric index give the same value. Reliability is also referred to as 'reproducibility' or 'precision'. It is important to recognize that a measurement may be reliable (reproducible or precise) and yet be inaccurate as a result of systematic measurement errors. The reliability or precision of a measurement procedure can be determined by including replicate measurements and can be expressed as the coefficient of variation (CV%).
- *Sensitivity* of an anthropometric index, i.e. the degree to which the index reflects nutritional status or predicts changes in nutritional status. Sensitive indicators show large changes in anthropometric measurement as a result of small changes in nutritional status of the individual. Sensitive indicators identify and classify those individuals within a population who are genuinely undernourished and respond to small changes in nutritional status resulting from nutritional intervention. Thus sensitive anthropometric indices can be applied for the identification of individuals with deviant anthropometry due to poor nutrition, in the past or present, and for the monitoring of responses to nutritional interventions.
- *Specificity* of an anthropometric index, on the other hand, is the ability of the index to identify and classify those individuals who are *not* undernourished. An index with 100% specificity will identify all well-nourished individuals in a popula-

tion and no well-nourished individual will be diagnosed as being undernourished.

- *Reference values*: Nutritional anthropometric indices can be evaluated by comparison with a distribution of reference values. A reference is a device for grouping and analysing data, and is obtained from a reference population. A reference population which is composed of reference individuals who are healthy and well-nourished is used to select a representative reference sample group, measurements made on whom will constitute the reference values. The distribution of the reference values may be used to derive reference limits. Comparison of individual data can be made against reference values, the reference distribution or even the reference limits. A reference has to be distinguished from a standard since the latter embodies the concept of a norm or a target which is essentially a value judgement. In many instances international references are widely used as standards.
- *Cut-off points*: The most useful way of presenting the nutritional situation of a population is to give an estimate of the proportion of individuals who may be considered to be at risk of an undesirable outcome. The undesirable outcome may be morbidity, mortality or impaired physical or psychological development. In principle such an estimate of individuals 'at risk' may be provided by the number outside the reference distribution. In practice, it is conventional to use cut-off points. Cut-off points are not the same as reference limits calculated from a reference distribution. Cut-off points as mentioned earlier are based on the relationship between nutritional anthropometric indices and functional impairment and/or clinical signs of nutritional deficiency, i.e. the risk of an undesirable outcome. Cut-off levels do not separate the 'undernourished' from the 'well nourished' without some misclassification. Misclassification occurs because of biological variation among individuals. The sensitivity and specificity of an indicator help determine the degree to which misclassification errors can occur and the choice of indicator could help reduce this problem.

Since the objective of nutritional anthropometric assessment at the community level is to provide an estimate of the prevalence and the severity of malnutrition, the choice of indices and indicators is subject to constraints. In practice, there are limits to the feasibility, accuracy and reliability of measurements, including that of age. The size of the representative sample and the number of measurements that can be obtained are also constrained by the availability of resources.

4.2 Severe Undernutrition and Changes in the Host's Defence Systems

Changes in the host's defence and the immune system are seen even if undernutrition occurs in infancy and childhood. Some of these changes are also observed in adults who are moderately or severely undernourished. Many of these changes – particularly those seen in the thymus and in thymus-dependent areas of other lymphoid organs – may be irreversible, while others are reversible and do respond to nutritional rehabilitation. The changes that occur in the host's defence and immunological systems in the undernourished individual are briefly discussed below and are summarized in Table 4.1.

The physical and chemical barriers to infection

The first line of defence is dependent on the physical and chemical barriers of the host that the infective agent has to overcome. This includes the skin, the mucous membranes and the various protective secretions provided by them. It is only when these barriers are breached that the host relies on the immune functions of the body to engage the pathogenic agent. In protein–energy malnutrition (PEM) impairment of most of the host barriers has been observed. Under normal conditions the host provides both a localized and a generalized response to

the entry of the pathogenic agent, manifested locally probably as an inflammatory infiltrate and as a fever in a generalized response to the infection. In severely undernourished individuals, both the localized and the generalized responses are diminished and may even be completely absent as a result of the immunocompromised state of the host.

Anatomic barriers such as the skin and mucous membranes are compromised in undernutrition. Skin lesions in severely undernourished children favour the penetration and entry of infectious agents. Changes in the mucosal epithelium of the gastrointestinal tract will favour pathogen colonization and bacterial translocation. There are marked changes during undernutrition in several non-specific host defence mechanisms. Lower levels of lysozyme are found in plasma, tears, saliva and other secretions, as a result of lowered production. The quantity of mucus secreted as well as its structure is altered. Salivary flow is reduced and its chemical composition altered in undernourished children. Gastric acid secretion is also significantly reduced. Metaplasia of mucosal epithelium, deficient mucus trapping and reduced movement of epithelial cilia all occur in undernutrition and influence the susceptibility of the individual to infections. Alterations in the intercellular materials and increased permeability of the intestinal and other mucosal surfaces have been demonstrated in experimental animals, confirming the increased risk of pathogenic infections in the undernourished state.

Undernourished states due to PEM (like in kwashiorkor and marasmus) are almost always accompanied by multiple micronutrient deficiencies and their consequences. The increased keratinization and metaplasia of epithelial surfaces and the loss of ciliated epithelium, especially of the respiratory tract, compromise an important protective function. The accumulation of cellular debris and mucus results in a favourable culture medium for organisms. The nutritional oedema of malnourished states like kwashiorkor and the increased fluid in the tissues favour the infective process while effectively impairing adequate circulation and the flow of nutrients and immune cells to the region. These changes also interfere with normal tissue replacement and repair, thus impairing the normal wound healing process. In the gastrointestinal tract the alteration of normal bacterial flora also contributes to infections. It is well documented that undernutrition alters the types, numbers and distribution of the normal gastrointestinal bacterial flora, which in turn contributes to a decreased resistance to intestinal infections in undernourished individuals.

Table 4.1. Summary of changes in host defence mechanisms in PEM. (Adapted from Jackson and Calder, 2004.)

Defence mechanism and immune function	Changes in PEM
Mucus structure	Altered
Mucus secretion	↓
Integrity of gut mucosa	↓
Leucocyte count	↓
Phagocytosis by neutrophils and macrophages	↔
Bacterial killing by neutrophils	↓
T lymphocytes	↓
CD4+ and CD8+ cells	↓
CD4+/CD8+ ratio	↓
Cytokine production	↓
NK-cell activity	↓
Interleukin production	↓
B lymphocytes	↔
Immunoglobulin levels	↔
Acute-phase proteins	↓

↓, decreased; ↔, no significant change.

Box 4.2. Malnutrition and Undernutrition – Are They Different Entities?

Malnutrition refers to all deviations from adequate nutrition, including undernutrition and overnutrition from inadequacy of food or excess of food relative to need, respectively. Malnutrition also encompasses specific deficiencies or excesses of essential nutrients such as vitamins and minerals. Conditions such as obesity, though not the result of inadequacy of food, also constitute malnutrition. The terms 'malnutrition' and 'undernutrition' are often used loosely and interchangeably, although sometimes a distinction is and needs to be made. Malnutrition arises from deficiencies of specific nutrients, or from diets based on the wrong kinds or proportions of foods. Goitre, scurvy, anaemia and xerophthalmia are forms of malnutrition, caused by inadequate intake of iodine, vitamin C, iron and vitamin A, respectively. Malnutrition and undernutrition mean more or less the same entity and refer to nutritional situations characteristic of relatively poorer socio-economic populations in developing countries.

Undernutrition is defined as the result of insufficient food caused primarily by an inadequate intake of food energy, whether or not any specific nutrient is an additional limiting factor. Undernutrition is defined as the fact of having a dietary energy intake below the minimum level required to maintain the balance between actual energy intake and acceptable levels of energy expenditure, while also accounting for the additional needs arising from: (i) growth in children; (ii) maintaining appropriate weight gain associated with fetal growth in pregnant women; and (iii) sustaining adequate milk production in lactating women. This emphasis on food energy as a general measurement of food adequacy seems pragmatically justified: increased food energy, if derived from normal staple foods, brings with it more protein and other nutrients, while raising intakes of such nutrients without providing more energy is unlikely to be of much benefit to the individual. Thus, in most situations, increased food energy is a necessary condition for nutritional improvement, even if it is not always sufficient in itself.

Table 4.2 summarizes the various changes associated with undernutrition that undermine the normal functioning of the external physical and chemical barriers to infection.

Morphological changes in immune organs

Clinical studies show significant morphological changes in undernutrition, with alterations in the size, weight, cellularity and architecture of the lymphoid organs. Most pronounced effects are seen in the thymus, which normally increases in size from birth until puberty and then involutes. Lesser effects are seen in the spleen, lymph nodes and other lymphoid organs in undernutrition. Severe undernutrition even causes atrophy of lymphoid organs such as the thymus, spleen, lymph nodes and tonsils. Since these changes manifest in the thymus and other lymphoid organs during severe undernutrition they have been referred to as 'nutritional thymectomy'.

Moderate to severe undernutrition in infants and children results in marked histomorphological changes in the thymus. The cortico-medullary regions of the thymus are more affected than the epithelial regions. In addition to a reduction in size and weight, depletion of lymphocytes, loss of cortico-medullary differentiation, swelling and degeneration within the thymus have been observed. The Hassal bodies in the thymus are enlarged, degenerated and even calcified occasionally. Paracortical regions of the lymph node and peri-arteriolar tissue in spleen exhibit similar changes. In lymph nodes the thymus-dependent paracortical areas show depletion of lymphocytes, while there is loss of lymphoid cells around small blood vessels in the spleen. These changes may be due to impaired cellular proliferation, or an increase in the level of free cortisol seen in undernutrition, or both. It is possible that

Table 4.2. Summary of changes in the physical and chemical barriers to infection in undernutrition. (Adapted from Scrimshaw *et al.*, 1968.)

Keratinization and metaplasia of epithelial surfaces
Alteration in intercellular substance
Loss of ciliated epithelium of respiratory tracts
Reduction or absence of secretion of mucus
Structural changes in mucus secreted
Reduced salivary flow and changes in composition
Reduced gastric acid secretion
Increased permeability of intestinal and other
  mucosal surfaces
Accumulation of cellular debris and mucus, providing
  a favourable culture medium for infectious agents
Nutritional oedema – increased fluid in tissue spaces
Reduced fibroblastic response
Interference with normal tissue replacement and repair

nutritional deprivation during intrauterine or neonatal growth may result in irreversible changes both in the thymus and in the thymus-dependent areas of other lymphoid organs.

Changes in T-lymphocyte responses and functions

Cell-mediated immunity is largely dependent on thymus-derived T lymphocytes. T-cell numbers can be specifically estimated by counting the number of lymphocytes that form rosettes with sheep red blood cells. Lymphoid atrophy and impaired maturation result in a decreased number of T cells in the peripheral blood in undernutrition – about 15% of children with moderate to severe undernutrition show low circulating lymphocyte numbers (lymphopaenia). This may be due to either a reduction in the number of precursor cells or impaired differentiation as a result of decreased thymic hormone (thymulin). The latter possibility is supported by the evidence that peripheral blood drawn from undernourished children mixed with the thymic hormone *in vitro* increases the number of rosetting lymphocytes (i.e. T lymphocytes).

In undernutrition, there is an increase in the number of uncommitted (or 'null') lymphocytes which bear neither B- nor T-lymphocyte markers. Many of these 'null' cells are immature T cells which may be associated with non-specific killing functions. The increase in uncommitted or 'null' lymphocytes in undernutrition may thus be the result of a reduced thymic inductive activity. The increase may be further boosted by the presence of circulating inhibitors or altered cell surface chemistry. Lymphocyte blast transformation, in response to a mitogen such as PHA or an antigen, is impaired in severely undernourished individuals. However, iron or folate deficiency can also reduce the lymphocyte response to mitogens. Lymphocyte-mediated cytotoxicity is increased in moderate undernutrition, a feature not seen in severe undernutrition. The levels of leucocyte and macrophage inhibition factors may be altered and the numbers of intraepithelial T lymphocytes are reduced in undernutrition.

Apart from the changes seen when undernutrition occurs during intrauterine or early postnatal life, most changes in T-cell-mediated immune responses are reversed on nutritional rehabilitation. DCH tests are valuable indices of T-cell-mediated immune function. DCH responses following a challenge with common antigens are decreased in undernutrition and improve following nutritional repletion. The exact mechanisms underlying this deficit in cell-mediated immunity are not known. A combination of factors (such as antigen recognition, antigen processing, efficient functioning of T lymphocytes, release of lymphokines, mobilization of polymorphs and macrophages) may influence the outcome of a cutaneous hypersensitivity test in undernourished individuals. DCH tests are often used to assess the immunological status of undernourished individuals and to assess the response to nutritional rehabilitation.

Changes in B-lymphocyte responses and functions

The numbers of circulating B lymphocytes are unaltered in an undernourished individual. Serum immunoglobulin levels may be normal in undernutrition or even modestly elevated, particularly during an infection. Antibody response to infectious agents is generally normal in undernutrition. However, if an antigen, especially a particulate antigen, requires the cooperation of Th cells then antibody responses to repeated infections are less satisfactory. This is largely the result of alterations in T-lymphocyte function since memory is a T-cell function. The impaired antibody responses seen in an undernourished individual improve with nutritional rehabilitation.

The finding that a decreased secretory immunoglobulin (IgA) response occurs over mucosal surfaces in undernutrition is of considerable fundamental and applied interest. Secretory IgA responses in nasopharyngeal and other external secretions are lowered and specific IgA production following vaccination with measles or polio viruses is markedly reduced. These changes may be due to a decrease in IgA-bearing cells or a lowered turnover of the IgA secretory component from an atrophied mucosal epithelium.

Changes in polymorphonuclear neutrophil functions

Although the total number of leucocytes and neutrophils may be unaltered, there are significant changes in neutrophil function in undernutrition. When the nutritional deficiency is complicated by an infection, chemotactic migration of neutrophils is markedly reduced; phagocytosis is normal but intracellular killing of bacteria and fungi is reduced. Intracellular killing is also reduced in iron deficiency states. Following phagocytosis, the neutrophil in an undernourished individual does not exhibit the characteristic 'respiratory burst'. Metabolic pathways such as the hexose monophosphate shunt, which demonstrate an increase in activity in normal neutrophils, are not seen in the neutrophils of undernourished individuals. These changes in neutrophils and their functions are reversed within a few weeks of nutritional rehabilitation.

Changes in complement functions

Several studies have demonstrated consistent changes in the complement system during undernutrition. Many of the complement components are produced by the liver, which is often affected as a result of protein deprivation. Undernourished children show reduced levels of C3, C1, C2 and C5, and occasionally of other complement components. The total haemolytic activity is also reduced. There is some evidence to show that the alternative pathways of complement production may also be affected during undernutrition.

Box 4.3. Indicators of Undernutrition in Infants, Children and Adults.

Infants

Birth weight is considered a good indicator of intrauterine growth retardation (IUGR). The definition of IUGR is an infant born at term (i.e. >37 weeks' gestation) with low birth weight (i.e. <2500 g).

The causes of IUGR are multiple and involve many different factors. The most important determinant of infant weight at birth is the maternal environment, of which nutrition is the single most important factor. Poor maternal nutritional status at conception and inadequate maternal nutrition during pregnancy can result in IUGR. Short maternal stature, low maternal body weight at conception and inadequate weight gain during pregnancy are factors that are associated with IUGR.

Children

Assessment of growth is the measurement that best defines the health and nutritional status of children in the community. Undernutrition is diagnosed using three anthropometric parameters, which are compared with an international reference standard such as the international growth standards developed by the World Health Organization (WHO).

- *Weight-for-age* is a convenient synthesis of linear growth and body proportion, and can be used for the diagnosis of underweight children.
- *Height-for-age* corresponds to linear growth, and can demonstrate long-term faltering of growth or stunting in children.
- *Weight-for-height* reflects body proportion, and is particularly sensitive to acute growth disturbances; a low value is indicative of wasting.

Values more than two standard deviations (SD) below the mean weight-for-age, height-for-age or weight-for-height of the reference population indicate under-

weight, stunting or wasting, respectively. When fed well and free of infection, children throughout the world tend to grow at similar rates whatever their ethnic or racial origin; when fed appropriately, healthy children everywhere can be expected to grow on average along the 50th centile of a reference population's weight-for-age and height-for-age. By expressing both height and weight as standard deviations or Z-scores from the median reference value for the child's age, the normal range will correspond to the 3rd to 97th centile (i.e. ±2 SD or ±2 Z-scores). By expressing data in this way it is possible to express the weight and height data for all children across a wide age range in similar Z-score units, and thereby produce a readily understandable comparison of the extent of growth retardation at different ages and in different countries.

A deficit in height is referred to as 'stunting' whereas a deficit in weight-for-height is considered as 'wasting'. These two measures are subsumed in the original designation of a child's failure to grow in terms of weight-for-age. Clearly this measure includes both the wasting and stunting features but fails to distinguish the important differences between the two. Wasting can occur on a short-term basis in response to illness with anorexia or malabsorption or because the child goes hungry for several weeks. Changes in weight-for-height therefore reflect the impact of short-term changes in nutritional status. Growth in height, however, is much more a cumulative index of long-term health because growth in length or height stops when a child develops an infection and the subsequent growth may be slow during the recovery period. Children normally grow in spurts intermittently and once children have failed to maintain their proper growth trajectory for stature they tend to remain on the lower centiles and 'track' at this low level for many years.

Mid-upper arm circumference (MUAC) is a simple measure of nutritional status in children, used particularly for screening in emergency situations. The MUAC of a pre-school child is almost age-independent. A circumference of more than 14 cm is considered normal; less than 12.5 cm indicates severe undernutrition. Measurements of 12.5–14 cm are suggestive of mild or moderate undernutrition.

Adults

One simple measure of undernutrition in adults is adult weight in relation to height, and the indicator body mass index (BMI) is considered the most suitable for both undernutrition and overnutrition in adults. BMI is a simple, reliable and easily obtainable measure of nutritional status in adults. The choice of BMI for the assessment of nutritional status of adults was based on the observation that BMI was consistently highly correlated with body weight and was relatively independent of the stature of the individual. BMI is obtained by dividing the weight of an individual (in kilograms) by the height (in metres) squared. Adults with BMI $<18.5 \, kg/m^2$ are considered to be chronically undernourished, while those with BMI >25.0 and $>30.0 \, kg/m^2$ are considered overweight and obese, respectively; the same BMI cut-offs apply to both males and females.

Table 4.3. Diagnostic criteria for the assessment of undernutrition in children and adults.

Childhood undernutrition	
Underweight	Low weight-for-age[a]
Stunted	Low height-for-age[a]
Wasted	Low weight-for-height[a]
Adult undernutrition	
Grade I	BMI = $17.0–18.49 \, kg/m^2$
Grade II	BMI = $16.0–16.99 \, kg/m^2$
Grade III	BMI $<16.0 \, kg/m^2$

[a]'Low' is defined as below −2 SD (Z-score) of the median reference value for the child's age, the reference being the National Center for Health Statistics/WHO or the new WHO international growth reference for age.

4.3 Changes in Immune Function in Intrauterine Growth Retardation

Undernutrition in pregnant women during the critical months of intrauterine life has far-reaching effects. Intrauterine growth retardation (IUGR) can be due to various causes, including maternal undernutrition, and is associated with involution of the thymus gland and impaired immunity in the newborn. IUGR and low birth weight (LBW) in infants are associated with compromise in immune function. Neonates generally tend to exhibit suboptimal immune function, and this picture in the newborn is complicated with IUGR and LBW as these infants demonstrate marked impairment of immunocompetence. The consequences of this are the increased risk of infection, higher morbidity and increased mortality seen among IUGR and LBW infants. These infants suffer from respiratory tract infections three times more frequently than appropriate-for-gestational-age and normal-weight infants.

IUGR infants show thymic atrophy and impaired cell-mediated immune function. DCH test responses are also impaired. Small-for-gestational-age infants continue to exhibit impaired cell-mediated immune responses for several months or even years after birth that often persists if the growth of these infants is poor and seems to correlate with the increase in infectious episodes seen clinically. It has also been shown that these infants may show a reduction in immunoglobulin-producing cells and in immunoglobulin levels. Since the immunoglobulins, in particular IgG, are transferred across the placenta from the mother after 32 weeks' gestation, IUGR infants show low serum concentrations of IgG associated with a higher risk of respiratory infections.

In contrast, LBW infants who are normal for gestational age show some differences from IUGR infants. LBW infants recover sooner from the impaired cell-mediated immune responses. Other investigations carried out in LBW infants show some derangement in phagocytic function, as well as a lower level of IgG at birth and a more prolonged and pronounced reduction in immunoglobulin levels compared with normal-weight infants. LBW infants show a decrease in circulating lymphocytes, T lymphocytes, CD4[+] cells and a decreased CD4[+]/CD8[+] ratio. They show a diminished lymphocyte proliferative response and a reduced killing ability of neutrophils. B lymphocytes may be normal, although most immunoglobulin levels apart from IgE show a reduction. Clinically, LBW infants show increased susceptibility to infections, diarrhoeal disease and pneumonia and increased mortality from infectious illness.

Box 4.4. Protein–Energy Malnutrition in Children.

Two classical syndromes of undernutrition in children have been recognized for several decades and although the clinical features may appear to be distinct and different, many children present features of both. These clinical presentations of severe childhood malnutrition often referred to as protein–energy malnutrition (PEM) are *kwashiorkor*, *marasmus* and the mixed condition of *marasmic kwashiorkor*. In marasmus there is severe loss of body weight as a result of severe wasting in infancy; the one additional characteristic other than the weight deficit which must be present for the diagnosis of kwashiorkor is the presence of oedema. Thus the severity of weight deficit and the presence/absence of oedema constitute two important criteria for both the diagnosis of undernutrition and its classification.

Kwashiorkor

The term 'kwashiorkor' was first introduced by Cecily Williams in 1933. In the language of the Ga tribe who live in Ghana, kwashiorkor was the name for the 'sickness of the older child when the next baby is born'. This childhood undernutrition manifesting with oedema was believed to be of dietary aetiology because of Cecily Williams' original observation that kwashiorkor developed in children weaned on to starchy food and was cured by milk. Subsequent observations made in Uganda seemed to confirm the belief that the chief cause of kwashiorkor was the lack of protein in the diet. Our understanding of the aetio-pathogenesis of kwashiorkor has changed little since and can be summarized as follows. Kwashiorkor develops when the diet has a low ratio of protein to energy, which may result in protein being a limiting factor for some children. The initial endocrine response to such a diet is a high insulin level and a low plasma cortisol level. This in turn promotes the uptake of amino acids by muscle, diverting them from the liver. As a consequence, there is a reduced synthesis of albumin (resulting in low circulating albumin levels, which cause oedema) and a reduced synthesis of lipoproteins (predisposing to a fatty liver). The presence of infections may divert amino acids for the synthesis of albumin by the liver. More recently, free radicals have been implicated in the causation of kwashiorkor; the free radical theory has attempted to explain the characteristic occurrence of oedema and skin lesions seen in children with kwashiorkor.

Kwashiorkor presents a variety of clinical features, with children characteristically appearing oedematous with a moon face and showing scaling, crazy pavement pigmentation and ulceration of the skin with sparse, thin, reddish hair. Clinically they are morose, lethargic and irritable, having large liver and often appreciable amounts of trunkal and limb fat which obscure an atrophied muscle mass. The condition, associated with growth failure and high mortality, is often accompanied by infections.

Marasmus

The term 'marasmus' is derived from the Greek word meaning 'dying away' and is applied to severe undernutrition in infants. The direct cause of marasmus seems to be different from that of kwashiorkor. When energy in the diet is limiting due to inadequate food intake, which may be precipitated or complicated by repeated infections, a hormonal response opposite to that seen in kwashiorkor emerges. The low insulin and high plasma cortisol result in amino acids being released from muscle and becoming available for the synthesis of protein, particularly albumin, in the liver. This results in severe muscle wasting with normal albumin levels, and hence there is no oedema. Absence of oedema in the presence of severe muscle wasting is characteristic of marasmus. Thus the 'marasmic infant lives on his own meat'.

Marasmus is a form of PEM which is characterized by marked wasting of muscle and subcutaneous tissue, presenting as a wizened, shrivelled, growth-retarded and skeletal infant or child who is often alert and irritable, with normal-coloured but shrivelled skin which may show some scaling and hypopigmentation. Marasmic children often have good appetite, unlike children with kwashiorkor who are generally anorexic. Mortality rates in marasmus are lower than in kwashiorkor.

Marasmic kwashiorkor

Marasmic kwashiorkor manifests with clinical features of both marasmus and kwashiorkor and is regarded as an intermediate form of severe PEM. Oedema is present alongside marked muscle wasting and underweight, with other skin and hair changes typical of kwashiorkor. When marasmic children are overfed early with too high a sodium intake, they often may become oedematous and simulate the mixed syndrome of marasmic kwashiorkor.

4.4 Changes in Immune Function seen in Protein–Energy Malnutrition in Children

PEM in children manifests as *kwashiorkor, marasmus* or even as *marasmic kwashiorkor*. Children with kwashiorkor manifest with oedema and skin changes while muscle wasting seems to be the dominant feature of marasmic children. Children with both forms of malnutrition demonstrate secondary immunodeficiency attributable to the poor nutritional status and hence are susceptible to frequent infections, some of them characteristic of opportunistic infections. Hence PEM can be considered a nutritionally acquired immunodeficiency state.

In children with kwashiorkor marked reduction is seen in the weight of the thymus, with histology of the thymus showing mostly epithelial and reticular tissue with marked depletion of lymphocytes. There is no distinction between cortex and medulla of the thymus, with few, poorly formed Hassal's corpuscles. Peripheral lymphoid organs show similar changes. Lymph nodes show decrease in numbers and a reduction in the size of lymphoid follicles, with paracortical areas depleted of lymphocytes. Lymphoid follicles in the spleen and appendix are smaller and lacking in small lymphocytes. Thymic atrophy seems a consistent finding. Spleens of children with PEM are also profoundly affected. The spleen is smaller in size and histologically shows a striking reduction in germinal centres and depletion of lymphocytes in paracortical and peri-arterial areas, regions considered to be thymus dependent. Gut-associated lymphoid tissue (GALT) is also affected, with decreased tonsillar and adenoid tissue in children and a reduction in the size of the intestinal Peyer's patches. Histological features in the gut lymphoid tissue are suggestive of a greater effect on cell-mediated than humoral immune systems.

Children with PEM also show significant to moderate peripheral lymphopaenia, i.e. reduced circulating levels of lymphocytes. The peripheral lymphocytes of children with PEM respond poorly to mitogens and there is a reduction in lymphocyte transformation. The clinical features related to the immune system seen in childhood PEM are suggestive of stress, the associated increased adrenocortical activity and the increased corticosteroid secretion. The high resting levels of plasma cortisol, the loss of normal diurnal variations in cortisol levels and the impaired cortisol catabolism seen (particularly high in marasmus) support this proposed mechanism as being responsible for the changes seen in PEM in children.

A more complex picture is evident with regard to humoral immunity in childhood PEM. The absolute numbers of B lymphocytes are normal or reduced but there are no changes in circulating B cells. The B lymphocytes from malnourished children show moderate spontaneous lymphocytotoxicity. In PEM although the level of serum albumin is reduced, the serum levels of gamma globulins are normal or elevated and the synthesis and turnover of gamma globulins is not affected. The synthesis of gamma globulins increases with concomitant infections in these malnourished children. There is a great variability in the levels of specific immunoglobulins, generally reflecting the particular or predominant infectious disease. In general, IgG, IgM and IgA levels show a wide scatter – suggestive of a normal range or a possible increase. Serum antibody responses after immunization suggest a normal response to bacterial (tetanus, diphtheria toxoids) but variable and generally lowered response to viral (polio, yellow fever, hepatitis) antigens. In general results indicate that although serum immunoglobulin levels are usually normal or even increased in PEM, the actual integrity of the humoral response may be normal or even decreased depending on the nature and dose of the antigen, the severity of undernutrition, or the state of nutritional repletion.

Secretory immunoglobulins (the first barrier encountered by a pathogen) are also altered in PEM. Abnormalities are seen in secretory IgA levels, with malnourished children responding to attenuated polio or measles virus by decreased frequency, delayed appearance and lower levels of secretory IgA. Decreased secretory IgA response is probably the result of a selective depression of IgA synthesis in submucosa or a reduction in synthesis of the secretory component of IgA, which would be consistent with the histopathological findings seen in the GALT in PEM children. This reduction in secretory IgA response may contribute to prolonging infections and increasing the severity of respiratory and enteric pathogens, thus increasing infectiousness and possibly leading to carrier status.

In summary, serum immunoglobulins may be normal or increased in childhood PEM but functional studies indicate that at least in response to antigens the quality of humoral response is impaired. This may result in qualitatively poor antibody responses or in the production of antibody molecules with low specific affinity for antigen. Thus susceptibility to infections may also be increased in PEM. Local mucosal immunity through secretory IgA may also be impaired, leading to increased frequency of infections and possibly of food allergies.

Cell-mediated immunity is also altered in children with PEM. This includes a decrease in peripheral blood T-lymphocyte levels (identified by their ability to form rosette configurations with sheep red blood cells). The depression of peripheral T-cell levels correlates with the degree of weight deficit in the child. Both the proportion and the absolute numbers of T cells are reduced and nutritional rehabilitation results in rapid improvement. Atrophy of the thymus-dependent areas of lymphoid tissue may be the likely mechanism responsible for this change. The relative proportions of T cells with markers for a component of the IgM molecule are decreased while those with marker for IgG are increased. CD4$^+$ Th cells are markedly deficient while CD8$^+$ cytotoxic or suppressor T cells are affected to a lesser extent.

DCH test responses are impaired, and defective DCH responses to a number of skin test antigens including tuberculin are seen. There is a good relationship between the degree of nutritional deficit and the impairment of DCH responses, and the response to these tests improves with nutritional rehabilitation. In summary, most studies with differing antigens and varying degrees of PEM have shown DCH to be impaired in PEM, in many cases proportional to the degree and severity of the undernutrition. In studies designed to assess the effect of nutritional rehabilitation on these immunological tests, the defects in DCH responses were shown to be readily reversible. When sensitized lymphocytes encounter an antigen they undergo blast transformation and synthesize DNA as a prelude to mitosis. Evaluation of this cellular response *in vitro* correlated well with DCH reactivity *in vivo*. The weight of evidence is suggestive of an *in vitro* lymphocyte transformation and an impaired proliferative capacity in PEM in children, which corresponds to the DCH responses observed.

Phagocytic cell function is also affected in children with PEM, although the findings are inconsistent and are largely attributable to the wide variation in patients studied. No firm conclusion can be drawn from the studies looking at chemotaxis and inflammation, as several studies have reported results consistent with depression, enhancement or no change in chemotaxis and the cellular inflammatory response. The phagocytic function appears to be normal in the case of both polymorphonuclear leucocytes and macrophages. Overall the reduction in phagocytic activity appears more due to the reduction in macrophages rather than their ability to phagocytose. The post-phagocytosis intracellular killing of pathogens that occurs is also altered and indicative of a deficit in the post-phagocytic metabolic burst of oxidative and glycolytic activity. Studies indicate that the infection rather than the poor nutritional status per se is the significant factor in impairment of bactericidal function.

Although precise correlation between *in vitro* assessment of the function of phagocytes and the susceptibility to infectious diseases is not firmly established, the weight of evidence suggests that the increased incidence of infection in undernourished children may be due in part to defective phagocytic function. Thus studies in childhood PEM suggest impaired chemotaxis, normal phagocytosis, defective bactericidal activity and abnormal metabolic function of phagocytic cells.

Complement function is also altered in children with PEM. In kwashiorkor and marasmus serum concentrations of almost all complement components are reduced. In moderate PEM, the level of C3 correlates with the degree of weight deficit in these children. Thus the overwhelming weight of evidence suggests that complement function is impaired in PEM and that this may be the result of a combination of decreased synthesis of complement and increased consumption due to complement activation. The reduced complement activity is likely to contribute significantly to increased susceptibility to infections, particularly of gram-negative infections, in children with PEM. This state is, however, reversible with nutritional rehabilitation.

Observations made in children with PEM show that there are definite changes in lymphoid organs and in the number and function of immune cells, as well as in the efficacy of humoral defence mechanisms (see Fig. 4.2). These are summarized in Table 4.4.

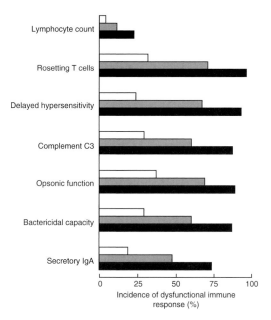

Lymphocyte count

Rosetting T cells

Delayed hypersensitivity

Complement C3

Opsonic function

Bactericidal capacity

Secretory IgA

Incidence of dysfunctional immune response (%)

Fig. 4.2. Bar graphs showing the percentage incidence of immune response dysfunction in mild (□, weight-for-height 70–80% of the reference growth standards), moderate (▨, weight-for-height 60–70% of the reference growth standards) and severe undernutrition (■, weight-for-height <60% of the reference growth standards) in children. (Adapted from Chandra, 1981a.)

Table 4.4. Summary of immune function changes seen in children with various forms of PEM. (Adapted from Chandra, 1981a, 1988.)

Atrophy of lymphoid tissues
Reduced thymidine uptake by T cells
Impaired maturation of T lymphocytes
Reduction in the ratio of Th cells to suppresser T cells
Depression of DCH
Reduction in IgA levels in plasma/serum and secretory IgA in tears
Impaired killing of bacteria by leucocytes
Reduction in secretory IgA response to viral vaccines
Reduction of complement component C3
Serum levels of IgG and IgM are normal or high
Humoral response to antigens is not reduced except in severe undernutrition

4.5 Undernutrition and the Increased Risk of Infection

The diminished and compromised immune function in undernourished individuals makes them more susceptible and increases their risk of infections. It is important to note that in moderate to severe undernutrition we are not dealing with a single nutrient deficiency but with multiple nutrient deficiencies that complicate the picture. The discussions here relate to the increased risk of a range of infectious diseases in clinically undernourished children or adults.

TB is the infection most studied, and the historical evidence from data obtained during wartime supports this association between poor nutritional status and increased risk of infection. Mortality from TB increased in Europe during both World Wars when diets were inadequate and nutritionally poor. During World War II, death rates from TB in Germany doubled and returned to pre-war levels a few years later when the food supply improved. Poor nutritional status was also linked to the increased incidence of TB in the Warsaw ghettos. US Navy recruits were found to have fourfold higher morbidity rates due to TB if they were 15% or more underweight compared with those with normal weight-for-height. Even in poor countries in Africa, those with a diversified diet consisting of meat products had a lower risk of infection from TB (1%) compared with those from predominantly cereal-eating tribes (6%) but from identical ecological environments.

There is a vast literature from developing countries showing that undernourished children have more frequent and longer-lasting episodes of acute diarrhoeal diseases and upper respiratory tract illnesses compared with well-nourished children. Similar observations of a higher mortality and morbidity due to infections with undernutrition have been reported for measles in children, amoebic dysentery and amoebiasis, schistosomiasis, malaria, trachoma, and typhus fevers. Severely malnourished children may even be susceptible to opportunistic infections like the fungus *Pneumocystis carinii*. Noma is another opportunistic infection occurring in malnourished children which evolves from gingival inflammation and may lead ultimately to oro-facial gangrene. Undernutrition often associated with multiple nutrient deficiencies lowers the resistance and increases the risk of a wide variety of infections – bacterial, viral and parasitic – in the undernourished individual.

4.6   Undernutrition, Morbidity and Mortality

The evidence that severely undernourished children have an increased incidence and prevalence of a range of infections even when growing up in a healthy and clean environment is well documented. The episodes of invasion with pathogens and the duration of illness – both of which are enhanced by the poor nutritional status of the child – result in marked increases in case fatality rates. A review and analysis of 15 studies examining the relationship between nutritional status and morbidity from diarrhoeal disease confirmed an association in 12 of the 15 studies.

Quantitative estimates of the impact of infection on weight gain and height increase have been made. Since the reduction in food intake is about 20%, the deficit in intake in a child has been estimated to be about 630 kJ (150 kcal) per day, which represents a calculated weight deficit of 30–40 g per day. Estimates have also been made, based on several clinical studies in developing countries such as Gambia and Sudan, of the deficit in weight gain over a period of time due to infections. This is likely to have a significant impact on growth even in well-nourished infants and in undernourished children it can interfere substantially with 'catch-up' growth, weight gain and growth, resulting in an increased risk of death.

Undernutrition was the principal cause of immunodeficiency worldwide among infants, children and even the elderly in the pre-HIV/AIDS era. Risk of four infectious diseases – diarrhoeal diseases, acute respiratory infections and pneumonia, measles and malaria – account for more than 50% of the deaths of children under 5 years of age and undernutrition is the underlying risk factor in nearly half of these (see Fig. 4.1).

It is reasonably clear from much of the earlier discussion that the predominant cause of mortality in undernourished children is largely the sequence of morbidity associated with infections caused by a wide range of pathogens. The most important causes of morbidity that may lead to case fatality include diarrhoeal disease, measles, acute respiratory infections, malaria, TB and HIV/AIDS. However, mortality statistics from several parts of the developing world do not provide a clear picture of the contribution of undernutrition to infant and child mortality largely as a result of inadequate or incomplete data collection.

The assumption is, however, that child mortality is closely associated with undernutrition and that this is largely the result of infections.

The contribution of undernutrition to mortality must vary with the disease, since the predisposition to infection and its impact in the undernourished state depend on the pathogen. Table 4.5 summarizes the various infective agents whose ability to cause infection is influenced by the host's nutritional status. There is reasonably sound evidence to show that deaths due to infectious diseases depend on the nutritional status of the child.

For example:

- in Uganda, the risk of death from diarrhoeal disease increased tenfold in children who were undernourished (measured as underweight and decreased arm circumference);
- in Bangladesh, children with body weight at 55% of the reference weight-for-age had a death rate of 14% within 3 months of discharge following diarrhoeal disease compared with 1% in children with weight-for-age at 75% of the reference value;
- in Senegal, the case fatality rate due to diarrhoea in hospitalized patients was increased twofold if weight-for-height was less than 80% of the reference value (and increased sixfold if the children had severe undernutrition with oedema, i.e. presented with kwashiorkor).

There are very few studies that have examined the relationship between adult undernutrition and morbidity. In moderately undernourished Rwandan women, 20% of days in a year are associated with sickness as compared with 4% in normal-weight women. Poor nutritional status in adult males in Bangladesh is also associated with high rates of loss of employment due to illness (over 50%) compared with less than 10% in adults with normal weight from similar social and economic backgrounds. However, since these are not actual records of infectious disease morbidity, it would be inappropriate to assume that they reflect increased risk of morbidity due to infections in undernourished men and women.

4.7   Tests of Immunocompetence in Undernutrition

DCH tests are useful clinical tools to assess the immunological status of undernourished individuals both at the bedside and in field

Table 4.5. Infectious and other diseases influenced by nutritional status. (Adapted from Chandra, 1983b.)

	Influence		
Infection	Definite	Variable	Mild
Bacterial	TB Bacterial diarrhoea Cholera Leprosy Pertussis Bacterial respiratory infection	Diphtheria Staphylococcal infections Streptococcal infections Syphilis	Typhoid Tetanus Plague Diseases caused by bacterial toxins
Viral	Measles Rotavirus diarrhoeas Viral respiratory infections Herpes	Influenza	Smallpox Yellow fever Arthropod-borne viral infection Encephalitis Poliomyelitis
Parasitic	*Pneumocystis carinii* infection Intestinal parasite infection Trypanosomiasis Leishmaniasis Schistosomiasis	*Giardia* infection Filariasis	Malaria
Fungal	*Candida* infection *Aspergillus* infection	Diseases caused by mould toxins	
Rickettsial		Typhus	

situations. DCH responses can also be assessed to follow up improvement during nutritional rehabilitation. DCH test responses to a range of antigens such as candida, trichophyton, mumps, tuberculin, etc. are generally depressed in individuals with PEM, both children and adults. The induration and cutaneous response seen with these tests is suggestive of impairment both in mild and moderate undernutrition and may even depend on the dose of the antigen. There is a range of other immunological tests (see Box 2.1) that can be used to study the alterations in immune function in undernutrition; the frequency of abnormalities in the various tests of immune function in mild, moderate and severe PEM in children is shown in Fig. 4.2.

Tests of immunocompetence can also be used to evaluate the response to nutritional repletion in undernourished individuals. The lowered levels of T-lymphocyte numbers return to normal on nutritional rehabilitation; an increase can be seen in numbers of rosetting lymphocytes within 5–15 days of nutritional therapy, long before clinical and biochemical indices show significant changes. Both complement levels and intracellular killing of bacteria (bactericidal action) by neutrophils are consistently reduced in undernutrition – and both respond rapidly to nutritional therapy. Although secretory IgA concentrations are reduced in undernutrition, they are not very sensitive indices for assessing the response to nutritional therapy.

Further Reading

Alleyne, G.A.O., Hay, R.W., Picou, D.I., Stanfield, J.P. and Whitehead, R.G. (1977) *Protein–Energy Malnutrition.* Edward Arnold, London. *A concise introductory textbook for postgraduate doctors and scientists concentrating on the scientific basis of PEM.*

Waterlow, J.C. (2007) *Protein Energy Malnutrition,* revised edn. Edward Arnold, London. *A recently updated reference book (original published in 1992) on the topic, aimed at physicians and public health workers.*

Case Studies

Case Study 4.1: Immune function test responses before and after nutritional rehabilitation.

The compromise of immunological function seen in the undernourished state is reversible with nutritional rehabilitation and good nutrition support. Examine Table 4.6, which outlines data on the responses to a delayed cutaneous hypersensitivity (DCH) test, one of the tests commonly used to assess immune function in young children with

Table 4.6. Percent positive DCH test responses. (Adapted from Chandra, 2000.)

	Candida	Trichophyton	Tetanus	DNCB
Baseline	38	29	43	68
After 8 weeks of nutrition support	63	59	78	92

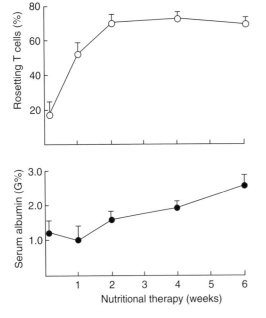

Fig. 4.3. Effects of nutritional therapy and rehabilitation on immune response (measured by the increase in number of T lymphocytes) and on serum albumin levels in undernourished patients. (This figure is reproduced with permission from Chandra, R.K. (ed.) *Primary and Secondary Immunodeficiency Disorders*, p. 200, Copyright Elsevier, 1983.)

protein–energy malnutrition (PEM), before and after 8 weeks of nutritional support and recovery.

Candida, trichophyton, tetanus (toxoid) and dinitrochlorobenzene are the recall and new antigens used to evoke a DCH response indicative of *in vivo* cell-mediated immunity of the host. The numbers represent the percentage of positive responses obtained and demonstrate that cell-mediated immunity is markedly depressed in PEM in children at baseline. The data also demonstrate that with nutritional rehabilitation, cell-mediated immunity reflected in DCH tests shows a marked improvement – suggesting that the depression of immune function is reversible when the nutrition of the host improves.

Take a careful look at Fig. 4.3, which shows the effect of nutritional rehabilitation of a group of undernourished patients. With 6 weeks of nutritional therapy there is marked increase in the percentage of T cells (T lymphocytes that form rosettes when incubated with sheep red blood cells); at the same time good nutrition provided to these undernourished patients improves their plasma protein levels, seen as an increase in serum albumin.

These examples demonstrate that the compromise of immune function observed in undernourished individuals is the result of poor nutrition and is reversed when the nutritional status of the patient improves. They also demonstrate the value of immune function tests in determining the immune status of the host and their use in assessing changes following nutritional interventions.

Reference

Chandra, R.K. (2000) Foreword. In: Gershwin, M.E., German, J.B. and Keen, C.L. (eds) *Nutrition and Immunology: Principles and Practice.* Humana Press, Totowa, New Jersey, pp. v–vii.

Case Study 4.2: Increased risk of morbidity and mortality in low-birth-weight infants.

Low birth weight (LBW) associated with intrauterine growth retardation (IUGR) is a serious public health problem in developing countries. According to UNICEF, 16% of children in developing countries are born with LBW at term, i.e. weighing <2500 g. More than 90% of LBW infants are born in developing countries and these infants are considered to be more susceptible to infection and death from infection. The present case study helps illustrate this point based on evidence from studies in LBW infants and children in developing countries.

Table 4.7 summarizes data reported in the literature from four cohort studies of full-term infants from four countries – Ethiopia, Brazil, India and Guatemala – showing the association of LBW with increased morbidity from infections.

The risk ratio is the ratio of the risk in the LBW infant divided by the risk in the normal-weight infant, which is considered to be equal to 1. Thus a risk ratio of 1.5 suggests a 50% increase in risk of illness, while a risk ratio of 2.4 implies a 240% increase of risk in the LBW infant. It is evident from the data in Table 4.7 that the risk of illness and morbidity and of hospital admissions is increased in LBW infants. Studying the data from India above also suggests that the risk of morbidity in LBW infants will vary with the type of infection– higher for instance due to acute respiratory tract infections compared with diarrhoeal disease. It is important to recognize that LBW infants may be disadvantaged in more ways than just their birth weight, such as their families' socio-economic circumstances and the household environment. An understanding of the multifactorial causality of undernutrition would explain this. The increased susceptibility may be the result of increased attacks and/or increased severity and duration of the infective episode in these undernourished infants.

Table 4.8 summarizes data from four cohort studies in three countries (Brazil, India and Guatemala) showing the associations between term LBW infants and increased risk of mortality.

The data in Table 4.8 illustrate the increased risk of death that LBW infants face during their first year of life from all causes. The increased risk of

Table 4.7. Data on LBW and morbidity from infections. (Adapted from Ashworth, 2001.)

Country	Age (months)	Risk ratio[a]	Outcome
Ethiopia	3–40	1.5	All infections
Brazil	0–6	1.3	Diarrhoea
India	0–3	2.4	Diarrhoea
		3.6	ALRTI
Guatemala	0–3	3.0	Sepsis and ALRTI

ALRTI, acute lower respiratory tract infection.
[a]Compared with infants of normal birth weight.

Table 4.8. Data on LBW and mortality. (Adapted from Ashworth, 2001.)

Country	Age (months)	Risk ratio[a]	Outcome
Brazil	0–6	10.2	All-cause mortality
India	0–11	2.6	All-cause mortality
India	0–11	1.7	All-cause mortality
Guatemala	0–3	1.7	All-cause mortality

[a]Compared with infants of normal birth weight.

death is from diarrhoeal disease, and respiratory and other infections like meningitis, sepsis and measles in the first year of life.

LBW infants with IUGR are undernourished infants and there is evidence that their immune functions are impaired compared with normal-weight infants. Hence LBW infants have increased susceptibility to childhood infections and this in turn contributes to their increased risk of morbidity and mortality.

Reference

Ashworth, A. (2001) Low birth weight infants, infection and immunity. In: Suskind, R.M. and Tontisirin, K. (eds) *Nutrition, Immunity and Infection in Infants and Children. Nestle Nutrition Workshop Series No. 45.* Lippincot, Williams & Wilkins, Philadelphia, Pennsylvania, pp. 121–136.

Case Study 4.3: Increased mortality in undernourished children.

Undernutrition in children is a major global problem of public health relevance. Underweight for age is the indicator universally used to assess the global burden of undernutrition. Undernutrition manifesting as low weight-for-age, i.e. underweight, is also associated with deficiencies of other micronutrients and contributes to the burden of morbidity in children. A significant proportion of the deaths in young children worldwide is attributable to low weight-for-age, as illustrated in the present case study.

Table 4.9 presents a compilation of data from ten cohort studies in children from different countries. It provides data on the relative risk of mortality from specific illnesses and from all causes in children with varying degrees of underweight, compared with normal-weight, well-nourished children of similar age ranges.

Table 4.9. Relative risk of mortality according to degree of underweight. (Adapted from Caulfield *et al.*, 2004.)

Cause of death	Normal weight	Mild underweight (Z-score = –1 to –2)	Moderate underweight (Z-score = –2 to –3)	Severe underweight (Z-score <–3)
Diarrhoea	1.0	2.3	5.4	12.5
Pneumonia	1.0	2.0	4.0	8.1
Malaria	1.0	2.1	4.5	9.5
Measles	1.0	1.7	3.0	5.2
All causes	1.0	2.1	4.2	8.7

Figures in Table 4.9 are the values of relative risk of mortality from a specific cause or from all causes in mildly, moderately and severely underweight children (low weight-for-age) compared with the risk that normal-weight children face (considered as equal to 1). Thus the relative risk is the probability of the event occurring in the various categories of underweight (i.e. undernourished) child as compared with that in a normal-weight, well-nourished child.

Mortality from specific infectious diseases like diarrhoeal disease, respiratory infections and pneumonias, from malaria and from measles is elevated in undernutrition and increases progressively with the severity of underweight. All-cause mortality also shows the same trend with increasing severity of low weight-for-age. Undernutrition in children increases the risk of infection and the risk of morbidity and mortality, and much of this is attributable to the children's impaired immune function and the environment in which they grow.

Reference

Caulfield, L.E., de Onis, M., Blossner, M. and Black, R.E. (2004) Undernutrition as an underlying cause of child death associated with diarrhea, pneumonia, malaria and measles. *American Journal of Clinical Nutrition* 80, 193–198.

5 Infections and Undernutrition: Causation and Consequences

- Infectious disease and episodes of frequent infections are often the immediate cause of undernutrition, particularly in children.
- Infectious disease influences the nutritional status of the host by affecting appetite, absorption of nutrients and by increasing body metabolism.
- Infections have several effects that can contribute to the deterioration of the nutritional status of the host.
- Repeated infective episodes, their intensity and duration, will affect the normal weight gain and growth in length of children.
- Several common infections such as measles, malaria, tuberculosis and HIV/AIDS predispose to poor nutrition and increase susceptibility to undernutrition.

5.1 Introduction

In developing countries in the tropics, there are many causes of undernutrition. The principal drivers are food and nutrition insecurity, whose determinants are poverty, poor environment and social exclusion. Poverty and disadvantage lead to deficient or inadequate availability of food, as well as to lack of access to food, hence hindering the consumption of a variety of foods as part of a diversified and healthy daily diet. The risk of infection is considerably increased by the unhealthy environment (e.g. urban slums) that poverty and disadvantage often force people to live in. Thus undernutrition in a community is the result of both social and biological causes. In addition, the psychosocial deprivation that goes with poverty worsens the situation. The importance of psychosocial factors explains why some children are worse off than others living in the same environment and with similar access to food. Poverty and social disadvantage thus play a prominent role in the aetiology of undernutrition. One of the crucial pathways by which this is mediated is the role played by infectious diseases in the causation of undernutrition (Fig. 5.1).

Poverty implies not merely lack of good food and nutrition; it also often means growing up in a poor environment that increases the risk of infections from a variety of infective agents. Infections affect appetite, increase intestinal loss of nutrients

and enhance nutrient needs, all of which increase the chances of undernutrition. Undernutrition, in turn, alters host defence and compromises the body's immunological response. This results in increased susceptibility to the entry of infective agents. Thus, a vicious cycle is set up in which undernutrition and infections promote each other and increase the risk of morbidity and mortality. This chapter outlines the role played by infection in the aetiology of undernutrition.

5.2 Infection and Immediate Causation of Undernutrition in Children

The interaction between infection and undernutrition is complex, and it is not always possible or easy to separate the effects of infection on undernutrition from the effects of nutrition on infection. However, it is often helpful to do so and in this section the role of infections as an immediate and direct cause of undernutrition is discussed. Many investigators have reported how an infective episode serves as a stimulus to precipitate frank undernutrition in a child who may either be well nourished prior to that, or marginally or mildly undernourished but growing normally in a poor environment. More often, in the latter case, the child may grow optimally for the first six months after birth as long as it is breastfed; but no

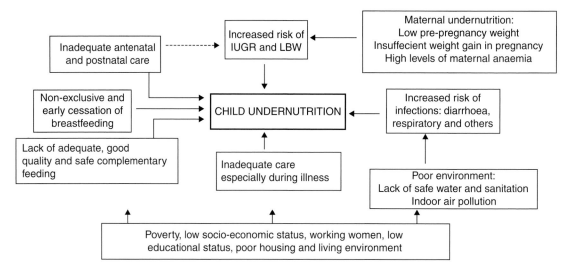

Fig. 5.1. Schematic diagram illustrating the roles of many of the multifactorial (food and non-food) causes of child undernutrition.

sooner are weaning foods introduced than the child develops infections and shows growth faltering. These patterns have been well recorded by Leonardo Mata and his colleagues from Guatemala and the body-weight record of one of the male children he followed up along with a record of the various infective episodes illustrates this very well (see Fig. 5.4 in Case Study 5.1).

In well-nourished children the deleterious effects of the usual infections of childhood rarely affect growth. A follow-up of children from birth until 5 years of age in Oxford showed that children who escaped all illness were 1 inch (25 mm) taller than those who had experienced severe illness during childhood and were 0.4 inches (10 mm) taller than those who suffered what was considered an average amount of sickness. Paediatricians in developing countries in the tropics have recognized for a long time that retardation and faltering of growth occurs with repeated infections in childhood. They have also known of the intimate association between infection and undernutrition in children who are at risk of poor nutrition resulting from poverty, inadequate food intake and growing up in a poor and unhygienic environment. Childhood infections, which result in loss of appetite, malabsorption and loss of nutrients, and the diversion of essential nutrients for the immune response, increase the risk of undernutrition. And if an infant or child is already undernourished due to inadequate food and inappropriate care, such an individual is at increased risk of severe and frequent infections in a poor and unhygienic environment which further aggravates the problem of undernutrition – thus setting into motion a vicious cycle of infection–undernutrition which results in increased morbidity and ultimately perhaps even death (Fig. 5.2).

5.3 Effect of Infection on the Nutritional Status of the Host

Infections and infective episodes can result in the deterioration of nutritional status in both children and adults. There are several mechanisms by which infection affects nutritional status (Fig. 5.3); they need to be understood to appreciate how the cycle of infection and undernutrition is perpetuated and may end up as a vicious cycle resulting in death.

Loss of appetite (anorexia) and reduced food intake

Anorexia, or loss of appetite, is a classical feature of infection in children and plays a major role in reducing food intake, thus leading to secondary undernutrition that drives the infection–undernutrition cycle. Food intake may be reduced by between 25 and 42% in children; this affects mostly intake of solid foods. The practice of 'starving a fever' is also an important factor that contributes to reduce

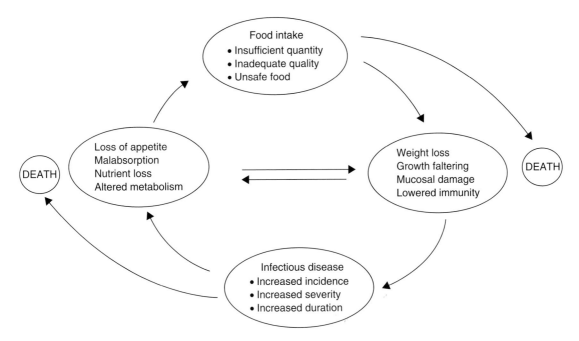

Fig. 5.2. The vicious cycle of 'infection–undernutrition'. (Adapted from Tomkins and Watson, 1989.)

Box 5.1. Characteristics of the Host and the Infectious Agent.

Characteristics of both the host and the infectious agent will determine the outcome of the entry of the agent into the host. The *characteristics of the host* include its immune function and hence the resistance it offers to the infective agent. These are determined by genetic variations and the environment, the latter including the diet and nutritional status of the host. Nutritional factors can modify the characteristics of both the host and the infectious agent. Thus the resistance offered by the host to the pathogen is likely to be high with a favourable genetic makeup in the presence of good nutrition, and the susceptibility greatest in a host with unfavourable heredity in the presence of coexisting poor nutritional status. Between these extreme situations lie a whole range of possibilities in which the nutritional status will be an important determinant of the ability of the host to resist infections. In addition, changes in the physiological status of the host, such as pregnancy and lactation in a mother, or the rapidly growing period in infancy and childhood with increased demands for nutrients, may tip this balance in favour of the pathogenic agent, thus increasing the susceptibility of the

host during these vulnerable periods. Previous exposure to the agent and the presence of acquired immunity to the agent is another factor that will influence the outcome of the interaction between the agent and the host.

Characteristics of the pathogen which will influence the outcome of the interaction with the host include the severity of the exposure, i.e. number of organisms and the virulence of the pathogen, as well as the effects induced by the infective agent in the host. The latter include the ability to act directly on the cells or tissues of the host (general or specific); the ability to produce and release toxins (exo- and endotoxins); the ability to alter and disrupt the normal functioning of the host's metabolic machinery; the ability to hide from or neutralize the defence systems of the host; and the deleterious side-effects that result from the host's response to the entry of the agent, which may benefit the pathogen. The requirement of the pathogen for essential nutrients from the host may also act as a factor that influences the outcome of the interaction between host and pathogen.

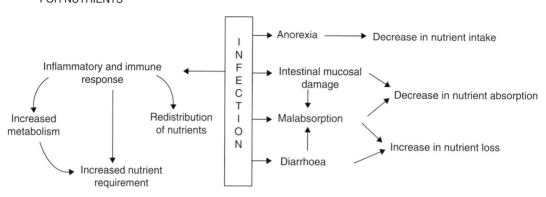

Fig. 5.3. Schematic diagram of the mechanisms by which infections can influence and alter the nutrient requirements and nutritional status of the individual.

food intake. Cultural trend and custom in different regions of the world to withdraw solid food from or to change the diet of a child during illness reduces energy and nutrient intakes and compounds the problem. Breast milk is well tolerated and hence breastfeeding is a must during episodes of infection in infants.

Several biological mechanisms – particularly those related to the increased production of cytokines – may be involved in reducing appetite during an infection. Cytokines are produced by a variety of immune and inflammatory cells and are now known to act directly within the central nervous system to induce anorexia and reduce food intake, resulting in weight loss in the host. Animal experimental studies suggest that IL-1β is possibly responsible for the anorexia, acting partly through down-regulation of the neuropeptide-Y pathway (neuropeptide-Y is an important neurotransmitter in the hypothalamic nuclei involved with feeding behaviour). Increased neuronal 5-hydroxytryptamine activity may also account for the depression of food intake seen in animal models of infection.

Physical and local causes contribute to the loss of appetite and reluctance to feed. Oral or buccal lesions in measles may contribute to loss of appetite, while vomiting after a meal in severe upper respiratory tract infections may also play an important role. Oral thrush (a fungal infection occurring in infants and children marked by white patches in the mouth), sore tongues, apthous ulcers and infected cheilosis (abnormal scaling of the lips and formation of fissures in the corners of the mouth,

due to deficiencies of B vitamins such as niacin and riboflavin), which frequently occur in malnutrition, may also make eating difficult and thus perpetuate the cycle of undernutrition and infection.

Fever (pyrexia)

Increase in body temperature of the host, i.e. a febrile response, is an invariable accompaniment of an infective process. A fever obviously has several biological advantages and the mechanisms involved in this response by the host are complex. Body temperature is well regulated in man by several structures in the central nervous system like the reticular formation, limbic system and lower brainstem, including some parts of the hypothalamus. These regions of the brain respond by increasing the rate of neuronal firing to a variety of cytokines, as well as other intermediary mediators like prostaglandins, released during an infection and the accompanying inflammatory process. These pyrogenic cytokines include interleukins (IL-1α and IL-1β, IL-6), TNF-α, and IFN-γ. The interactions are complex and since cytokines do not cross the blood–brain barrier, they alter the thermoregulatory set-point by inducing phospholipase A_2 to release prostaglandin E_2 which acts on these neurons in the brain. It is now believed that the fever-induced anorexia is also mediated by prostaglandin E_2. However, since antipyretics inhibit the fever response but not the anorexia it has been postulated that the anorexia-inducing effects of endotoxin are possibly mediated directly by IL-1. It is probable that the other manifestations of an infection, apart from fever and anorexia, may also probably be related to IL-1 effects.

It is important to note that hypothermia (rectal temperature <35°C) is often a clinical feature of undernourished children, and is related to the severity of the undernutrition. Children with marasmus who have marked reduction in their skinfold thickness suffer hypothermia more than those with kwashiorkor in whom the presence of oedema and the relatively well-preserved subcutaneous tissues provide relatively better insulation. In addition, marasmic children have grossly depleted energy stores and are more at risk of hypothermia. Hypothermia is an important consideration since infants and children with pre-existing undernutrition may not readily manifest clinically with a febrile response during an infection, which may then be missed and thus early treatment not carried out. It is now recommended that routine antibiotic cover be provided to severely undernourished children during their nutritional rehabilitation.

For every 1°C rise in temperature, the basal metabolism of the child with an infection rises by 10–15%. Hence, energy expenditure of the body is higher at rest and the requirement for energy is increased under conditions such as during an infection when food intake may have dropped. This is partly compensated for by the marked reduction in physical activity in a child with an infection. In general, children who are ill are in negative energy balance.

Effects on body metabolism

The infective process induces a number of metabolic changes that alter the nutritional status of the host (Table 5.1). Both anabolic and catabolic processes occur at the same time although the latter are generally more dominant in the host during an infection, resulting in loss of body tissues. The increase in body temperature raises energy requirements above basal levels at a time when the host is generally anorexic. Since carbohydrate stores of the body, mostly as glycogen, are limited and inadequate to meet the increased needs over a long time and lipid stores are not effectively utilized by an infected host, the body relies largely on protein as a principal source of energy. The supply of energy is hence dependent upon the production of glucose by the liver from amino acids (i.e. gluconeogenesis) released from the contractile proteins present in muscle.

Thus an infective episode is characterized by increased protein breakdown with an increased excretion of nitrogen and a negative nitrogen balance. There is a temporary increase in circulating amino acid levels and an increase in urea formation and excretion. Infections thus result in increased protein metabolism, which is largely due to an increase in protein breakdown rather than protein synthesis. This marked increase in muscle protein breakdown leads to the branched-chain amino acids released by the breakdown being oxidized *in situ* to provide energy, while other amino acids are taken up by the liver for new protein synthesis and for metabolic repair and stress responses. Protein synthetic activity is specifically driven towards synthesizing acute-phase proteins and other inflammatory peptides in preference to the synthesis of albumin and other plasma proteins. There is also an increase in several of the metal-binding proteins such as lactoferrin, metallothioneine and caeruloplasmin.

Protein catabolism hence dominates the infective process and the amino acids released are taken up by the liver and deaminated during gluconeogenesis, resulting in the excretion of nitrogen as urea and other nitrogenous products in the urine and other body fluids. The carbon skeleton of the protein is also lost as carbon dioxide as a result of its utilization for energy. These metabolic features can be demonstrated in patients with sepsis in whom infused amino acids like alanine are increasingly converted to glucose and a non re-utilizable end product, i.e. 3-methyl histidine, which is excreted in the urine and considered a marker of muscle protein breakdown.

Some infections result in a shift from use of glucose to increased use of fat for the release of energy. The changes in lipid metabolism during an infection hence depend on the nature, duration and severity of the infection. Thus depending on the activity of the enzyme systems involved with lipid metabolism such as lipoprotein lipase, fatty acid synthetase and acetyl-coA carboxylase, the levels of free fatty acids and triacylglycerols may be increased or decreased. An example is how defective lipid clearance results in increased triacylglycerol levels in gram-negative bacillary infections. There is also a reduction in the production and utilization of ketone bodies, implying an inefficient use of the host's lipid stores, increasing further the reliance on the endogenous protein stores of the body. It has been suggested that some of these effects on lipid metabolism (such as inducing increase in triacylglycerol levels and

Table 5.1. Metabolic changes in the host during an infection.

Macronutrient metabolism	Changes during infection
Protein metabolism	Breakdown of muscle protein Temporary increase in amino acid pool and increased urea synthesis. With prolonged infections, amino acid levels fall Decrease in branched-chain (i.e. gluconeogenic) amino acids like valine and alanine Increased nitrogen loss and negative nitrogen balance Increased synthesis of acute-phase proteins and metal-binding proteins Reduced synthesis of albumin Increased gluconeogenesis (amino acids used as fuel source)
Carbohydrate metabolism	Increased glucose oxidation Increased glucose and insulin levels Functional insulin resistance in muscle
Lipid metabolism	Levels of free fatty acids and triacylglycerols may increase or decrease Some infections characterized by increased triacylglycerol levels Reduced production and utilization of ketone bodies like hydroxybutyrate and acetoacetate Tendency to fatty liver in severe infections
Vitamin metabolism	Fall in circulating levels of vitamin A, vitamin C and riboflavin
Mineral metabolism	Decrease in circulating levels of plasma iron and zinc Reduced gastrointestinal absorption of iron Removal of iron to liver cells Uptake of zinc by reticulo-endothelial cells Increase in circulating copper levels resulting from increased synthesis of copper-carrying protein Increased loss of magnesium, potassium, phosphorus and sulfur in urine and other body fluids
Hormonal changes	Increase in insulin Increase in glucocorticoids; loss of diurnal changes in glucocorticoids Increase in glucagon and growth hormone

suppressing lipoprotein lipase activity) are the actions of a compound resembling IL-1, called cachectin, which is also secreted by macrophages during an infection.

Infections thus induce a complex hormonal adaptation characterized by changes, particularly those affecting protein and energy metabolism, which seem to be principally related to increases in cortisol and insulin secretion. Glucocorticoid levels are elevated and their normal diurnal variations are lost or dampened. The high levels of circulating insulin in a predominantly catabolic state indicate that the body cells, in particular muscle cells, are resistant to the actions of insulin (i.e. functional insulin resistance). Increased gluconeogenic activity is evident in fasting hyperglycaemia, abnormal glucose disappearance, an exaggerated insulin response to a glucose load and an increased glucose oxidation rate. Other hormones like glucagon and growth hormone are also elevated as a part of this complex response to an infection.

Vitamin and mineral metabolism of the host is also affected as a result of an infection. Circulating levels of several vitamins (vitamin A, riboflavin, vitamin C) fall during an infection. Decreases in levels of iron and zinc are seen due to an increase in their uptake by the liver and by phagocytes. Iron is taken up by the cellular iron-binding protein, lactoferrin, which is released from activated neutrophils into the plasma during an infection. Since these proteins are cleared from the circulation, plasma iron levels drop during an infection. Zinc levels decrease as a result of the synthesis of the metal-binding protein, metallothioneine, which is one of the intracellular acute-phase proteins synthesized during the infection. Copper levels rise, largely the result of increases in synthesis of the copper carrier protein, caeruloplasmin. It is postulated that these changes in minerals may be beneficial to the host during an infection. The reduced availability of iron may impair bacterial growth and the production of virulence factors. Zinc is present in several enzymes and may play an important role in priming the host to turn on cellular proliferation. The increase in copper and caeruloplasmin levels may increase efficiency of iron utilization for haemoglobin synthesis at a time when iron availability is reduced to compromise the viability of the infective agent.

Effects on gastrointestinal function

Intestinal function is affected during an infection, and this affects the availability and absorption of nutrients even when the infection is not directly related to the gastrointestinal tract. Gut permeability may be altered in viral infections such as measles. Gastrointestinal function is most compromised in the presence of intestinal pathogens; the changes include alteration in digestion and absorption if the infective agent alters the intestinal mucosa and villi. Malabsorption of macro- and micronutrients and of water and electrolytes may result in poor nutrition of the individual, increasing the chances of becoming undernourished.

The effects of infection on gastrointestinal function are best illustrated for infective agents that act directly on the gut. From the host's perspective they include the host elements of epithelial and mucosal defences, the bacterial mechanisms of virulence that influence the function of the gut, and the interactions between host and the agent. The main physical barrier of the gut consists of the epithelial cells and the intercellular junctional complexes that maintain the integrity of the barrier. This epithelial cell barrier is covered by a mucous coating which can bind a wide range of molecules. It is now well recognized that the normal bacterial flora of the intestine helps maintain the gastrointestinal barrier against pathogenic agents. Furthermore, antimicrobial agents are secreted by the intestinal cells such as soluble immunoglobulins, lysozymes and two groups of antimicrobial peptides, i.e. defensins and cathelicidins. The leucocytes in the gut mucosa also secrete an antimicrobial peptide called bacterial permeability increasing protein. Gut epithelial cells respond to the presence of a pathogen by producing various inflammatory mediators, some of which increase fluid secretion and intestinal motility to help mechanically flush out the pathogenic agent, manifesting as diarrhoea. Others mobilize innate and adaptive immune mediators which include host cytokine responses to the pathogen.

Pathogenic bacteria use a variety of strategies to promote their survival and transmission to initiate the infective process. The pathogenic virulence strategies of the infective agent include toxin production in the intestinal lumen; adherence to and invasion of the epithelial cells, resulting in their death; translocation across the epithelial layer; and finally the induction of systemic effects by entry into the host through the blood or lymphatic system. Maintenance of fluid and electrolyte balance is an important function of the gut; enteropathogens interfere with these gastrointestinal functions of the epithelial cells by enhancing or inhibiting absorption or secretion in the gut.

Growth

Growth in children, both increase in body weight and increase in height/stature, is influenced strongly by infections. Growth faltering in infants and children, as illustrated from studies in Guatemala (see Fig. 5.4 in Case Study 5.1), is due to the combination of interactions between severe and frequent infections and poor nutrition which constitute the undernutrition–infection cycle. The host responses to an infection discussed above, including reduced food intake, increased nutrient losses from the gut, the increased energy expenditure due to pyrexia and the metabolic alterations, all contribute to diversion of nutrients from the normal growth process and contribute to nutrient wastage. The activation and amplification of the host's defence mechanisms result in inappropriate partitioning of nutrients, and the diversion and redistribution of ingested and endogenous nutrients away from preserving and maintaining the host's nutritional status and body composition and away from the contributions needed for the accretion of tissues for optimal growth. The catabolic losses during an infective episode are not readily replaced even when normal dietary intake is restored, and return to normal nitrogen balance is a slow process.

The anabolic effect of growth hormone on muscle and bone is mediated through IGF-1. Chronic overproduction of cytokines, in particular IL-1, during the infective process influences circulating IGF-1 levels. The reduction in IGF-1 is probably mediated by impairing hepatic *IGF1* gene expression or by reducing the amount of IGF-binding protein. The diversion of essential nutrients like amino acids from the growth process for the synthesis of acute-phase proteins accounts for some of the nutrient wastage. In addition, since the type of amino acid required for synthesis of acute-phase proteins (which are relatively rich in aromatic amino acids) is different from skeletal muscle protein (which is rich in branched-chain amino acids), imbalances in amino acids required may also contribute to nutrient wastage. Either way, the host's nutrient needs for optimal growth are compromised by infection.

5.4 Infections that Predispose to Poor Nutrition Status and Undernutrition

Several infections that commonly occur in developing societies, mostly in the tropics, play an important role in the aetiology of childhood undernutrition (see Table 5.2). These include bacterial, viral and

Table 5.2. Common infections that predispose to undernutrition in the host.

Measles
Diarrhoeal disease
Acute respiratory infections and pneumonias
Intestinal parasitic infestation
Malaria
TB
HIV/AIDS

Box 5.2. Infective Agents.

A wide range of infective organisms are responsible for infections in the human host. They are arranged below not in order of importance to human disease, but based on the size of the organisms.

- *Viruses*: These are the smallest of microorganisms responsible for human infections, being composed of either a DNA or an RNA strand, and are obligate intracellular pathogens. RNA viruses include those that cause measles, mumps, poliomyelitis, HIV/AIDS and rabies among other diseases. DNA viruses include those that are responsible for hepatitis B, herpes infections and the poxes – chicken pox and small pox.
- *Chlamydiae and Rickettsiae*: Chlamydiae are small organisms which, like viruses, grow inside cells and have a cell wall, but unlike viruses have both DNA and RNA. They include the organism responsible for trachoma and psittacosis. Rickettsiae are smaller than bacteria and are intracellular pathogens growing in living cells. Rickettsiae are responsible for typhus fever and trench fever.
- *Bacteria*: A range of bacteria are responsible for an even wider range of infections, in man. Bacteria are round, elongated or comma-shaped microorganisms that grow in aerobic or even anaerobic environments and can enter the body through a variety of routes. These include the organisms that are responsible for diarrhoeal disease, respiratory infections and pneumonia, meningitis and skin infections, as well as conditions like plague,

anthrax, tuberculosis, leprosy and food poisoning among others.
- *Spirochaetes*: These organisms infect human hosts and are responsible for diseases such as leptospirosis, Lyme disease and syphilis.
- *Fungi*: These are much larger, multi-nucleated and branched organisms. They are responsible for skin conditions like ringworm infections, subcutaneous infections like mycetoma of the foot, and systemic infections like histoplasmosis, aspergillosis, cryptococcosis and candidiasis.
- *Protozoa*: Protozoa are unicellular organisms, larger and more complex than bacteria and generally motile. These include the organisms responsible for malaria, amoebiasis, giardiasis, leishmaniasis and toxoplasmosis.
- *Helminths*: These include the trematodes or flukes responsible for diseases like schistosomiasis; the cestodes or tapeworms causing intestinal tapeworm diseases like *Taenia saginata* and the tissue-dwelling cysts or worms in diseases like cysticercosis and hydatid disease; and the nematodes or roundworms causing infestations like hookworm or guinea worm and filarial infections.
- *Arthropods*: These larger organisms are responsible for illness directly by stings or bites, which may result in allergic reactions of variable severity; or indirectly by acting as a vector for other infective agents like the mosquito, which is responsible for malaria, filariasis, yellow fever and dengue infections.

Box 5.3. Infant and Child Nutrition and Risk of Infections.

Nutrition is an important determinant of the optimum growth and health of infants and children. Prevention of undernutrition in children requires ensuring availability of and access to an adequate quantity of good-quality and safe food to meet the child's nutrient needs. The 'food–care–health' conceptual framework developed by UNICEF shows that the causes of undernutrition are multifactorial; they embrace food, health and caring practices; and operate at immediate, underlying and basic levels, where factors at one level influence other levels. While inadequate dietary intake may be an immediate cause of childhood undernutrition, the underlying causes at the household or family level may be responsible for insufficient access to food, inadequate maternal and child care, poor water or sanitation, and inadequate access to health care services. The basic causes are much broader and include the political, social, cultural, religious and economic systems in which the community or household exists.

Breastfeeding

Initiation of early breastfeeding and the promotion of exclusive breastfeeding for at least 6 months are crucial for the health and optimum growth of the infant. This includes preparing the pregnant mother and helping her to decide to breastfeed the child. It also includes support in the postpartum period, through formal and informal activities, which may help women to have confidence in their ability to breastfeed and relieve any doubts and anxieties they may have about it. Protection of breastfeeding should be aimed at guarding women who normally would successfully breastfeed against situations that might cause them to alter this healthy practice. Promotion of breastfeeding is becoming increasingly difficult with the changing work patterns of women in developing societies and the changing demands on their time. The Baby Friendly Hospital Initiative expects to help protect, support and promote breastfeeding by addressing problems in hospitals. However, this may be less relevant for communities where most babies are born outside hospital settings.

Complementary or supplementary feeding

With a healthy mother providing adequate breast milk, breastfeeding alone should ensure optimal growth and good nutrition of an infant up to 6 months of life. Continued breastfeeding with the addition of appropriate and safe high-quality complementary foods up into the second year of life provides the best nourishment and protects children from infections. Thus, at 6 months of age, complementary feeding should be introduced gradually while the infant continues to be breastfed. The introduction of complementary feeds is a critical period in a child's life, since breast milk is no longer able to provide all the nutrients the child needs. Hence delaying the introduction of complementary feeds can cause a child's growth to falter. However, too early introduction or the provision of unsafe complementary feeds, where the preparation and storage of food are not hygienic, can increase the risk of infection and consequently undernutrition. From 6 to 18 months of age the child needs frequent feeding and will require frequent meals that are dense in energy and nutrients and also easily digestible. Foods the rest of the family normally eat will have to be adapted to suit the need of a growing child. Emphasis on hygiene in the preparation and storage of complementary feeds is essential.

Care

Of the three underlying causes of undernutrition, namely food, health and care, care is the one least investigated and understood, and also least emphasized. Adequate care is not only important for the child's survival but also for optimal physical and mental development. Care also contributes to the child's general well-being and happiness. Child care may be influenced by external factors; by local factors such as equity and access to health services; and by factors within a family or household, such as adequate housing, safe water, household hygiene and the mother's knowledge and educational achievement, as well as the demand for work and income outside the home. Nutritionally, care encompasses all measures and behaviours that transmit available food and health resources into good child growth and development. In most developing countries the mother is the caregiver for the infant and the very young child, although in extended families older and young relatives (older siblings) often play an important role. Care-giving behaviour is often assumed to be solely the responsibility of mothers; it should in fact be the responsibility of the entire family. Identification of child caring practices that are desirable should be the first step in any health promotion strategy that involves care. Protection of good practices that promote child care from erosion or loss due to the developmental process is essential. Support is essential when good traditional practices of mothers or families are threatened or eroded by changes in society.

Thus the UNICEF 'food–care–health' conceptual framework provides an understanding of the multifactorial nature of child undernutrition and helps address the crucial issues relevant to preventing the infection–undernutrition cycle.

parasitic infections. A brief discussion of the role played by each of these infections follows.

Measles

Measles is a viral infection that is responsible for high mortality among children in developing countries, and is also an important infective episode that precipitates severe undernutrition in children. This infection has a profound effect on the child's appetite and food intake is depressed for several weeks. The high fever and the accompanying lesions in the buccal mucosa contribute to the severe loss of appetite. In some societies, this is compounded by the belief that withholding of food is necessary during a period of acute illness. There is also damage to the mucosa of the small intestine, and if a secondary infection occurs during a measles episode, this could further damage the intestinal mucosa. There is severe catabolism with breakdown of tissues and the negative energy balance that children attain results in growth faltering and weight loss. Even children who are well nourished before the infection can end up showing marked weight loss, growth faltering and impending undernutrition.

Measles imposes an unusual and severe nutritional stress on children and more so if they are already undernourished. Measles is often responsible, as an immediate precipitating cause, for severe clinical forms of undernutrition in young children. It is well documented that about a quarter of children admitted to hospitals with severe undernutrition in tropical Asia have suffered from measles in the immediate past. Hospital-based studies have also documented the significant weight loss that occurs in children during an episode of measles. These children end up with severe post-measles morbidity which is ten times more frequent than in children who have not had measles but have been exposed to the same environmental conditions. The children with measles show a marked retardation in growth, and poor nutritional status. Post-measles, these children demonstrate much reduced body-weight gain and growth. The phenomenon of marked weight loss during the acute episode of measles (2–12% loss of their pre-measles body weight) and slower weight gain in the post-measles period is seen in all children with measles, irrespective of their pre-measles body weight. These observations clearly demonstrate both the adverse effects of measles on growth and nutritional status of children, and the importance of pre-measles nutritional status on the subsequent nutritional consequences.

Measles is often associated with vitamin A deficiency in children. Infective episodes, particularly of severe infections like measles, affect the vitamin A status of the child. The general metabolic response to infection results in a reduction in plasma retinol, while urinary excretion of the metabolites of vitamin A is increased. There is a decrease in synthesis of retinol-binding protein (RBP) – the carrier protein for retinol – by the liver, and a temporary reduction in vitamin A absorption may also occur. The damage that the measles virus inflicts on epithelial surfaces such as the conjunctiva and other mucosal surfaces increases the requirement for vitamin A to help in the repair of these tissues. Thus, measles infection not only predisposes to general undernutrition, but can also specifically precipitate vitamin A deficiency. This explains why a combination of measles and vitamin A deficiency is the commonest cause of blindness in children in parts of Africa.

Cell-mediated immunity plays an important role in recovery from measles infection. Since undernutrition is associated with the suppression of cell-mediated immune responses, pre-existing undernutrition (i.e. poor nutrition pre-measles) and the post-measles compromised nutritional status can result in adverse responses in a child. Studies on the nature of the immune responses in measles further indicate that measles produces a general immunosuppression, particularly with respect to T-cell-mediated immune functions. The suppression of T-cell-mediated responses following measles may persist for 3 to 6 months. However, the humoral immune responses appear to be adequate and independent of the nutritional status. The non-specific suppression of some of the immune responses is believed to be responsible for the high morbidity due to secondary infections, observed during and after the measles episode in most children.

Diarrhoeal disease

Diarrhoea is characterized by an abnormally rapid passage of food along the gastrointestinal tract. The total content, and particularly the water content, of the stools increase and there is frequently undigested food present. The stools are semi-fluid or liquid in consistency and the frequency of passing stools is increased. For epidemiological purposes, diarrhoea is defined as the presence of three or more liquid stools in a day. If diarrhoea continues for 14 days or more, it is termed persistent diarrhoea syndrome (PDS). It is estimated that between 3% and 20% of diarrhoeal episodes become persistent and that PDS accounts for about 50% of diarrhoea-related deaths. PDS is more common in younger children and particularly in those with poor nutrition.

Diarrhoea is the commonest illness in pre-school children in the tropics. Exclusive breastfeeding during the first six months of life protects a child from diarrhoeal disease, and the introduction of weaning foods (in a contaminated environment) usually marks the point at which the disease manifests. The episodes of diarrhoea increase in prevalence thereafter and peak towards the end of the first year and during the second year of life.

Many organisms – bacterial, viral and parasitic – are responsible for diarrhoeal disease, although in many instances no pathogens are isolated. The common pathogens which cause diarrhoeal disease in children in developing societies in the tropics are shown in Table 5.3.

Diarrhoea is induced either by the tissue destruction within the small intestine or by the stimulation of the adenylate cyclase system within the mucosal cells by the production of toxins by pathogens. In a well-nourished child, the rapid loss of fluids along with nutrients reduces the availability of nutrients to meet the child's daily requirements. Thus, repeated episodes of diarrhoeal disease or persistent diarrhoea over long periods can compromise the nutritional status of even a previously well-nourished infant or child, predisposing it to undernutrition. On the other hand, acute episodes of severe diarrhoea can cause rapid loss of fluids and electrolytes and lead to dehydration and electrolyte imbalances that may compromise the survival of the child even before undernutrition sets in.

In an already undernourished child, however, several changes associated with the poor nutritional status enhance the risk of infections by pathogens that cause diarrhoeal disease. In addition, it is now well recognized that changes in the organ systems, particularly the gut, can enhance the deleterious effects of diarrhoeal disease. For example, the secretory responses, with faecal loss of fluids and electrolytes, are highest in those who are severely undernourished, probably due to changes in the morphology of the intestinal mucosa as a result of both the undernutrition and the increases in resident bacteria in the upper gastrointestinal tract. The latter is attributed to the achlorhydria (lack of acid secreted) in the stomach, which favours colonization of the upper intestine by bacteria. Most severely undernourished children have much increased numbers of bacteria in the upper intestine and these may induce several effects. For instance, their metabolic products may be toxic to the mucosal epithelium of the upper intestine. The bile acids produced by the action of these bacteria on the constituents of the bile secreted into the gut may damage the intestinal mucosa. There is evidence that the intestinal secretions, which are full of these bacteria, cause increased secretion of fluids even from the normal intestine of experimental animals when perfused into them. These effects may increase secretory activity of the colonized small intestine of an undernourished child when an intestinal pathogen enters the gut. Bacteria also alter the concentration of bile salts (which are essential for fat absorption) and thereby increase fat loss from the intestine. This reduces availability of fat-soluble vitamins to the individual. There is also evidence to suggest that accompanying micronutrient deficiencies (for instance, of vitamin A) increase susceptibility to diarrhoeal disease, and that deficiencies of trace elements (such as zinc) contribute to additional fluid losses from the intestine during a diarrhoeal disease infection.

It thus appears that diarrhoeal disease is an important precipitating cause of undernutrition in children. Several studies have shown that admissions to hospital of children with undernutrition are greatly increased during seasons when diarrhoeal

Table 5.3. Common pathogens causing diarrhoeal disease in the tropics.

Pathogens in the small intestine	Pathogens in the large intestine
Viral	
Rotavirus	
Bacterial	
Vibrio cholerae	Shigella
Escherichia coli	Escherichia coli
(enterotoxigenic – ETEC)	(enteroinvasive – EIEC)
(enteropathogenic – EPEC)	
Campylobacter	Campylobacter
	Salmonella
Parasitic	
Giardia lamblia	Entamoeba histolytica

disease is most common – during a warm summer rather than a cold winter. Studies also show that signs of vitamin A deficiency, such as xerophthalmia and keratomalacia, are precipitated by gastroenteritis (as well as measles).

Acute respiratory infections and childhood pneumonias

Acute respiratory infections (ARIs) and pneumonias are the second most common infective episodes in children in developing societies in the tropics after diarrhoeal disease. It is estimated that between one-fifth and one-third of deaths are due to or associated with ARIs. They are important infections that increase vulnerability to undernutrition in childhood and particularly affect children in the first year of life, and can often lead to middle-ear infections. In developing countries the risk of ARI and pneumonia is linked to indoor air pollution from the use of unprocessed solid fuel. In addition to indoor air pollution, the other risk factors for ARI and pneumonia are lack of measles immunization and overcrowding in the household. Undernutrition is also an important risk factor which contributes through the presence of LBW, underweight of the child and poor breastfeeding practices. With the increased risk of ARI in an undernourished child, the undernutrition–infection cycle is perpetuated. Other risk factors for ARI include parental smoking, and zinc and vitamin A deficiency in the child.

ARI and pneumonia are caused by bacterial pathogens and some viruses. The commonest agent in bacterial infections is pneumococcus (*Streptococcus pneumoniae*), accounting for 30–50% of pneumonia cases. The second most common organism responsible is *Haemophilus influenzae* (10–30% of cases), followed by *Staphylococcus aureas* and *Klebsiella pneumoniae*. Among viruses, respiratory syncytial virus is the leading cause followed by influenza A and B, parainfluenza and adenovirus. TB infection is often detected during an illness; and in children with HIV, bacterial infections are a major cause of pneumonia-related mortality.

ARIs have an indirect effect on the nutritional status and growth of the child, largely by affecting the child's appetite and consequent food intake. A child with respiratory illness may readily feel breathless, and have difficulty in swallowing solid foods and drinking fluids. In pertussis, for instance, vomiting very often follows eating and makes it difficult to feed a child and to ensure that the food is kept down after a difficult feed. A child with pneumonia will show all the characteristics of a child with severe infection and the consequent fever and anorexia, which in turn will compromise its nutritional status.

Intestinal parasites

Parasites that infest the gastrointestinal tract of man are not only pathogenic but also result in the loss of a wide range of nutrients, and this predisposes to poor nutritional status in both children and adults. There are several intestinal parasites that are important in developing societies in the tropics and need to be considered here.

Roundworm (Ascaris lumbricoides)

Roundworm is one of the commonest intestinal parasites seen in children. It is thought that *Ascaris* infestations may interfere with the absorption of proteins and fat because increased absorption is seen following treatment with anti-*Ascaris* drugs in children who are heavily infected with the parasite. *Ascaris* also causes lactose deficiency in the gut, resulting in malabsorption. While in the human body, *Ascaris* induces systemic effects; there is evidence that during the part of the life cycle outside the gut but still within the body, the parasites induce immunological reactions with the production of cytokines. These immune products may be responsible for the loss of appetite frequently seen in children with *Ascaris* infection.

The epidemiological evidence for the importance of *Ascaris* infection in increasing vulnerability to undernutrition is variable. In India, Tanzania and Kenya, improvement in growth has been seen in children with mild to moderate undernourishment who were de-wormed by anti-*Ascaris* drugs. In children in Brazil and Papua New Guinea, on the other hand, there was no improvement in nutrition following de-worming. The children in Brazil and Papua New Guinea were well nourished prior to anti-*Ascaris* treatment – this may be an important factor since it appears that while *Ascaris* may be a significant contributor to moderate undernutrition, its role in mild undernutrition is not clear.

Hookworm (Ancylostoma duodenale and Necator americanus)

Hookworms cause intestinal blood loss and although it appears that most of the protein in the lost blood may be recovered lower down in the intestinal tract, there is always significant loss of iron. Hookworms are a major cause of iron deficiency and anaemia in many countries. It is estimated that the daily faecal blood loss per 350 hookworms may be 10 cm^3, which represents 2 mg of iron. Hookworms are more prevalent in older children, adolescents and adults, and infections take some time to affect general nutrition, apart from the anaemia. In areas where it is endemic, severe, prolonged hookworm infections may lead to undernutrition with oedema of the feet in older children.

Whipworm (Trichuris)

Whipworm is now recognized as an important parasite since it is associated with loss of body weight, stunted growth and anaemia in St Lucia and Malaysia. Substantial loss of blood and mucus can occur during a severe infection, and although malabsorption rarely occurs, loss of nutrients from the gut can be serious. There may also be a loss of appetite, leading to reduced food intake and increased vulnerability to undernutrition.

Schistosoma infections

Infections with *Schistosoma* can considerably compromise nutrition. However, the effects depend on the species responsible. *Schistosoma haematobium* infection in Nigerian children is associated with thinness, while treatment with drugs improved the nutritional status of Kenyan schoolchildren infected with *S. haematobium*. Infection with *Schistosoma mansonii* is more serious, being associated with severe weight loss and lowered serum protein levels. Chronic infections with either species can result in impaired growth and the children are typically both thin and short.

Giardia infections

Infections with *Giardia lamblia* are common in poor environments in the tropics and subtropics, and most children in such circumstances become infected during the first year of life. Infection with

this parasite damages the intestinal mucosa and results in malabsorption of nutrients, particularly fat. It seems to be commonly seen in children with undernutrition, and there is some evidence that *Giardia* infection results in impaired growth and weight loss in children.

Entamoeba infections

Infections with the parasite *Entamoeba histolytica* occur mostly in adults, although they are seen in children too. Since the parasite infects the large intestine, severe infections result in serious loss of blood and mucus, and may also cause systemic problems such as liver abscesses due to infection of the liver by the parasite. Amoebiasis can cause nutrient loss and can lower the levels of circulating proteins; this sometimes leads to undernutrition.

Cryptosporidium infection

Cryptosporidium is now recognized as an important pathogen causing diarrhoeal disease in well-nourished children. It affects the mucosal morphology and hence can cause malabsorption of nutrients and so predispose to undernutrition. It has been reported to be present in nearly half the children with undernutrition presenting with post-measles diarrhoeal disease in Rwanda.

Malaria

Malaria is an important infection that results in iron deficiency and generalized undernutrition. Malarial infections lead to a decrease in red blood cell production and at the same time there is increased red blood cell destruction due to haemolysis; this combination leads to anaemia. Infections with the malarial parasites have similar metabolic effects to other systemic infections. They increase protein metabolism, with more protein breakdown than synthesis, thus resulting in protein depletion. There is loss of appetite, and the frequent episodes of fever increase the energy needs of the infected individual. Malarial infections also compromise placental function and can result in LBW.

Severe malaria and bacterial septicaemia may have a common cytokine-mediated pathology which may account for the changes manifest in the host. Cytokine concentrations are high in some forms of malaria and so too are levels of TNF, although much of the TNF is bound to soluble receptors and hence demonstrates little bioactivity. Cytokines are involved in the fever in malaria, in the suppression of erythropoiesis contributing to the anaemia and in the placental dysfunction resulting in placental insufficiency, which probably contributes to IUGR.

The pathogenesis of anaemia in malaria is multifactorial and is contributed by the destruction of red blood cells with the malarial parasite, the shortened lifespan of red blood cells which had parasites once and which were extracted by the spleen, and by the suppression of erythropoiesis. There is even contribution from the accelerated destruction of non-parasitized red blood cells. Anaemia is a particular problem in children with malaria. The degree of anaemia and the rapidity with which it appears vary and the fall in haemoglobin may occur at the rate of 2 g per day. In children with severe anaemia other factors such as bacteraemia, hookworm infestation and vitamin A deficiency may be the principal cause even in malaria-endemic regions.

Tuberculosis

Infections with the tubercle bacillus can manifest as very poor 'catch-up' growth or growth faltering in children, which does not respond to intensive feeding. It is crucial to remember that, in children, TB can be an important cause of severe undernutrition that fails to respond to nutritional rehabilitation. Very often, in the absence of a firm diagnosis, a therapeutic trial with anti-TB drugs can result in improvement in the nutritional status of the child. Infections such as TB not only have systemic metabolic effects, resulting in protein breakdown and loss of appetite, but are also important causes of anaemia in severe undernutrition.

HIV/AIDS

Wasting and failure to thrive have long been recognized as important features of HIV infection. Wasting and undernutrition are associated with HIV infections in both children and adults, and wasting is one of the three major symptoms in the clinical definition of AIDS. Infants born with HIV infection who then develop AIDS very often show features of undernutrition characteristic of kwashiorkor or marasmus.

Several factors contribute to undernutrition and wasting during an infection with HIV; they include anorexia, diarrhoeal episodes, fever, malabsorption and intestinal atrophy. The increased susceptibility to opportunistic infections makes the situation worse and promotes the process that results in severe undernutrition.

Both TB and HIV/AIDS are dealt with in detail in Chapter 9.

The two case studies that follow illustrate the close links between nutrition and infection, and the role of breastfeeding and supplementary feeding in this interaction on the growth profiles of both normal-weight and LBW infants.

Further Reading

Mata, L.J. (1978) *The Children of Santa Maria Cauque: A Prospective Field Study of Health and Growth.* MIT Press, Cambridge, Massachusetts. *An extraordinary account of a 9-year prospective incidence observation study of infection and nutrition in a community living in a Guatemalan highland village.*

Scrimshaw, N.S., Gordon, C.E. and Taylor, J.E. (1968) *Interactions of Nutrition and Infection.* World Health Organization, Geneva, Switzerland. *A comprehensive review of the then literature on the interrelationships of infectious disease and malnutrition, drawing attention to its public health importance.*

Tomkins, A. and Watson, F (1989) *Malnutrition and Infection. Nutrition Policy Discussion Paper No. 5.* United Nations Administrative Committee on Coordination, Sub-committee on Nutrition, Geneva, Switzerland. *A dated but state-of-the-art review on the interaction of malnutrition and infection that is the cause of most of the preventable deaths among children in developing countries.*

Case Studies

Case Study 5.1: Interactions of infection and nutrition.

Study Fig. 5.4 (from Leonarda Mata's work) carefully. This illustrates the growth and weight gain of a male child. His birth weight was normal (>2.5 kg) although it was lower than the expected standard for children of that region. The weight gain in the first 6 months is indicative of good growth despite the occasional illness noted in the chart. A succession of repeated infections after that, precipitated by an episode of cellulitis and upper respiratory infections between the ages of 6 and 9 months,

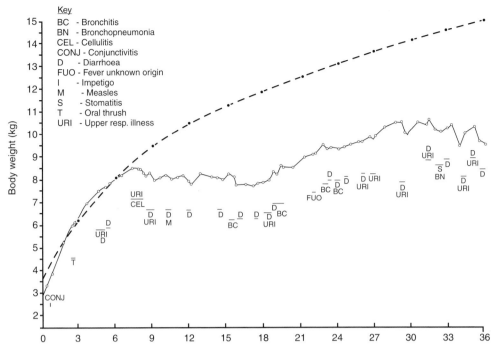

Fig. 5.4. The longitudinal changes in body weight of a male child (—o—) and the impact of episodes of infection on his growth (– –•– – indicates median of the growth reference). (Adapted with permission from Mata *et al.*, 1971.)

resulted in growth faltering thereafter. The increase in infective episodes seems to occur at the onset of weaning and the introduction of supplementary feeding. The growth chart also illustrates that the number and duration of the frequent infections cause growth faltering and prevent 'catch-up' growth, leading to underweight and resulted in undernutrition.

From birth to 6 months of age, the child demonstrated normal weight gain despite some infective episodes such as diarrhoea and upper respiratory tract illness. Between the ages of 6 and 12 months the child experienced repeated bouts of diarrhoea, respiratory infections and an episode of measles that served to halt his weight gain and resulted in undernutrition. From 12 to 36 months of age the child continued to have several bouts of serious illness which did not permit him to regain a normal trajectory of weight gain and growth. This case illustrates how frequent infections can undermine normal growth of children.

The impact of illness after 6 months and following the introduction of weaning and supplementary feeds is important here. The exclusive breastfeeding recommended in the first six months of life protects the child and reduces exposure to infective agents. Even when infections occur they do not perturb much the normal growth and weight gain of infants. The process of weaning and introduction of supplementary feeds represents a crucial period for children. This process can contribute to infections and poor nutrition both by the introduction of unsafe and contaminated feeds as well as the provision of inadequate nutrients in the supplementary feeds. The emphasis is rightly on exclusive breastfeeding for 6 months and for safe and adequate supplementary feeds while encouraging breastfeeding after 6 months for as long as possible. Encouraging lactation may also help contraception and delay the conception and birth of the next child.

Reference

Mata, L.J., Urrutia, J.J. and Lechtig, A. (1971) Infection and nutrition of children of a low socioeconomic rural community. *American Journal of Clinical Nutrition* 24, 249–259.

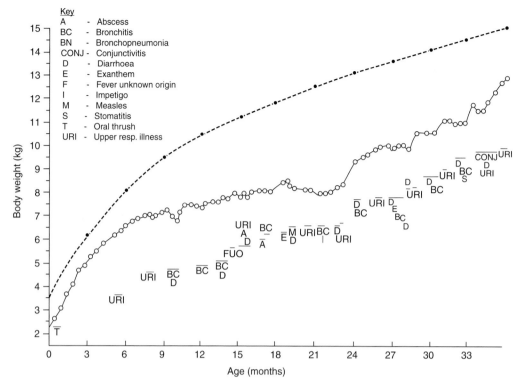

Fig. 5.5. The longitudinal changes in body weight of a male child with LBW (—o—) and the impact of episodic infections on his growth (– –•– – indicates median of the growth reference). (Adapted with permission from Mata *et al.*, 1971.)

Case Study 5.2: Interactions of infection, nutrition and low birth weight.

Figure 5.5 (again from Leonardo Mata's work) shows the growth curve of a male child who was born with low birth weight (LBW) (<2.5 kg). Despite his LBW and a few episodes of respiratory infections he grew relatively well in the first six months, tracking parallel with the standard growth curve for children of that region. LBW infants can catch up and even demonstrate growth rates along the normal trajectory.

With weaning at 6 months growth faltering occurred; the supplementary feeds provided were found to be deficient in energy and protein, possi-

bly also in micronutrients. Marked weight loss occurred at 9 months when an episode of bronchitis and measles was combined with diarrhoeal illness. Infective episodes became frequent thereafter and the child's weight stagnated, never catching up with growth after that. His height also departed from the normal standard and the child was both underweight and stunted at 3 years of age.

Reference

Mata, L.J., Urrutia, J.J. and Lechtig, A. (1971) Infection and nutrition of children of a low socioeconomic rural community. *American Journal of Clinical Nutrition* 24, 249–259.

6 Vitamin A Deficiency and Risk of Infection

- Micronutrient deficiencies such as vitamin A deficiency compromise several aspects of the immune response and the body's defence mechanisms.
- Review of the evidence that suggests that vitamin A deficiency increases risk of infection in children; in particular, the risk of respiratory illness and diarrhoeal disease is increased substantially in a vitamin A-deficient child.
- Vitamin A supplementation reduces infectious disease morbidity in children.
- Vitamin A deficiency results in increased mortality in children. Mortality in children with vitamin A deficiency is higher than that observed in non-deficient children in the same environment.
- Vitamin A supplementation trials have consistently shown a reduction in mortality in children.

6.1 Introduction

Vitamin A plays an important role in the body's immune response, having a role in the maintenance of the integrity of epithelial surfaces and in the development of the lymphoid system. The earliest observations that suggested a link between vitamin A and the body's defence mechanisms were made even before its structure was identified. These were animal experiments showing that malnourished animals fed only on fats, protein and starch failed to grow normally and were susceptible to infections, whereas animals fed butter and cod liver oil were protected from infections. Several subsequent studies in human subjects supported these early observations. Follow-up of the growth and development of children in an orphanage in Denmark showed that children fed generous portions of butter fat and whole milk grew better and were less susceptible to infections of the urinary and respiratory tracts and the middle ear. Hence vitamin A was soon considered an 'anti-infective' factor and clinical trials were conducted. The earliest was one done near London and showed that when children with measles admitted to the Grove Fever Hospital were given vitamin A, they had only half the case fatality rates of children who received no vitamin A. Although subsequent studies supported the benefits of vitamin A in infections from common cold to puerperal sepsis, the importance of the anti-infective role of vitamin A was superseded by the interest in antimicrobials and antibiotics, which revolutionized the treatment of infections.

High rates of mortality in undernourished children who also had xerophthalmia were observed over 30 years ago. Interest in the role vitamin A deficiency plays in increasing the mortality due largely to infectious diseases in children was reactivated more recently with a study in Indonesia that demonstrated a 34% reduced mortality following supplementation with vitamin A. Investigations of the illnesses or events prior to death suggested that the reduction in mortality with vitamin A supplements was largely attributable to a reduction in mortality from measles, diarrhoeal disease and severe undernutrition. There was apparently little impact on mortality due to ARI in any of these trials.

Interest in the important role that vitamin A plays in reducing susceptibility to infections thus re-emerged from the studies conducted in Indonesia in the 1980s. Some of the clinical and epidemiological evidence that supports the role of vitamin A deficiency in increasing infectious disease risk as well as morbidity and mortality, especially in children, is presented in this chapter. It is clear that the risk of both diarrhoeal disease and ARI is increased considerably when a child has vitamin A deficiency. Other studies have also confirmed the impact of vitamin A status on morbidity associated with infections. Some of the best evidence to support this is obtained from intervention studies that have supplemented vitamin A and monitored the impact on subsequent morbidity. Vitamin A supplementation appears to reduce the severity of infections such as measles, persistent diarrhoea and malaria. The protective effect is greater, the more severe the infectious episode. Vitamin A treatment of measles leads to fewer and less severe complications, and enhanced immunological and clinical recovery.

6.2 Vitamin A and Its Role in Immune Function

Vitamin A is integral to a host's defence mechanisms preventing the entry of pathogenic agents into the body. Although deficiency of vitamin A causes thickening and increased keratinization of the skin (hyperkeratosis) it does not compromise the barrier function of the skin. However, vitamin A is fundamental to maintaining the integrity of the epithelium of the gastrointestinal, respiratory and genitourinary tracts, and vitamin A deficiency affects the normal functioning of the mucosal epithelial lining of these organs. Squamous metaplasia with abnormal keratinization takes place in the respiratory and genitourinary tracts, but not in the gut. Loss of mucus from goblet cells of the mucosal epithelium of the respiratory, gut and genitourinary tracts results in reduced mucus production and secretion. There is loss of cilia in the epithelial lining of the respiratory tract and loss of microvilli in the gastrointestinal epithelium. These changes result in compromising the first line of defence against potential pathogens. The reduced mucus secretion reduces its ability to adhere to pathogenic bacteria, trapping them in the mucus, and the loss of cilia results in the inability to move them out of the airways. Pathogenic bacteria that are ordinarily cleared by the mucus seem to adhere to the damaged epithelium and the patches of squamous metaplasia seen in vitamin A

deficiency. The same feature is seen in the gastrointestinal tract, with reduced mucus secretion unable to move the pathogen rapidly downwards. The damage to the villi increases the permeability of the gut. There is evidence that pathogens are translocated from the gut into the regional lymphoid tissue, suggesting that pathogenic penetration of the gut has occurred in vitamin A deficiency states. Vitamin A deficiency also impairs the process of repair and regeneration of these normal mucosal epithelial barriers. These changes obviously increase the risk of infections in children with vitamin A deficiency.

Similar changes with loss of mucus-producing goblet cells of the ocular epithelial surfaces along with squamous metaplasia of the lining of the conjunctiva and cornea are well documented. The loss of mucus in vitamin A deficiency is a serious breach of the mucosal immune mechanisms. There is also an impairment of mucosal-associated immune cell function and alterations in the antigen-specific secretory immunoglobulin concentrations. Thus the secretion of mucosal immune factors and anti-infective or inflammatory markers in saliva, genital tract and breast milk may be affected. Vitamin A supplementation studies have shown an improvement in gut permeability, but the results with regard to the concentrations of the secretion of mucosal immune markers in breast milk, saliva and genital fluids have not been consistent.

The functions of neutrophils, which provide an important defence by non-specific immune responses, are impaired significantly in vitamin A deficiency states. Neutrophils are attracted to, phagocytose and kill pathogenic agents like bacteria and parasites. In vitamin A-deficient states neutrophil function is characterized by impaired chemotaxis, adhesion and phagocytosis. Their compromised ability to generate active oxidant molecules results in their impaired ability to kill pathogens following phagocytosis. While the numbers of neutrophils seem to increase in vitamin A deficiency, the impairment of normal neutrophil development and compromise in their normal function diminish the protection against bacterial and other infections.

Vitamin A deficiency also manifests with similar paradoxical responses with regard to macrophages. While their numbers increase, their ability to phagocytose and kill bacteria after ingestion is impaired. In vitamin A-deficient

Box 6.1. Physiological and Nutritional Aspects of Vitamin A.

Vitamin A is a generic term used for all retinoids and related structures with 20 carbon atoms and their precursors, the pro-vitamin A carotenoids with 40 carbon atoms. The biologically active vitamin A retinoids include retinol (alcohol form), retinal (aldehyde form) and dehydroretinol, as well as their oxidized forms like retinoic acid. Of the precursor forms of vitamin A the ones biologically important are α-carotene, β-carotene and β-cryptoxanthin. These precursor carotenoids are cleaved by enzymes in the small intestine and the liver to release the active form of vitamin A. Of the carotenoids, β-carotene is the one biologically most active as it releases two molecules of vitamin A compared with only one from the other carotenoids.

Sources of vitamin A in the diet

Vitamin A is found as retinol palmitate in foods of animal origin such as liver, fish-liver oils, milk, butter, cheese, egg yolk and some fatty fish. Pro-vitamin A carotenoids are present in both animal and plant foods. Plant sources of vitamin A, a main source in the diets of the poor in developing countries, are yellow- and orange-coloured fruits (mango, papaya, etc.) and vegetables (carrot) and dark green leafy vegetables (spinach). Red palm oil and cooked yellow sweet potatoes are also good sources of carotenoids. Pro-vitamin A carotenoids are converted to the active form of the vitamin, i.e. retinol, and the efficiency of this conversion is better with coloured fruits and vegetables than from green leafy vegetables. It is now generally agreed that the conversion factor for carotenoids from plant sources to retinol is 12:1 and that this applies only to fruits; for vegetable sources of carotenoids the conversion factor is even poorer at 26:1. Thus less of the active vitamin A is available from carotenoids in vegetables as compared to fruits. Processing of food and the food matrix will also influence the bioavailability of vitamin A from the diet. In industrialized countries many food sources such as margarines are fortified with vitamin A.

Vitamin A absorption

The bioavailability of vitamin A from a mixed diet depends on the food matrix, the release of preformed vitamin A from precursor carotenoids and on the fat content of the diet. Pro-vitamin A carotenoids are released from vegetables in the diet if they are well cooked and masticated to allow the carotenoids to be freed from the cellulose in these plant foods. The released vitamin A and carotenoids are fat soluble and will aggregate with the lipid globules in the intestinal contents, then being subject to the action of the lipid digestive enzymes secreted into the gut. Bile salts will enable the process of emulsification and the retinoids and carotenoids will be absorbed along with the lipids across the intestinal epithelial cells. A specific cellular binding protein may be involved and accounts for the high efficiency of absorption that occurs. Within the intestinal cell (enterocyte) the retinol is esterified to retinol palmitate and, together with triacylglycerols and other fat-soluble nutrients, is packaged into chylomicrons which are then carried to the liver. The retinyl esters are converted to retinol in some liver cells and stored as retinol palmitate in other liver cells, while being transported across bound to retinol-binding protein (RBP). Hence the liver is the main store for vitamin A, normally accounting for 80% of the total body store of vitamin A.

Mobilization and transport of vitamin A

Retinol is released from the liver store bound to RBP and this retinol–RBP complex is bound in turn to another larger protein called transthyretin. About 95% of retinol transported in the plasma/blood is found in the retinol–RBP–transthyretin complex, and the rest as retinol–RBP complex. Very little (less than 1%) retinol is present in plasma/blood as free retinol. The retinol–RBP complex is taken up by specific cell surface receptors and the retinol is transferred into the cell where it binds with RBP present inside the cell, i.e. cellular RBP. The RBP released from the receptor of the cell surface is recycled and now available to transport other molecules of retinol. Evidence from individuals who have a genetic disorder and cannot synthesize RBP but have no signs of vitamin A deficiency apart from some night blindness, suggests that retinol bound to the chylomicrons can be taken up directly by cells apart from the eye. There is thus the possibility of another metabolic pathway for retinol, implying that the role played by RBP in transporting retinol is not an absolute requirement to meet nutritional needs. However, RBP fulfils several important functions. RBP facilitates the transport of a fat-soluble vitamin such as retinol in an aqueous plasma/blood environment. It also protects retinol from oxidative damage during transport. In addition it probably regulates the mobilization of retinol depending on the body's needs and can help deliver the retinol to specific target sites depending on the presence of the cell surface receptors to which the retinol–RBP complex binds. Plasma carotenoids are transported in the lipoproteins, both low-density (mostly carotenes) and high-density lipoproteins.

In a healthy person no vitamin A is excreted from the body although oxidized metabolites are excreted in the urine. Both RBP as well as the RBP–transthyretin complex are excreted by the kidney. Excess retinol and more so β-carotenes may be retained in enterocytes which are shed into the intestinal lumen, with the rapid turnover of enterocytes resulting in loss in faeces.

Table 6.1. Host defence and immune function changes in vitamin A-deficient states. (Adapted from Semba, 2002.)

Abnormal keratinization of epithelial surfaces, e.g. respiratory tract, genitourinary tract, conjunctival and corneal surfaces
Loss of cilia from respiratory epithelial lining cells
Loss and flattening of microvilli in the gastrointestinal tract
Loss of mucin and goblet cells in epithelial linings of respiratory, gastrointestinal and genitourinary tracts
Impaired mucosal-associated immune function
Impaired neutrophil functions related to chemotaxis, phagocytosis and intracellular killing
Impaired lymphopoiesis by bone marrow, resulting in reduced production of total lymphocytes and decreased
 CD4+ cell numbers
Decreased numbers of NK cells and impairment in their normal functioning
T-lymphocyte function shifted towards a dominant Th1 type response
Decrease in numbers and functions of B lymphocytes
Impaired antibody responses to TD and Ti antigen exposure

states there is enhanced macrophage-mediated inflammatory response due to increased production of interleukins and INF-γ. Thus vitamin A deficiency results in increased pathogen replication and also enhanced inflammatory responses. The impaired macrophage response is unable to control the pathogen/bacterial proliferation while the enhanced production of pro-inflammatory cytokines exacerbates the inflammatory response of the host. Vitamin A supplementation has been shown to down-regulate the secretion of pro-inflammatory cytokines like TNF-α and IL-6 in response to infections with some pathogens.

NK cells are part of the first line of defence and play an important role in innate immunity by killing virus-infected cells (as well as tumour cells), but they are also affected by vitamin A deficiency. Studies have shown that NK-cell numbers and their ability to kill pathogens (by lytic activity) are diminished in vitamin A deficiency states.

T-lymphocyte function is affected by vitamin A and vitamin A supplements increase total T-cell numbers in children, particularly CD4+ cells. T lymphocytes recognize the antigen or the antibody produced by the host in response to the pathogen. APCs play an important role in exposing the T cells to the antigen and in the initiation of proliferation and maturation of these lymphocytes (see Chapter 2). The naïve Th cells recognize the antigen via the T-cell receptor and with the help of IL-12, result in the development of the Th1 memory cells which mediate immunity to intracellular pathogens. Th2 memory cells, on the other hand, originate in the presence of IL-4 and stimulate immunity to extracellular pathogens. Th1 cells respond to intracellular pathogens like viruses and produce INF-γ and

IL-2, stimulate cytotoxic lymphocyte responses and macrophage activation, and enhance DCH responses with limited effects on B-lymphocyte function. Th2 cells respond to extracellular pathogens and produce interleukins like IL-4, stimulate lymphocyte production of immunoglobulins (IgG, IgE and IgA) and promote eosinophil and mast cell development. Vitamin A deficiency impairs antibody responses (IgG and IgE decreased) which are dependent on Th2 cells. These effects are due to decreases in the numbers of antigen-specific plasma cells while the ability of each cell to secrete antibodies is not altered. Supplementation of vitamin A has been shown to increase antibody response to tetanus toxoid and diphtheria vaccine in vitamin A-deficient children.

Vitamin A status also changes the pattern of Th1 and Th2 response and cytokine production. Vitamin A deficiency shifts the immune response towards the Th1-cell-mediated activity and impairs Th2 response, while supplementation with vitamin A tends to boost Th2 type responses. The production of Th2 cytokines is diminished whereas the production of Th1 cytokines is increased in vitamin A deficiency. It is apparent that vitamin A may affect the balance of Th1/Th2 responses through multiple mechanisms. It also appears that the immunological mechanism through which vitamin A exerts an effect are pathogen specific and this is not entirely due to the Th1/Th2 balance. There is no conclusive evidence from supplementation studies in human subjects that vitamin A has a direct effect on cytokine production or lymphocyte activation. Vitamin A supplementation however, seems to confer greater DCH responses in some studies and not in others.

Vitamin A may modulate the activity of B lymphocytes, although the antibody response of B lymphocytes may be normal when the antibody response does not require the help from T cells. While vitamin A deficiency impairs the capacity of the host to mount an antibody response to T-cell-dependent antigens, it is probably true to state that B-lymphocyte development is unaffected in vitamin A deficiency states.

The mechanism of the action of vitamin A on the immune system is still not clear. It is probably mediated through active metabolites like retinoic acid, which act via specific nuclear receptors regulating gene transcription. Retinoic acid is produced by the cells of the intestines such as dendritic cells and provides an intestine-specific environmental cue to differentiate immune cells. This important action may also contribute to protecting the gut from pathogens.

The main changes in host defence and immune function associated with vitamin A deficiency states are summarized in Table 6.1.

6.3 Vitamin A Deficiency and Risk of Morbidity and Mortality due to Infections

Vitamin A has long been recognized to reduce the risk of infections in animals and man, and was considered an 'anti-infective' factor. Since early in the 20th century, vitamin A was administered to treat or prevent a variety of infections until the era of antimicrobials and antibiotics which were dramatically more effective than the administration of vitamin A. There are several reports in the early literature dating from the 1920s implicating poor vitamin A status with increased risk of morbidity and mortality due to infectious diseases. All of these reports between the two World Wars were from developed countries. For instance, it was observed among patients with xerophthalmia that nearly two-thirds had severe infections. In another report of individuals with xerophthalmia, infections were frequent and there was 25% mortality due to bronchopneumonia. In vitamin A-deficient infants with xerophthalmia, respiratory and genitourinary infections were common and often fatal. In another report on infants more than half the number with xerophthalmia and keratomalacia died of secondary infections. The frequency of otitis media, pneumonia and other severe infections doubled in children whose diets were deficient in vitamin A.

Studies in developing countries in the tropics since the 1950s also support these earlier observations from Europe and North America. None of the children who had xerophthalmia were free of respiratory infections in Papua New Guinea; and African adults on low vitamin A intakes were more commonly infected with the helminth, *Onchocerca* (a parasitic worm causing river blindness).

Two large-scale studies, one in Indonesia and the other in India, examined the risk of diarrhoeal disease and ARIs in children with and without clinical evidence of vitamin A deficiency (xerophthalmia). The risk of getting an infection in a vitamin A-deficient child was compared with the risk that a child with no evidence of vitamin A deficiency has (which is considered equal to 1). The ratio is termed the relative risk. The study in Indonesia was a follow-up of pre-school children for 18 months and showed that children with mild xerophthalmia had twice the risk of diarrhoeal disease and had ARI twice as frequently as children with no evidence of vitamin A deficiency. The results from India, involving a similar group of children, supported the findings of the Indonesian study, although the impact on respiratory infections was more dramatic than on diarrhoeal disease. Table 6.2 summarizes some of the findings from these two studies.

Although the increased mortality among children with xerophthalmia was noted in the 1970s, importance at that stage was accorded to the blindness and visual impairment that are associated with vitamin A deficiency since they were considered to be of greater public health importance. Interest in the association between vitamin A deficiency and risk of infections was prompted by the observation that rural pre-school children in Indonesia with mild xerophthalmia had higher rates of mortality than children with no xerophthalmia growing up in the same environment. The direct relationship between mortality rates and severity of xerophthalmia suggested that subclinical deficiency of vitamin A may

Table 6.2. Relative risk of ARI and diarrhoeal disease in children with xerophthalmia.

	ARI	Diarrhoea
Age 1–2 years		
Indonesia	2.3	3.4
India	4.0	0.9
Age 2–3 years		
Indonesia	1.9	3.4
India	2.0	1.5

Box 6.2. Physiological Functions of Vitamin A.

In addition to the role that vitamin A plays in immune function, it also has important functions related to vision and reproduction in the body. In the retina, retinaldehyde combines with light-sensitive opsin proteins to form rhodopsin in the rods and iodopsin in the cones. Retinol (all-*trans* form) is isomerized to *cis*-retinol in the retina and then oxidized to *cis*-retinaldehyde, which reacts with the opsin to form rhodopsin. When light falls on the retina the absorption of light by rhodopsin causes isomerization of the retinaldehyde bound to opsin from *cis* to *trans* form and a conformational change in the opsin. This results in initiation of the nerve impulse in the retina and the release of retinaldehyde. The all-*trans* retinaldehyde released is reduced to all-*trans* retinol which is now available for regeneration of rhodopsin. The key to this visual or rhodpsin cycle for rhodopsin regeneration is the ready availability of retinol and hence vitamin A. Vitamin A deficiency thus manifests with night blindness since the rods are responsible for vision in dim light or at dusk.

Vitamin A is essential for cellular differentiation, embryogenesis and growth; a role fulfilled by retinoic acid. Cellular differentiation accounts for the morphological changes that the epithelial lining of the body undergo until it matures. When vitamin A is lacking, the mucus-secreting cells of the lining of the gut and respiratory tracts are replaced by keratin-producing cells. A similar change also occurs in the lining to the eyes – the cornea and conjunctiva, with their epithelial lining drying up and becoming rough resulting in *xerosis*. Vitamin A in the form of retinoic acid is also responsible for embryogenesis through the control of genes linked to development and growth. Retinoic acid binds to nuclear receptors which in turn influences the expression of several genes. Thus retinoic acid functions as an important regulator of gene transcription and influences a wide range of functions during embryogenesis. Hence vitamin A in excess during pregnancy can result in lethal consequences to the fetus (see Box 6.4).

Vitamin A plays an important part in the synthesis of mucopolysaccharides, glycoproteins and glycosaminoglycans. Mucopolysaccharides are an important component of mucus secretions. Vitamin A plays a crucial role in the transfer and incorporation of sulfate which is essential for the synthesis of mucopolysaccharides. Hence vitamin A deficiency can result in impaired mucopolysaccharide synthesis which manifests as reduced mucus secretion by the mucous membranes of organs such as the respiratory tract, thus increasing the susceptibility to infections. It reduces the production of tears, thus contributing to dryness and reduced wettability of the eye surface (*xerophthalmia*). These effects of deficiency on mucopolysaccharide synthesis also contribute to changes in the skin (*follicular hyperkeratosis*) and changes in the ground substance of bone and cartilage, thus causing deformities during growth. Retinoids are also implicated in the synthesis of glycoproteins which are important components of mucus and receptors on cell surfaces and of glycosaminoglycans which constitute the viscous extracellular matrix on cell surfaces.

Vitamin A is required for normal growth of the body and participates in the growth and maturation of cells in the cartilage of bones. Vitamin A supplementation in Indonesia and Nepal has promoted better growth in children in several studies but not in others, probably the result of the fact that vitamin A is just one of the nutrients that is essential for normal growth in children. Vitamin A may also facilitate the production of red blood cells by the bone marrow, possibly by influencing the absorption and utilization in the body by reducing infection and inflammation. Vitamin A's role in immunity, infection and disease is discussed in the main text of this chapter.

Apart from functioning as precursors of preformed vitamin A, carotenoids also act directly on the body. β-Carotene functions as an important antioxidant in the body. The xanthophyll carotenoids – zeaxanthin, mesozeaxanthin and lutein – are constituents of the macula lutea of the retina and are responsible for its yellow colour. Macular degeneration occurs in ageing populations and this seems to be related to the concentration of xanthophyll carotenoids, especially lutein, in the macula. Lycopene, a red pigmented carotenoid present in tomatoes, is not a precursor of vitamin A. It functions as a good antioxidant like β-carotene and seems to be linked with reducing the risk of prostate cancer in men.

Box 6.3. Vitamin A Deficiency States.

Vitamin A deficiency manifests with signs of xerophthalmia (dry eyes) and there are, according to WHO, several stages of this clinical condition: (i) conjunctival xerosis with patches of dryness in the conjunctival epithelium (X1A) and with Bitot's spots, i.e. foamy deposits on the surface of the conjunctiva (X1B); (ii) corneal xerosis with extension of the dryness and non-wettability to the surface of the cornea (X2); (iii) corneal ulceration (X3A) usually minimal at the edges of the cornea leading on to more extensive corneal ulceration (X3B) that can lead to blindness; and resulting finally in (iv) corneal scarring (XS) and blindness.

These changes seen in the conjunctival and corneal epithelial linings are also evident elsewhere. In the skin it manifests as increased keratinization resulting in follicular hyperkeratosis. It also affects the lining of the respiratory, gastrointestinal and genitourinary tracts. In the gut, the epithelial lining and the villi are flattened and mucous glands reduced while in the respiratory tract the changes lead to loss of cilia and reduced mucus secretion.

Since retinol is required for the synthesis of the visual pigments in the retina of the eye, vitamin A deficiency results in visual impairment which manifests as 'night blindness'. Individuals with marginal vitamin A deficiency are unable to see in dim light because the rods in the retina are unable to synthesize the visual pigments due to reduced availability of the active form of vitamin A, retinol. These changes are reversible with the administration of vitamin A.

Vitamin A deficiency impairs immune function and increases risk of infectious morbidity and mortality. It also contributes to nutritional anaemia since it influences iron metabolism, haemoglobin synthesis and red blood cell production.

---

be associated with higher mortality in children. The study, carried out in a large number of pre-school children, showed that mortality was four times higher in children with mild xerophthalmia (night blindness and or Bitot's spots), i.e. mild vitamin A deficiency state, and in some age groups increased eight- to 12-fold. The mortality increased linearly with the severity of vitamin A deficiency state (night blindness alone, Bitot's spots alone or both) and was attributable for at least 16% of the deaths in children aged 1–6 years. The study was significant in that it established the association between low vitamin A status and the increased infectious disease risk, and generated interest in vitamin A supplementation studies which have provided the evidence for an important role for vitamin A in immune function and susceptibility to infections.

6.4 Vitamin A Supplementation on Mortality, Morbidity and Resistance to Infections

The first large-scale supplementation trial with vitamin A was carried out in Indonesia a few years after the initial report of the association between mild vitamin A deficiency and increased mortality in children. There are now over 100 field trials with vitamin A which seem to show that vitamin A supplementation reduces morbidity and mortality from a wide range of infections in man.

Intervention trials with vitamin A and mortality

Several large community intervention trials in children aged 6 months to 5 years in several countries in Asia and Africa showed an overall decrease in mortality of 30%. The benefits of vitamin A supplements to infants less than 6 months of age was less certain. Not all the studies showed a significant benefit and the differences between different study sites in the nutritional status of the children, their morbidity patterns and access to health care were obviously crucial in influencing the mortality rates. Comparison of the studies also indicated that the decrease in mortality observed was more marked with frequent small doses than with infrequent high doses of vitamin A. Most of the deaths were due to infectious diseases and the deaths averted in the supplemented group were mostly from measles and diarrhoeal diseases but not from ARI or pneumonia. The reduced mortality in measles and diarrhoea cases was attributed to the less severe clinical manifestations in the children who received vitamin A supplements.

Studies in pregnant women in Nepal who have vitamin A deficiency characterized by night blindness demonstrated a higher risk of infectious disease morbidity and mortality. Vitamin A or β-carotene supplementation reduced the infectious disease morbidity and mortality in these women. Studies on pregnant mothers showed that supplements reduced childbirth-associated deaths but not the subsequent infant survival. Dosing pregnant mothers with vitamin A in communities with low vitamin A status and high maternal mortality rates dramatically reduces maternal mortality rates and dosing the newborn infant with vitamin A within 2 days of birth significantly reduces neonatal mortality.

Table 6.3 summarizes data from the literature on vitamin A supplementation and reduction of mortality in children. It shows that in seven out of eight studies a significant reduction in mortality was observed. Meta-analyses of all the available data from these trials have estimated the reduction in mortality to range from 23% to 34%. Investigations of the illnesses or events prior to death suggest that the reduction in mortality with vitamin A supplements was largely attributable to a reduction in mortality as a result of measles, diarrhoeal disease and severe undernutrition. There was apparently little impact on mortality due to ARIs in any of these trials.

Analysis of all the community intervention trials suggested that while vitamin A deficiency increases overall mortality, particularly from measles, improving vitamin A status reduces overall mortality. Treating children who were ill with measles with high doses of vitamin A was also effective in reducing their risk of complications and death. The obvious conclusion was that vitamin A deficiency increases risk of some infections and supplements of vitamin A diminish the risk of mortality from infectious diseases, although the benefits are evident with some infections but not with others.

Vitamin A supplementation and resistance to infections

Vitamin A supplementation trials in several countries in the developing world in Africa and Asia have shown that vitamin A can reduce risk of infection and the morbidity and mortality due to common childhood illnesses like diarrhoeal disease and measles, while it does not appear to reduce morbidity and mortality due to acute lower respiratory tract infection (ALRTI). Vitamin A supplementation also reduces the morbidity of malaria and influences HIV/AIDS.

Vitamin A and diarrhoeal disease

Diarrhoeal disease in children in developing countries is caused by a number of pathogens, both bacterial and viral. The characteristics of the pathogen such as its ability to produce toxins or invade tissues or influence water and electrolyte absorption will determine the manifestation of the diarrhoeal illness. Clinically evident vitamin A deficiency states have been shown to be associated with increased risk of diarrhoeal diseases in children. In Ghana, vitamin A supplementation was associated with a decreased attendance at clinics for illness, reduced hospitalization rates for severe disease, and decreased severity of illness due to diarrhoeal disease. In Brazil, vitamin A supplementation increased the protection against diarrhoeal episodes of longer than 3 days in children. Vitamin A supplementation has also been shown to reduce the incidence and duration of diarrhoeal episodes and is of particular benefit in children who are not breastfed.

Supplementation of vitamin A or fortification of foods with vitamin A has been shown to reduce morbidity and mortality due to diarrhoeal disease in children, with the overall reduction in child mortality being attributed largely to the reductions in mortality associated with diarrhoeal illness. The severity of diarrhoeal disease is also reduced with vitamin A supplementation. While vitamin A supplementation shows a remarkable and significant

Table 6.3. Summary of vitamin A supplementation trials on childhood mortality.

Location	Number of children	Percentage change in mortality
Aceh, Indonesia	29,236	−34
West Java, Indonesia	11,220	−45
Tamil Nadu, India	15,419	−54
Hyderabad, India	15,775	−6
Sarlahi, Nepal	28,640	−30
Jumla, Nepal	7,197	−29
North Ghana	21,906	−19
Khartoum, Sudan	29,615	+6

impact on diarrhoeas, it has no effect on pneumo-nias in pre-school children. Although community interventions with vitamin A supplements protect against diarrhoeal diseases by reducing the risk of this illness, it is not clear whether it has a general-ized effect against all infectious agents or only against some of the pathogens.

Vitamin A and acute lower respiratory tract infections

Like diarrhoeal diseases, a wide group of pathogens – both bacterial and viral – are responsible for ALRTI in children in developing countries. In addition, often secondary bacterial infections follow viral infections of the lungs. In community intervention trials with vitamin A, the risk of symptomatic respi-ratory infection increases. A study in Ecuador seems to suggest that low-dose weekly supplements of vitamin A are beneficial to undernourished children by reducing significantly the risk of respiratory infections in those who are underweight compared with those who are normal weight and who show an increasing ALRTI risk. Community trials with vitamin A also failed to influence the morbidity and mortality associated with ARIs.

Vitamin A and measles

Studies on increased risk of measles with poor vita-min A status or studies showing resistance to mea-sles infection in children if they were being supplemented with vitamin A are not common, and are complicated by the fact that many of these chil-dren were probably immunized against measles. However, a study in Zaire showed that children with low plasma levels of vitamin A and hence with a likelihood of vitamin deficiency had higher mor-tality from measles. Vitamin A supplementation reduces the morbidity and mortality from acute measles in infants and children in developing coun-tries. The effects of administration of vitamin A during an acute illness of measles are discussed separately below (section 6.5).

Vitamin A and malaria

Poor vitamin A status is associated with malaria in several studies from Africa. There is evidence that vitamin A supplementation may help to reduce the morbidity of *Falciparum* malaria, which is esti-mated to contribute to over 1 million deaths worldwide per annum. A well-controlled clinical trial in Papua New Guinea with vitamin A sup-plementation significantly reduced the incidence of malaria in pre-school children by 20–50%. The number of febrile incidents, parasitic load and the proportion of subjects with enlarged spleen were reduced. In this study clinic-based relapses of malaria were also found to be reduced. The effects of vitamin A supplements were best observed in children aged between 1 and 3 years, while chil-dren less than 1 year old had the least benefit from the vitamin supplementation.

Vitamin A, tuberculosis and HIV infection

Vitamin A has been considered more as an adjunct therapeutic agent based on the long and extensive historical record, mostly in the pre-antibiotic era, of its use in the treatment of pulmonary and mil-iary TB in Europe and the USA.

Vitamin A supplementation may provide benefits to HIV-infected pregnant mothers and children in developing countries. Low plasma vitamin A status is possibly associated with higher mother-to-child transmission of HIV, although two trials in Africa with vitamin A supplementation did not reduce the vertical transmission of HIV from mother to child. However, it did seem to reduce the incidence of preterm births. Low vitamin A status and poor intakes also seem to increase disease progression and mortality in HIV-infected individuals although there is no evidence that vitamin A supplements influence the viral load of HIV in blood. Periodic high doses of vitamin A reduce morbidity in chil-dren born to HIV-infected mothers as well as reducing the morbidity from diarrhoeal diseases in HIV-infected children and AIDS-related death. Vitamin A supplements may thus reduce the sever-ity of opportunistic infections while not in any way affecting the HIV specific-immune impairment.

6.5 Vitamin A Supplementation during Acute Illness

Vitamin A supplementation in diarrhoeal disease

Several beneficial actions of vitamin A on the host defence mechanisms may account for the positive benefits of vitamin A supplementation to prevent or manage diarrhoeal disease. These include the role of vitamin A in: (i) the regeneration of the intestinal mucosa following damage due to the invasive pathogens; (ii) intact phagocytic responses against the invasive pathogens; and (iii) Th2-mediated secretory IgA antibody response and serum IgG antibody response, both against bacterial toxins. The results of clinical studies are variable however, and seem to depend on the type of diarrhoea and the pathogen involved. Vitamin A does not benefit watery diarrhoeas while invasive diarrhoeal disease does benefit from vitamin A administration.

A clinical trial in Brazil showed that the severity of the diarrhoea was reduced when vitamin A was supplemented. In *Shigella* dysentery urinary losses of vitamin A are substantial and vitamin A supplementation has been shown to reduce the morbidity in children. Therapeutic administration of vitamin A in hospitalized children with diarrhoeas seems to manifest with paradoxical responses depending on the dose of vitamin A and the nutritional status of the child. Low-dose daily administration of vitamin A seems to benefit children with PEM by decreasing the incidence of severe nosocomial diarrhoea, while a single high dose of vitamin A administered to children with no PEM seems to increase the risk of nosocomial diarrhoeas. The reason for this observation is unclear.

Vitamin A supplements and respiratory infections

Clinical interventions with vitamin A have failed to show any improvement in the recovery from respiratory infections; in fact it appears that vitamin A supplementation may have resulted in more severe disease. As in the case of diarrhoeal disease, even with respiratory infections, children who are underweight and have underlying PEM seem to benefit since vitamin A supplements enhance their recovery. The question whether vitamin A in some manner increases pulmonary inflammation in healthy children has been raised in order to explain the contradictory findings seen in healthy children given vitamin A during respiratory illness.

Vitamin A supplementation in measles

Measles is an acute viral infection. Children with severe measles are at increased risk of secondary, opportunistic bacterial infections (like pneumonia and diarrhoea) since the measles virus compromises the normal immune response of the host. Clinical trials with vitamin A in measles have been carried out in children hospitalized with severe illness. High doses of vitamin A have been shown to improve recovery, decrease the duration of the illness, reduce the risk of complications and decrease mortality from measles. It is not clear whether vitamin A supports the immune system which is suppressed by the measles virus infection or prevents the onset of secondary bacterial infections and thus favours the host's defence during this illness. While the evidence that vitamin A supplements enhance measles-specific compromised immune function is inconclusive, vitamin A does seem to enhance recovery of the mucosal integrity, antibody response to bacterial antigens and the recovery of neutrophil function. These mechanisms do help prevent secondary bacterial infections and restoration of the body's defence mechanisms may help speed up recovery from this illness in children.

A clinical trial conducted in the 1930s in London showed that vitamin A supplementation reduced mortality in children with acute measles. Several more recent clinical trials in children with an acute measles infection have confirmed that high-dose vitamin A reduces morbidity and mortality. Vitamin A administration also reduces the opportunistic infections such as pneumonia and diarrhoea associated with the measles virus-induced immune suppression. Vitamin A supplementation has been shown to reduce risk of complications due to pneumonia after an acute measles episode. A study in South Africa showed that the mortality could be reduced by 80% in acute measles with complications, following high-dose vitamin A supplementation.

Vitamin A supplementation appears to modulate antibody responses to measles and it increases total lymphocyte counts. Administration of high doses of vitamin A to children with measles resulted in significantly higher IgG responses and higher circulating lymphocyte counts. When vitamin A and measles vaccine are administered together the response seems to suggest interference which was dependent on the level of maternal antibodies present, although the overall seroconversion to measles was affected.

6.6 Effects of Infections on Vitamin A Status

The common observation that children with clinical evidence of vitamin A deficiency often present with concurrent or recent history of infection raises the issue of whether and how recurrent infections may alter the vitamin A status of the host. Experimental evidence in animals shows that acute viral infections can deplete liver stores of vitamin A. Thus severe or recurrent infections can precipitate vitamin A deficiency, particularly in those with marginal status of vitamin A or on low intakes in their habitual diets.

Several of the mechanisms responsible for the poor nutritional status that results from severe and recurrent infectious episodes have been discussed in an earlier chapter (Chapter 5). In this brief section, more specifically, the role of infections in predisposing to micronutrient malnutrition is discussed.

Loss of appetite (anorexia) during an illness decreases energy intake significantly and thus reduces the intakes of other nutrients. Breast milk intake, which is a good source of vitamin A, is not generally affected when infants and young children have diarrhoea or fever, even when non-breast milk sources of intake are reduced by 20–30%. Encouraging breastfeeding during illness will ensure good vitamin A intakes.

Malabsorption associated with diarrhoeal illness can specifically affect vitamin A absorption. Often competition with parasites in the gut may decrease the availability of vitamin A for the host. In Nepal, risk of xerophthalmia increased with infection with roundworms (*Ascaris*). In a study in Indonesia diarrhoeal diseases increased the risk of vitamin A deficiency while in Peru children with longer episodes of diarrhoea had lower serum retinol levels. Isotopic studies with vitamin A tracers have shown that children with diarrhoea absorb 70% of the tracer and those with *Ascaris* infection absorb 80%, compared with normal healthy children who absorb 99%. The worm load in the gut is bound to influence the level of malabsorption of vitamin A, which should generally improve with the treatment of the infestation.

Significant loss of vitamin A in the faeces can occur during invasive diarrhoeal disease such as *Shigella* dysentery or even with hookworm infestation which results in significant blood loss. During an illness or fever, urinary losses of vitamin A can be significant and substantial. An episode of severe infection can precipitate xerophthalmia in a child with marginal reserves of vitamin A. RBP, which is a low-molecular-weight protein, is normally reabsorbed on filtration by the renal tubules. However, during febrile episodes this reabsorption is impaired and RBP is lost in the urine. RBP is normally bound to transthyretin which reduces its filtration, but during a fever this association is disrupted and the production of transthyretin is also impaired, with more amino acids being mobilized to synthesize acute-phase proteins. Thus increased quantities of retinol may be lost in the urine during an illness, which will affect the vitamin A status of the host.

An infective episode may accompany a period of increased requirement for a nutrient such as vitamin A since retinol and retinoic acid play an important role in immune mechanisms. The acute-phase response following an infection may also contribute to impair utilization of vitamin A by decreasing the mobilization and transport of retinol from the liver stores to the sites where they are needed. It has been observed that serum retinol levels drop during an infection; however, this may not be a true reflection of the vitamin A status of the host as this response may be part of the acute-phase response induced in the host by the infection. This raises the important question of how much serum retinol levels reflect the vitamin A status of individuals who live in environments in developing countries with constant exposure to pathogens that can cause frequent and recurrent infections.

Further Reading

Semba, R.D. (2002) Vitamin A, infection and immune function. In: Calder, P.C., Field, C.J. and Gill, H.S. (eds) *Nutrition and Immune Function.* CAB International and The Nutrition Society, Wallingford, UK, pp. 151–169. *A good review on the interaction between immune function and vitamin A with emphasis on the mechanisms of action of the nutrient and their impact on infections.*

Sommer, A. (2008) Vitamin A deficiency and clinical disease: an historical overview. *Journal of Nutrition* 138, 1835–1839. *A historical review of vitamin A deficiency including its recent resurgence in influencing morbidity and mortality in children in developing countries.*

Stephensen, C.B. (2001) Vitamin A, infection and immune function. *Annual Review of Nutrition* 21, 167–192. *This review provides an overview of the infection–undernutrition cycle as it applies to vitamin A and provides valuable information on how vitamin A influences the immune response.*

Villamor, E. and Fawzi, W.W. (2005) Effects of vitamin A supplementation on immune responses and correlation with clinical outcomes. *Clinical Microbiology Reviews* 18, 446–464. *A critical review of the impact of vitamin A supplementation on indicators of immune function measured in clinical trials and population studies.*

Case Studies

Case Study 6.1: Vitamin A deficiency and bacterial adhesion to cells.

Epithelial cells, particularly those lining the respiratory and gastrointestinal tracts, act as barriers to prevent entry of pathogenic organisms. Bacteria must adhere to these mucosal epithelial cells before systemic invasion begins. In this case study, nasopharyngeal secretions were collected from three groups of children with more or less similar levels of undernutrition expressed as weight-for-height. The groups were: (i) an otherwise apparently healthy group; (ii) a group with mild vitamin A deficiency; and (iii) a group with moderately severe vitamin A deficiency. In the second group 40% had evidence of xerophthalmia while 75% of the children in the last group had xerophthalmia.

The epithelial cells isolated from the nasopharyngeal secretions were incubated with labelled *Klebsiella pneumoniae* bacteria and their adherence to the cells was estimated by a standardized bacterial adherence technique. The data in Table 6.4 show that bacterial adhesion to epithelial cells in the nasopharyngeal secretions is significantly much higher in children with low vitamin A status

Table 6.4. Bacterial adhesion to epithelial cells in nasopharyngeal secretions according to vitamin A status. (Adapted from Chandra, 1988.)

	Vitamin A deficiency		
	None	Mild	Moderately severe
Serum retinal (µmol/l)	2.2	1.1*	0.4*
Dietary vitamin A intake (retinol equivalents)	321	201*	186*
Weight-for-height (percentage of standard)	81	77	74
Proportion with xerophthalmia (%)	0	40	75
Number of bacteria adhering per epithelial cell	4.8	7.9*	10.3*

*Statistically significant difference compared with the 'no vitamin A deficiency' group.

as indicated by low dietary intakes and low serum retinol suggestive of vitamin A deficiency. Poor vitamin A status is associated with features suggestive of an increased cell adhesion of bacteria. This is indicative of compromise in the defence mechanisms of the body and an increased susceptibility to bacterial infections in vitamin A-deficient individuals.

Reference

Chandra, R.K. (1988) Increased bacterial binding to respiratory epithelial cells in vitamin A deficiency. *British Medical Journal* 297, 834–835.

Case Study 6.2: Randomized trials with vitamin A and immune function.

The data provided in Table 6.5 come from a selection of randomized trials where vitamin A was administered and changes in some aspect of immune function was examined and compared with groups not administered vitamin A supplements. The clinical trials were all conducted in infants and children and are from several developing countries.

These studies tested a variety of immune responses and need to be looked at carefully. The first two studies (from South Africa and Indonesia) show that vitamin A supplementation affects T-cell function by increasing T-lymphocyte counts, particularly the CD4[+] subpopulation and thus altering the CD4[+]/CD8[+] ratio. The next two clinical trials from Bangladesh assessed delayed cutaneous hypersensitivity (DCH) test responses and found no differences in the vitamin A-supplemented infants and children to a wide variety of antigens. DCH responses are an indicator of T-cell-dependent macrophage activation.

The last two studies from Indonesia and Bangladesh show that antibody production is significantly affected by vitamin A administration. Although this is a B-lymphocyte function, there is very little other evidence to support a potential beneficial effect of vitamin A supplementation on the proliferation and activation of B lymphocytes. The effect of vitamin A on antibody production has been attributed to the influence of vitamin A on antigen-presenting cells, thus boosting antibody production.

Reference

Villamor, E. and Fawzi, W.W. (2005) Effects of vitamin A supplementation on immune responses and correlation with clinical outcomes. *Clinical Microbiology Reviews* 18, 446–464.

Table 6.5. Data from randomized trials on vitamin A administration and immune function. (Adapted from Villamor and Fawzi, 2005.)

Country	Subjects	Intervention	End point	Vitamin A group	Placebo group
South Africa	Infants with measles	Vitamin A versus placebo (4 doses)	Lymphocyte count (10^9/l)	8.1	6.45*
Indonesia	Children (3–6 years)	Vitamin A versus placebo	CD4[+]/CD8[+] ratio	1.32	0.97*
Bangladesh	Children (1–6 years)	Vitamin A versus no intervention	Percentage with positive DCH test	29.5	31.9
Bangladesh	Infants (6–17 weeks)	Vitamin A versus placebo	Percentage with positive response to:		
			Tetanus	30.6	32.8
			Diphtheria	30.6	22.4
			PPD	59.7	46.6
Indonesia	Children (3–6 years)	Vitamin A versus placebo	Anti-tetanus IgG (µg/l)	62	24*
Bangladesh	Infants	Vitamin A versus placebo	Anti-diphtheria IgG (µg/l)	22.9	11.0*

DCH, delayed cutaneous hypersensitivity; PPD, purified protein derivative.
*Statistically significant difference compared with the vitamin A-supplemented group.

Case Study 6.3: Mild vitamin A deficiency and increased risk of respiratory illness and diarrhoeal disease.

This case study is based on a study reported in the literature conducted in rural Indonesia. Children of pre-school age, i.e. less than 1 year to over 5 years of age, 3135 in all, were followed up every 3 months for 18 months, i.e. for six 3-month intervals. The specific objective of the study was to examine whether or not the risk of developing respiratory and diarrhoeal disease is higher among children with mild xerophthalmia (either with night blindness or the presence of Bitot's spots, indicating mild vitamin A deficiency) as compared with non-xerophthalmic children in the same environment. Each 3-month interval was subject to recording the incidence of respiratory illness and diarrhoeal disease; however, the significant comparisons were made only between children who had stable ocular status at the start and the end of each 3-month interval, i.e. they were either normal at the start and end of the interval (N–N) or had ocular signs suggestive of mild vitamin A deficiency at the start and end of the interval (X–X). The investigators chose the N–N and X–X categories as representing stable, but contrasting vitamin A status in these children. The data on respiratory illness and diarrhoeal disease are presented in Tables 6.6 and 6.7, respectively.

The risk of respiratory disease was almost twice as frequent among xerophthalmic children compared with normal children (relative risk of 1.8), while the risk of diarrhoeal disease was almost three times as frequent among xerophthalmic children compared with normal children (relative risk of 2.7). One can hence conclude that children with stable vitamin A deficiency are at increased risk of both respiratory illness and diarrhoeal disease. This relationship held constant even if the children had differing general nutritional status. When children were separated by their general nutritional status (weight-for-length either >90% of the standard or <90% of the standard) the incidence of respiratory disease and diarrhoeal disease was

Table 6.6. Data on respiratory illness according to xerophthalmia status. (Data compiled and adapted from Sommer *et al.*, 1984.)

Age (years)	No. of 3-month child intervals		Cases of respiratory illness		
	N–N group	X–X group	N–N group	X–X group	Relative risk
<1	5,484	42	470	8	2.2
2	2,993	143	257	31	2.3
3	3,051	188	176	21	1.9
4	3,031	164	100	13	2.4
>5	3,644	191	89	5	1.1
Total	18,203	728	1092	78	1.8

Table 6.7. Data on diarrhoeal disease according to xerophthalmia status. (Data compiled and adapted from Sommer *et al.*, 1984.)

Age (years)	No. of 3-month child intervals		Cases of diarrhoeal disease		
	N–N group	X–X group	N–N group	X–X group	Relative risk
<1	5,425	36	421	9	3.2
2	3,414	135	202	31	3.4
3	3,018	160	151	27	3.4
4	2,958	147	93	14	3.1
>5	3,624	183	87	14	3.2
Total	18,039	661	954	95	2.7

higher among xerophthalmic children than normal children at each age interval. This suggested that well-nourished children with mild vitamin A deficiency were at greater risk of morbidity than poorly nourished children with no ocular signs of mild vitamin A deficiency. The investigators of the study linked this probable causal association between risk of respiratory and diarrhoeal disease and mild vitamin A deficiency in children in Indonesia with the increased mortality they had reported earlier in pre-school children with vitamin A deficiency.

Reference

Sommer, A., Katz, J. and Tarwotjo, I. (1984) Increased risk of respiratory disease and diarrhoea in children with pre-existing mild vitamin A deficiency. *American Journal of Clinical Nutrition* 40, 1090–1095.

7 Iron Status and Risk of Infection

- Iron deficiency compromises several aspects of the immune response and increases the risk of infection.
- Iron deficiency is caused by both a poor dietary intake of iron and parasitic infections that result in iron loss from the body.
- Iron deficiency increases the risk of infections such as influenza, and iron supplementation reduces the risk of these infections.
- Excess iron can also increase the risk of some infections like malaria.
- Evaluation of the effects of iron deficiency or its supplementation on risk of infection has to be carried out by separating the effects observed in areas which are endemic for malaria.
- Iron overload affects immune function and can be reversed by the administration of iron chelators.

7.1 Introduction

Iron is an essential nutrient present in the diet and fulfils several physiological functions, the most important of which is to transport oxygen from the lungs to the cells with the aid of haemoglobin, an iron-containing protein present in the red blood cells (see Box 7.1). Iron deficiency states are among the commonest micronutrient deficiencies in the world, especially in the tropics. Iron deficiency of varying degrees may be a significant but relatively minor public health problem in developed, industrialized countries. Among the populations of developed countries some groups, such as infants, young children, adolescents, women, the elderly, vegetarians, and minority or migrant groups, are at risk of iron deficiency. Iron deficiency states (see Box 7.2) affect over 2 billion people in the world, the vast majority in developing countries, nearly half of whom may be pregnant women, and estimates suggest that 500 to 600 million people may suffer from iron deficiency anaemia. Hence iron deficiency is a major global public health problem with adverse consequences especially for women of reproductive age and for young children. In pregnant women, iron deficiency contributes to maternal morbidity and mortality, and increases risk of fetal morbidity and mortality and LBW. Iron deficiency leads to changes in behaviour, such as attention, memory and learning, and thus impairs cognitive development of infants and small children. Poor iron status reduces the physical working capacity and productivity of adults in both agricultural and industrial work situations. These functional impairments are economically important: it is estimated that productivity losses due to iron deficiency in poor countries may range from 2% to nearly 8% of Gross Domestic Product.

The predominant cause of iron deficiency states worldwide is nutritional, i.e. the diet failing to provide for the body's requirements of iron. In tropical countries, intestinal parasitic infestations exacerbate iron deficiency by increasing the loss of blood from the gastrointestinal tract. Malaria more specifically, but TB and HIV/AIDS as well, also contribute to the iron deficiency state. A low intake of iron in the diet and its poor absorption then fail to meet the enhanced demands for iron, resulting in anaemia. Cereal-based diets have less bio available iron and the frequent infections and common parasitic infestations among those living in poor environments may reduce absorption of iron and increase iron loss from the body.

Iron deficiency is associated with increased incidence of infections. Iron-deficient subjects showed increased incidence of malaria in Tanzania, while in Indonesia iron deficiency was associated with an increased number of episodes of diarrhoea and respiratory illness. Iron supplementation has varied effects on infections. The results seem to depend on

Box 7.1. Physiological and Nutritional Aspects of Iron.

Iron in the human body is present mainly in the protein haemoglobin of red blood cells or erythrocytes (about 60% of total body iron) and in body stores (about 25%) mainly in the liver but also in the spleen and bone marrow; the rest occurs in the protein myoglobin of muscle as well as in some enzymes and iron-transporting proteins. The main physiological function of iron is to transport oxygen and also carbon dioxide. This ability to carry oxygen from the lungs to the cells and carbon dioxide from the tissues back to the lungs is due to the protein haemoglobin present in erythrocytes, which then transfers the oxygen to the myoglobin present in skeletal muscle. Iron is also present in enzymes like peroxidase, catalase and cytochromes, thus playing an active role in the electron transport systems of the body which release energy in the cells. Iron is required for the continued production of red blood cells by the bone marrow and plays an important role in the immune functions of the body.

Sources of iron in the diet

Iron is present in a wide variety of foods of animal and plant origin. Dietary iron is of two types: (i) *haem iron* from the haemoglobin and myoglobin present in meat and animal products; and (ii) *non-haem iron* available as soluble iron, in iron salts, in metalloproteins and even as contaminants present in staple cereal grains, fruits and vegetables. Haem iron is present in meat, liver, poultry and fish. The important sources of non-haem iron are cereals like rice, maize and wheat and their flours. A wide variety of fruits and vegetables are good sources of non-haem iron. Non-haem iron is also available from milk and milk products like cheese and from eggs. Breast milk is an important source of non-haem iron; human breast milk provides more readily available non-haem iron than cow's milk.

Iron absorption

The absorption of iron in the gut is a complex process influenced by the nature of the iron in the diet, the presence of promoters and inhibitors in the diet, and the important role played by proteins that are responsible for the transport of iron across membranes. Iron absorption is said to occur in four stages. In the *luminal phase* dietary iron is rendered soluble by the gastric acid secretion. The solubility is retained as the digested food enters the small intestine where the contents become increasingly less acidic, influenced by mucus secretion and by the action of vitamin C (ascorbic acid) which reduces the effects of chelators (substances that bind ions and

removes them from solution) like phytates and tannins. The nature of the soluble iron, i.e. whether it is present as ferric (Fe^{2+}) or ferrous (Fe^{3+}) iron, also determines bioavailability since ferrous iron is better absorbed. Iron absorption occurs in the duodenum and jejunum. In the next, *mucosal phase* of iron absorption, iron is transported via the brush border of the apical cells of the duodenum and jejunum into the cell. In the third, *intracellular phase*, depending on the iron status of the host, iron is either transported directly across the mucosal cell and released on the other side or bound to a storage protein, *ferritin*, present in the mucosal cell. In the final *release phase*, iron is released into the portal circulation and bound to *transferrin*, a transport protein. The amount of iron absorbed is regulated by the state of the iron stores of the body and the rate of red blood cell proliferation, i.e. erythropoiesis. Iron uptake and mucosal release are increased when the iron stores in the body are low or depleted, or when the rate of erythropoiesis is increased. A polypeptide called *hepcidin* secreted by liver cells is now known to regulate iron absorption depending on the body iron stores.

While haem iron is readily absorbed, the absorption of non-haem iron in the gut is influenced by the coexistence of promoters and inhibitors in the diet. Promoters include ascorbic acid (vitamin C), other organic acids and some spices. Ascorbic acid facilitates bioavailability by converting ferric to ferrous iron which is more soluble and more easily absorbed. Some protein digestion products rich in the amino acid cysteine are also shown to enhance the absorption of non-haem iron. Polyphenols present in vegetables and cereal grains are strong inhibitors of iron absorption. Foods rich in polyphenols demonstrate low bioavailability of non-haem iron and include tannins in tea and other beverages. Phytates found in the husks of grains also inhibit iron absorption, and thus increasing the content of bran decreases iron bioavailability. The presence of ascorbic acid and meat can overcome this inhibitory effect.

Physiological regulation of body iron stores

Iron needs of the body including for the synthesis of haemoglobin are met by body iron stores, the absorption of iron from the diet as well as by the re-use of iron released by the breakdown of haemoglobin following the death of red blood cells. It is important to recognize that most of the iron entering the circulation is from recycled iron and not from dietary sources. It is equally important to appreciate that once iron enters the system it is unlikely to be

Continued

Iron Status and Risk of Infection

Box 7.1. Continued.

lost from the body except through blood loss or the transfer of iron from the mother to the fetus.

A number of protein molecules are involved in the transportation of iron from both haem and non-haem sources in the diet into the upper intestinal cell or enterocyte, and these processes are all regulated tightly. The release of iron into the portal circulation from the enterocyte and from the reticulo-endothelial system (such as the spleen), from where recycled iron is obtained, is mediated by a trans-membrane protein called *ferroportin*. Ferroportin production in turn is regulated by hepcidin. Once across the enterocyte and in the portal circulation, iron is bound to the transport protein transferrin, which transfers the iron to the bone marrow for incorporation into haemoglobin. The uptake of iron by these newly developing red blood cells involves specific receptor molecules on the surface of these cells. The transferrin molecule is available to mop up more iron entering the circulation once it has downloaded the iron into the cell where iron is needed.

It now appears that the iron-transporter protein, ferroportin, and its regulator, hepcidin, is the main mechanism by which the body responds to changing iron needs, by increasing or decreasing both absorption of iron from the gut and the release of iron from the reticulo-endothelial system. Hepcidin not only senses the demand for iron, possibly by detecting the level of iron saturation of transferrin, but also participates in immunological responses mediated by cytokines like interleukin-6 (IL-6). Although the mechanisms are not well understood it would appear that there are other proteins involved which may all be concerned with sensing the body's iron needs. These in turn are able to activate the synthesis of hepcidin by the liver, which in turn binds to ferroportin, leading to the resulting complex being internalized inside the cell and thus inhibiting iron release. This elegant feedback mechanism operates to increase or decrease iron release depending on the physiological need for iron.

The links between hepcidin and cytokines are also important. Injection of IL-6 rapidly increases hepcidin and consequently causes a drop in circulating iron levels. Thus the release of cytokines, IL-6 in particular, during an inflammatory response sequesters iron from the circulation and the hypoferraemia limits the iron supply to the invading pathogen. These mechanisms also account for the anaemia associated with chronic infections, as the continued production of cytokines leads to reduced iron availability for normal red blood cell production. While proteins like hepcidin play an important role in regulating circulating iron levels, other proteins are involved in regulating the levels of intracellular iron, emphasizing the fact that the iron needs of the body are carefully regulated.

the route of administration of the iron supplement, as well as the dose of iron administered. Increased mortality was reported when children received high doses of iron by mouth in Nigeria. The mortality rates were also higher when iron supplements were given to children who were hospitalized for treatment of undernutrition. Children in Papua New Guinea and New Zealand who received iron by routes other than by mouth (e.g. intramuscular iron) had higher morbidity, mainly due to respiratory illness. Thus iron seems to play a crucial role in infectious morbidity and understanding its role both in iron-deficient states and during therapeutic interventions is crucial, as iron compounds are one of the most widely administered compounds worldwide both for preventive and therapeutic reasons.

7.2 Iron Deficiency and Immune Function

The important role that iron plays as a nutrient in the immune functions of the body has been outlined briefly in Chapter 3. In this section a summary of the important effects of iron deficiency states on functional immunity is provided. One significant problem encountered when critically reviewing the role of iron on functional immunity in man is the fact that almost all human studies lack adequate control of other coexisting nutrient deficiencies including undernutrition, which complicates the picture and often leads to the inability to attribute specific changes in immune responses to iron deficiency per se. It is clear however that iron deficiency states compromise humoral immune response to a much lesser extent than functional changes in cell-mediated immunity, which are evident even with latent iron deficiency. But even these changes are not comparable in severity to the impact of other nutrient deficiencies on immune function. Some of the important actions of iron on immune function based on animal experimental and human studies of iron deficiency are summarized in Table 7.2.

The immune function changes seen in iron deficiency that are probably responsible for the impaired

Box 7.2. Iron Deficiency States.

Iron deficiency progresses in stages from normality to sequential changes in the amount of stored iron in the various compartments of the body. In stage 1, iron stores are depleted and the adequacy of iron for erythropoiesis results in normal haemoglobin levels. When the iron stores are depleted and circulating levels of iron fall the iron deficiency state moves to stage 2, wherein although erythropoietic function is compromised it is not reflected in a change in haemoglobin level. In the final stage, i.e. stage 3, the exhausted iron stores and low circulating iron affect erythropoiesis considerably and are reflected in the drop in haemoglobin levels, which indicates the presence of anaemia. Serum ferritin levels fall and transferrin saturation drops as the iron deficiency state progresses. Serum transferrin levels rise, but more recently an elevation in soluble serum transferrin receptor levels has been shown to be indicative of iron deficiency anaemia as opposed to anaemia associated with chronic disease.

Table 7.1 shows the changes in measures and markers of iron status associated with the three stages of iron deficiency.

There exist clinical conditions when excessive amounts of iron accumulate in the body. These clinical entities of *iron overload* can vary from minor excess of iron in the body to very severe and life-threatening iron overload where excessive iron is deposited over a period of time in vital organs such as the heart and liver. Chronic iron overload is generally the result of genetic abnormalities involving the many proteins involved in iron metabolism.

Table 7.1. Stages of iron deficiency and the associated changes in measures and markers of iron status.

Stage 1: Depleted iron stores	Tissue iron depleted
	Absent bone marrow iron
	Low serum ferritin ($\downarrow\downarrow$)
	Normal serum iron
	Normal transferrin saturation
	Normal haemoglobin
Stage 2: Latent iron deficiency (iron-deficient erythropoiesis)	Tissue iron absent
	Low serum ferritin ($\downarrow\downarrow\downarrow$)
	Low serum iron ($\downarrow\downarrow$)
	Low transferrin saturation ($\downarrow\downarrow$)
	Normal haemoglobin
	Raised serum transferrin
Stage 3: Iron deficiency anaemia	Tissue iron absent
	Low serum ferritin ($\downarrow\downarrow\downarrow$)
	Low serum iron ($\downarrow\downarrow\downarrow$)
	Low transferrin saturation ($\downarrow\downarrow\downarrow$)
	Low haemoglobin ($\downarrow\downarrow$)
	Raised serum transferrin
	Elevated serum transferrin receptors

$\downarrow\downarrow$, moderately decreased; $\downarrow\downarrow\downarrow$, severely decreased.

immune response seen in iron-deficient states are summarized below. It is important to note that all of them are not consistently observed in iron-deficient states in human subjects for the reasons mentioned earlier.

- T-lymphocyte functions are impaired along with the depression of T-lymphocyte numbers. There is a reduction in the proportion and absolute numbers of T cells. There is also a defective T-lymphocyte-induced proliferative response, i.e. an impaired mitogen-induced proliferation. Th-cell responses are altered.
- Humoral immune responses are generally unaltered.
- Immunoglobulin production and function are normal.
- Serum concentrations of complement are normal.

- Phagocytic function is normal, but there is reduced bactericidal activity of polymorphonuclear neutrophils, which is reversed with iron therapy.
- NK-cell activity is decreased (in animal studies).
- Impaired IL-2 production by lymphocytes is observed.
- Reduced production of macrophage migration inhibition factor.
- DCH responses including tuberculin responses are reduced; and these are reversible with iron repletion.
- Decreased activity of several iron-dependent enzymes.

The activity of cellular and extracellular iron-binding proteins like transferrin has also been considered as providing host defence against pathogens as they inhibit bacterial growth by withdrawing iron from the circulation. Proteins in milk such as lactoferrin have a similar effect as they

inhibit bacterial growth by withdrawing iron. While this is the case for cow's milk, in breast milk the bulk of the iron is not attached to lactoferrin and yet is highly bioavailable for the infant. The inhibition of the growth of a variety of bacteria by both transferrin and lactoferrin *in vitro* has lead to the concept of 'nutritional immunity', according to which the lowering of iron saturation of transferrin (and lactoferrin) in iron-deficient states enhances functional immunity and furthers the host's defence against a pathogen. However, this mechanism may not be effective against virulent invasive pathogens which have efficient and powerful mechanisms (like siderophores) to remove iron from transferrin. It is likely that this may be true even of less virulent opportunistic infections. The one important organism which may have a specific disadvantage in iron-deficient states is the malarial parasite (*Plasmodium*). Hence a critical evaluation of the relationship between iron-deficient states and infections needs to be carefully carried out by separating studies in regions endemic to malaria from the others.

7.3 Iron Deficiency and Increased Risk of Infection

As mentioned earlier, clarity in the association between iron-deficient states, risk of infection and infectious morbidity is confounded by the fact that iron deficiency alone without other forms of nutritional deficiencies is rare and hence complicates the observations in human studies. In addition, the impact that some endemic infections like malaria have on this relationship complicates the picture further. The topic of iron deficiency and infectious disease risk is controversial and has to be dealt with carefully, preferably from a historical perspective to make sense of it all.

From a historical perspective, it is true to state that the evidence from epidemiological studies and clinical observations supports the general belief that susceptibility to infections, especially due to bacterial pathogens, increases in iron-deficient subjects. It has been observed from studies in industrialized country settings that infants receiving iron supplements have a lower incidence of gastrointestinal and respiratory infections, and infants from a low socio-economic group fed iron-fortified milk formula had significantly lower levels of respiratory and gastrointestinal infections. In developing country settings too, studies are generally supportive of this relationship, as for

Table 7.2. Iron deficiency states and immune function.

Cell-mediated immune function	Impaired
Thymus weight	↓
Total T lymphocytes	↓ or ↔
CD4+ cells	↓ or ↔
CD8+ cells	↓ or ↔
CD4+/CD8+ ratio	↓ or ↔
Cytotoxicity	↓
Interleukin secretion	↓ or ↔
IFN-γ secretion	↓
DCH response	↓
Humoral immunity	Some B-cell functions impaired
B lymphocytes	↓, ↑ or ↔
Immunoglobulin levels	↑ or ↔
Antibody response to tetanus toxoid	↔
B-cell proliferation	↓
Other immune functions	
Macrophage phagocytosis	↓
Macrophage killing capacity	↓
Neutrophil migration	↓
Neutrophil phagocytosis	↔
Neutrophil bactericidal activity	↓
NK-cell activity	↓
TNF-α secretion	↓
Complement	↓

↓, decreased; ↔, no significant change; ↑, increased.

instance in Indonesia, where iron-deficient planta- tion workers showed higher prevalence of acute and chronic infections; although other studies in children who received iron and folate supplementation showed no difference in the incidence of respiratory or gastrointestinal infections compared with children receiving a placebo. All these studies in addition suf- fered from one or another methodological problem which made establishing this relationship from epi- demiological observations more tenuous.

Clinical observations from developed countries are generally supportive of this relationship, how- ever tenuous it may appear. Two-thirds of infants and pre-school children hospitalized for anaemia had evidence of an infection. Children hospitalized for an infection had sixfold higher rates of iron deficiency anaemia compared with children in the general population. Preterm infants who received early iron supplements seemed to be protected against both anaemia and risk of infection. In these industrialized country settings clinical studies dem- onstrate the increased risk of opportunistic infec- tions among iron-deficient individuals, thus supporting the hypothesis that iron deficiency states have altered functional immunity and increase susceptibility to infection. Reports include the recurrence of oral lesions from herpes simplex virus in iron-deficient young adults who were otherwise well. A majority of patients with chronic mucocu- taneous candida infections were found to be iron deficient and almost all of them improved with iron therapy alone. In another prospective study of

surgical patients, infections after abdominal sur- gery were significantly more common among those with low pre-operative levels of serum ferritin.

7.4 Iron Deficiency and Reduced Risk of Infection

While, in general, almost all nutrient deficiencies compromise immune function and affect the host adversely by increasing the risk of infections, iron status of the host presents a paradox. While iron deficiency may increase the susceptibility of the host to infection, a situation which can be amelio- rated by the administration of iron, iron deficiency can also reduce the likelihood of an infection. Microbial pathogens need iron for survival and correcting the deficiency may harm the host by promoting the replication and growth of the patho- genic agent since free iron is essential for microbial growth. These observations pose the paradox of the role of iron and risk of infection and may present what appears to be a controversy, resulting in having to weigh the benefits against the likely dangers of providing iron to the infected human host. This paradox is also probably responsible for the controversy in this subject resulting from the weak association observed between risk of infec- tion and iron deficiency states (see Box 7.3). It also needs to be recognized that it is not always easy to draw firm conclusions to resolve this paradox from available studies, given their design limitations and the presence of several confounding factors.

Box 7.3. The Paradox of Iron Status of the Host and Risk of Infection.

Iron plays a crucial role in the interaction of the host with the pathogenic agent. Iron deficiency increases the susceptibility of the host to infections. Iron defi- ciency can also reduce the risk of infections since microbial pathogens need free iron for replication and growth in the host. These issues need to be consid- ered carefully to resolve the controversies in the litera- ture in this field and to understand the paradox of iron status of the host and infectious disease risk.

Role of iron in host–pathogen interaction
The key features of this interaction are as follows.

- Iron is a highly insoluble compound at the physi- ological pH of the host and hence can be consid- ered as a scarce resource within the body.

- Iron is present in large number of enzymes, pro- teins, and oxygen carrying and delivery systems.
- Free iron is potentially harmful because of its reduction–oxidation (redox) characteristics and can result in the generation of harmful free radicals.
- The host has a range of transport, sequestration and storage proteins for iron that helps prevents potential tissue damage due to free iron.
- The host responds to the entry of a pathogen during an infection by depleting iron from the cir- culation, thus denying iron to the pathogen.
- Free availability of iron neutralizes the bacterio- static and bactericidal activity of the host.
- Several pathogenic agents have potent iron- acquisition systems (like siderophores) which are

Continued

Box 7.3. Continued.

capable of extracting iron from bound forms even when levels are low.

Iron deficiency promotes risk of infection

The evidence that favours this view is as follows.

- Oral supplementation of non-hospitalized infants with iron increased haemoglobin and reduced attacks of respiratory illness and diarrhoeal disease by approximately 50% compared with untreated controls.
- When infants from a low socio-economic group were fed iron-containing milk formula for a period of 6–9 months and compared with controls, both groups had similar growth rates but the formula-fed infants had a striking reduction in the incidence of respiratory infections.
- Children with anaemia principally due to iron deficiency had significantly higher prevalence of gastroenteritis compared with non-anaemic controls.
- Administration of parenteral iron during the first few days of life reduced hospital admission rates over 2 subsequent years from respiratory and gastrointestinal illness compared with untreated controls.
- In a placebo-controlled trial on infants with prophylactic parenteral iron, the death rate from infectious diseases was significantly reduced.
- Children with malnutrition showed a reduction in gastroenteritis after iron deficiency was corrected with iron supplements.
- Diarrhoeal disease rate decreased in urban children after introduction of iron-fortified milk formula.
- Anaemic, iron-deficient hospitalized infants showed that meningitis and pneumonia were more common in the presence of iron deficiency.
- In adults, an association was reported between urinary infection and anaemia during pregnancy. Urinary infections were twice as common in anaemic pregnant women compared with non-anaemic pregnant controls.
- Supplementation of infants and children with iron and folic acid, while showing no difference in death rates compared with controls, demonstrated modest protective effects against diarrhoea, dysentery and respiratory infections.

Iron deficiency protects against infections

Based on apparently contradictory observations, a hypothesis has emerged that relative or absolute iron deficiency may reduce susceptibility to certain infections. This is supported by evidence that provision of iron exacerbates the infective process and risk of infection as follows.

- Iron supplementation of patients with quiescent tuberculosis (TB) resulted in clinical recurrence of the disease.
- A minority of patients (7%) with iron deficiency anaemia had bacterial infections compared with 65% of patients with anaemia from causes other than iron deficiency. Malaria was common among those with iron deficiency and the incidence of clinical attacks of malaria increased after iron therapy in these patients.
- Iron-deficient nomads had no clinical evidence of infection, while 30% of those with normal iron status had several infections such as malaria and TB. When iron was administered to iron-deficient individuals, 38% had an occurrence of episodes of fever compared with 7.6% of those not administered iron.
- Neonatal sepsis rates were 17 per 1000 births when prophylactic iron was provided and fell to 2.7 per 1000 live births when the iron supplementation of newborns was suspended.
- Parenteral iron supplementation of infants resulted in more hospital admissions for malaria, respiratory infections, measles and middle-ear infections compared with those who were not given iron.
- Children with anaemia treated with oral iron had an increased risk of clinical malaria.
- Treatment of anaemic adults with oral iron increased the risk of clinical malaria.
- Oral supplementation trials of pre-school children with iron and folic acid in a population with high rates of malaria showed that those supplemented had a higher risk of death and admission to hospital for an illness compared with controls.

The constant competition for nutrients between the host and the pathogenic agent underlies this paradox and raises the question of who benefits from the iron administration – the host or the pathogen. Nearly identical studies from developing countries in high malaria transmission settings, as opposed to countries where the risk of malaria is low, illustrate quite different health outcomes of iron administration. This highlights the fact that intervention with micronutrients like iron by supplementation or fortification to address the huge challenges of global micronutrient deficiencies may not be universally applicable and may need to be undertaken with caution, as they could result in adverse health outcomes.

It was observed that Somali nomads entering a feeding camp had no infections if they were iron-deficient whereas those with normal iron status had high rates of infection. In Papua New Guinea, infants with lower haemoglobin levels at birth were found to be less likely to have contracted malaria and less likely to have been admitted to hospital at 1-year follow-up, implying again that iron deficiency was protecting the individual from malaria and other infections. In the same country it was observed that individuals with thalassaemia (a genetically inherited blood disorder which manifests with anaemia) were much less likely to develop severe malaria or to be admitted to hospital for non-malarial infections.

These observations of a paradoxical relationship between iron status of the host and the risk of infection are also supported by studies examining the response to iron intervention and therapy in developed country situations. There are several reports incriminating iron therapy with an increase in infections. Increase in sepsis due to *Escherichia coli* infections was seen in neonates who received parenteral iron. The high incidence of neonatal *E. coli* meningitis was reduced when this preventive iron therapy was discontinued or selectively used. Studies in poor countries also support the adverse role played by iron therapy in increasing risk of infectious morbidity, possibly by exacerbation of pre-existing or latent infections. Somali nomads with iron deficiency anaemia who improved their haematological status with iron therapy had an increased number of clinical attacks of malaria compared with a non-treated group. Fevers were also more common in the former group and some of them demonstrated the presence of pathogens in their urine.

7.5 Iron Deficiency, Iron Supplementation and Risk of Infection

In earlier discussions the complexities related to risk of infection and iron deficiency states were mentioned along with the paradox of the host's iron status and infection. Given the problem with the early observations and the controversies generated in this field, the subsequent sections deal with these issues by examining the data from carefully conducted, prospective and long-term iron intervention/supplementation trials separately for developed country settings and developing country settings. In the case of developing countries it may

also be useful to separate those studies which are from endemic malarial regions.

In developed country settings

A study of premature infants in Texas, USA found no differences between a control group and an intervention group (administered intramuscular iron dextran) for hospital admissions. A placebo-controlled study of infants with oral iron in Bristol, UK showed no differences in illnesses between control and supplemented groups and small differences in haemoglobin levels. These two studies demonstrated no benefit.

Parenteral iron administration to premature infants in Finland reduced the incidence of infections to half that of a comparable control group. Although parenteral iron dextran increased the risk of severe sepsis and meningitis in neonates in New Zealand, follow-up of the same population up to 2 years demonstrated a beneficial effect with lower risk of hospitalization due to respiratory, gastrointestinal and other infections in the treated groups. In Chicago, USA, 18-month follow-up of infants randomized to formula milk with or without iron showed a significantly lower percentage with anaemia and a significantly reduced risk of respiratory infections in the iron-supplemented group. These studies demonstrated a beneficial effect of reduced risk of infection with better iron status following iron intervention.

Long-term iron intervention studies in developed country settings were based on either parenteral iron or oral iron. Both routes of intervention showed either benefit by reducing risk of infection or no significant effect; the latter can be interpreted as no evidence of harm. The only exception to this is the increased risk of severe sepsis and meningitis seen immediately in the neonatal period with parenteral iron administration.

In developing country settings

In a controlled intervention trial in Cape Town in South Africa, controls received standard milk formula while the intervention group received an iron-fortified milk powder which provided five times more iron than the control formula. The intervention group had better haematological outcomes after 9 months compared with controls, but the infectious morbidities were similar. In Santiago, Chile, a complicated study on infants using iron-fortified milk and followed up to 15 months showed no significant differences in respiratory or gastrointestinal morbidity between controls and test groups. This study also showed that the group that benefited most with significantly lower morbidity rates was the one that had breast milk alone. In a complex study in Pakistan, milk cereals with and without iron were used as weaning foods and comparison made with neighbouring communities where there was no nutritional intervention. The haematological characteristics of children receiving the iron-fortified cereals showed measurable improvement. However, all groups receiving the cereal weaning food had reduced infectious morbidity compared with the controls, and this was attributed to the general improvement in nutrition due to the weaning food supplement rather than the beneficial effect of iron per se. Daily administration of iron to children aged 2 to 48 months in Bangladesh showed no differences in attack rates from diarrhoea, dysentery or ARIs compared with a control group. Careful examination of the outcomes of this study showed that a subgroup of children aged less than 1 year in fact had a higher risk of infection with oral iron, demonstrated by significantly more episodes of dysentery in this subgroup. These studies in non-malarial settings from developing countries showed little or no benefit from iron supplementation, one small group actually showing detrimental effects of oral iron supplementation.

Administration of oral iron in a well-conducted trial in Indonesian schoolchildren who were initially either anaemic or non-anaemic showed most benefit in the anaemic group of schoolchildren, who demonstrated better haematological status, significantly reduced infectious morbidity and improved growth with just 12 weeks of iron supplementation. Another study also from Indonesia, where anaemic malnourished pre-school children were given oral iron, showed reduced rates of fever, respiratory infections and diarrhoea. These two Indonesian studies demonstrated positive benefits with reduced morbidity from infections following oral iron administration to anaemic children. In a recent well-conducted prospective trial supplementing a large number of pre-school children with iron and folic acid daily in Nepal, the supplementation had no effect on the risk of mortality but showed modest, non-significant protective effects, implying that oral iron and folic acid may protect against diarrhoea, dysentery and acute respiratory illness. In summary, it would appear that the correction of iron deficiency by oral iron repletion may reduce risk of infection and infectious morbidity and mortality.

In developing countries with endemic malaria

A large well-designed prospective study from Papua New Guinea used parenteral iron supplementation of infants (2 months of age) who were followed up to when they were 12 months old. The results showed that infants in the iron treatment group were admitted more frequently for clinical symptomatic malaria, severe respiratory infections, measles and acute otitis media (middle-ear infection). The risk of malarial episodes was high in the iron-supplemented group among those who were not hospitalized. The infectious morbidity associated with pneumonia was high in the iron group – higher rates of admission, more time spent in hospital and more deaths due to pneumonia. It was also observed that nearly 90% of the children admitted due to pneumonia had evidence of concurrent malaria. Two other studies in pre-school children (one in Ethiopia and the other in Gambia), but using oral iron to treat anaemia, have shown an increased risk of clinical malaria.

A study of 6-month oral iron supplementation of 6- to 26-month-old children in Togo, West Africa showed high relative risk for malarial parasitaemia and diarrhoeal disease compared with controls, although these differences were not significant statistically. The lack of significant morbidity does not imply that there was no risk of iron intervention. A recent well-designed study in Zanzibar, East Africa, a high malaria transmission setting, provided daily oral iron and folic acid supplements to infants and pre-school children up to 3 years of age. The iron-supplemented group demonstrated a higher risk of clinical malaria, cerebral malaria and hospital admissions related to malaria. This group also had a significantly higher risk of other febrile illnesses like pneumonia, sepsis, meningitis, measles and pertussis. The iron-supplemented group had a 12% rate of higher adverse events which required hospitalization and the case fatality ratio for individuals who were admitted to hospital was higher in the iron/folic acid group compared with the un-supplemented children. The same has been observed in adults: treatment of anaemic adults with oral iron in Ethiopia also increased the risk of clinical malaria.

A careful summary of iron intervention studies from developing countries in malaria-endemic regions can be interpreted as showing a significant increase in clinical malaria and a significant increase in pneumonia and non-malarial infections, but no differences in diarrhoeal disease morbidity. These results are contrary to the other studies in developed and non-malarial regions of developing countries, where iron supplementation seems to be beneficial to the host by reducing the risk of infections. This link between malaria and iron is important. It shows that risk of malaria increases with iron administration in endemic regions and also that the coexistence of malarial infection has a promoting effect on other infectious morbidity, especially respiratory infections. The reduction in malaria as well as non-malarial infections seen following the use of insecticide-treated bed nets would support this view. It would also explain the beneficial effects on respiratory disease of iron supplements in non-malarial settings. The link between iron status and malaria is further supported by evidence from clinical trials demonstrating an enhanced parasite clearance following the administration of iron chelators like desferrioxamine. Administration of the iron chelator desferrioxamine along with standard anti-malarial treatment improves recovery time from coma in cerebral malaria and doubles the rate of parasite clearance from the host.

It now appears that malaria is not the only tropical infection to interact in a deleterious manner with iron status of the host. Iron administration to HIV patients increases the mortality associated with opportunistic infections. Treatment with the chelator desferrioxamine affects the rate of progression of HIV in individuals with thalassaemia. Experimental evidence is supportive of the hypothesis that iron therapy enhances pathogens that spend part of their life intracellularly and these include malaria, HIV/AIDS and TB. While iron-deficient states may have a negative effect on most infections, they decrease susceptibility to malaria, HIV and TB.

7.6 Iron Overload and Immunity

Immune functions are also affected in states of iron overload, usually resulting from multiple blood transfusions in clinical conditions like thalassaemia and sickle cell disease. Patients with iron overload have fewer T lymphocytes and $CD4^+$ cells, reduced $CD4^+/CD8^+$ ratios and reduced lymphocyte proliferation responses to mitogens. These patients also show reduced DCH responses.

While it is reasonable to attribute some of these features of impaired cell-mediated immunity seen in iron overload states to coexisting undernutrition as in PEM, and with nutrient deficiencies like those of vitamin A and zinc, the fact that administration of iron chelators such as desferrioxamine improves T-cell function confirms that iron overload is largely responsible for this phenomenon.

Iron overload seems to have no effect on humoral immunity in man. It also has no apparent effect on TNF-α secretion. However, IL-1 secretion is reduced in iron overload patients and is reversed on administration of desferrioxamine. While iron overload has no effect on macrophage phagocytosis and the subsequent intracellular killing of the microbes, it has deleterious effects on neutrophil function. Reduced phagocytosis and decreased bactericidal activity of neutrophils are seen in patients with iron overload.

Further Reading

Dhur, A., Galan, P. and Hercberg, S. (1989) Iron status, immune capacity and resistance to infections. *Comparative Physiology and Biochemistry* 94, 11–19. *Reviews the role of iron on immune function and deals with the consequences of iron deficiency on resistance to infection in man and animals.*

Farthing, M.J. (1989) Iron and immunity. *Acta Paediatrica Scandinavia Supplement* 361, S44–S52. *This review discusses the lack of consensus on the relationship between iron status and immunity, highlighting the fact that man can tolerate both deficiency and excess of this nutrient.*

Kuvibidila, S. and Baliga, B.S. (2002) Role of iron in immunity and infection. In: Calder, P.C., Field, C.J. and Gill, H.S. (eds) *Nutrition and Immune Function.* CAB International and The Nutrition Society, Wallingford, UK, pp. 209–228. *Provides an excellent summary of the current knowledge of the effects of iron deficiency and iron overload on immune function, and the implication for risk of infection.*

Prentice, A.M., Ghattas, H., Doherty, C. and Cox, S.E. (2007) Iron metabolism and malaria. *Food and Nutrition Bulletin* 28, S524–S539. *Summarizes the data from ecological studies and intervention trials related to iron and malaria, discussing this in the light of current understanding of host–pathogen interactions involving iron metabolism.*

Oppenheimer, S.J. (2001) Iron and its relation to immunity and infectious disease. *Journal of Nutrition* 131, 616S–635S. *A recent, extensive and excellent review of the literature on the unresolved debate over the interaction of iron and infection.*

Case Studies

Case Study. 7.1: Iron deficiency in adults in Indonesia – causes and consequences.

Iron deficiency is a major global micronutrient deficiency of public health relevance and is a serious nutritional problem in the developing world. This case study is based on a report from Indonesia on iron deficiency in adult plantation workers and provides information related to its causes and consequences.

Adult male workers in a rubber plantation in West Java, Indonesia were the subjects in the study. About 45% of these adult males were anaemic with a haemoglobin value of <13.0 g/dl, 6.3% had haemoglobin levels <6.3 g/dl and 88% of these plantation workers had parasitic infestation with hookworm. Other parasites like *Ascaris* (in 49%) and *Trichuris* (in 63%) were also seen, as well as *Giardia lamblia* (in 4.3%). These parasites may have contributed to loss of many nutrients.

Stool examination carried out in these subjects focused on estimation of the intensity of the hookworm infestation (by estimating the number of eggs per milligram of faeces) and was used to grade the intensity of the infection to correlate it with haemoglobin and haematocrit (packed cell volume, PCV), as summarized in Table 7.3.

Hookworm infestation is a serious public health problem in developing countries and is estimated to contribute to 22 million disability-adjusted life years lost. Hookworm infestation is due to two different parasites: *Necator americanus* and *Ankylostoma duodenale*. These parasites live in the gut and produce respectively 5000–10,000 and 10,000–25,000 eggs per female per day, each worm being responsible for 0.03 ml and 0.15–0.23 ml of blood loss per day respectively. Since the species of hookworm probably responsible for the infection in Indonesia is *Ankylostoma*, both the egg production and the blood loss are likely to be high.

However, the correlation between the intensity of the hookworm infestation and the severity of the anaemia in Table 7.3 is suggestive of the fact that frank anaemia does not manifest itself until the worm load is high. Nevertheless, it is safe to assume that the parasite load in the less intense categories is also associated with blood loss and hence iron loss in the faeces. There is thus little doubt that the haemoglobin and haematocrit level in this study may not reflect the true extent of the level of iron deficiency in the presence of the infestation in these adult plantation workers.

The anaemia and iron deficiency appear to be caused largely by the parasitic infestation, although poor diets may also contribute. Estimation of dietary intakes in a sample of the studied workers showed that while the intakes of iron and other nutrients in anaemic individuals were lower than those seen in the non-anaemic subjects, the intakes of iron in both groups were suggestive of poor iron intakes.

Results of physiological tests (step tests) reflecting work capacity were found to be lower among the anaemic subjects. Work output in the plantation was also significantly lower and so was the monthly payment received by these labourers. There was a linear correlation between haemoglobin levels and the monthly payments received by the plantation workers as this was based on the work output in the rubber plantation.

Risk of infection and morbidity was also higher among the anaemic individuals. Period prevalence of illness over a 4-week period was higher among the anaemic compared with the non-anaemic. It was 8:5 for influenza and 3:1 for bronchitis. The anaemic had one-third more cases of diarrhoeal illness. Infectious disease morbidity scores were significantly higher in the anaemic and there was a significant correlation between morbidity scores and haemoglobin levels.

This study illustrates some of the causes of iron deficiency states in developing countries and provides some insights into the consequences of iron

Table 7.3. Data on intensity of hookworm infestation and haemoglobin and haematocrit levels. (Adapted from Basta *et al.*, 1979.)

Intensity of hookworm infestation (no. eggs/mg faeces)	Haemoglobin (g/dl)	Haematocrit (PCV) (%)
100	13.2	40.6
100–699	13.6	40.8
700–2,599	13.3	39.6
2,600–12,599	12.9	38.9
12,600–>25,000	7.9	26.7

deficiency, including both infective and non-infective outcomes.

Reference

Basta, S.S., Soekirman, M.S., Karyadi, D. and Scrimshaw, N.S. (1979) Iron deficiency anaemia and productivity of adult males in Indonesia. *American Journal of Clinical Nutrition* 32, 916–925.

Case Study 7.2: Iron supplementation of schoolchildren in Kenya – effect on appetite and growth.

Iron supplementation of schoolchildren was carried out in Kenya. The objective of the study was to provide further support to earlier observations that provision of iron to iron-deficient children improves their growth. Since iron deficiency in man is associated with loss of appetite, it was also aimed at evaluating whether the improvement in growth was due to improvement in the appetite of these children.

A randomized, double-blind, placebo-controlled iron supplementation was conducted in primary-school children aged between 6 and 11 years. Baseline characteristics evaluated included haematological, anthropometric and assessment of parasitic infestation in these children. A daily supplement of placebo or iron was then provided for 14 weeks and measurements made again. The differences in the various parameters examined are summarized in Table 7.4.

Appetite was evaluated based on the consumption of a culturally appropriate food snack (maize porridge) as well as using a self-perceived appetite score in both the placebo and iron-supplemented groups, before and 14 weeks after the supplementation. The data related to appetite of the primary-

Table 7.4. Change in haematological and anthropometric parameters and morbidity following placebo or iron supplementation. (Adapted from Lawless *et al.*, 1994.)

	Placebo group	Iron treatment group
Haematological		
Haemoglobin (g/l)	−2.4	3.2*
Ferritin (µg/l)	0.3	16.5*
Anthropometric		
Weight (kg)	0.7	1.6*
Height (cm)	1.1	1.4*
Morbidity[a]		
Diarrhoea	9	−7
Cough	−1	8

[a]Morbidity presented as percentage with diarrhoea or cough during the week before the examination.
*Statistically significant difference compared with the placebo group.

school children from this study are summarized in Table 7.5.

The study demonstrates that both the consumption of the culturally appropriate test meal and the self-perceived appetite scores improved only in the iron-supplemented children. The improvement in appetite observed, that contributed to a 10.6% increase in energy consumed, may have accounted for the improvement in growth in the iron-supplemented children. It is however difficult to attribute the improved growth observed in the study solely to the improvement in appetite.

Reference

Lawless, J.W., Latham, M.E., Stephenson, L.S., Kinoti, S.N. and Pertet, A.N. (1994) Iron supplementation improves appetite and growth in anemic Kenyan primary school children. *Journal of Nutrition* 124, 645–654.

Table 7.5. Change in parameters related to appetite following placebo or iron supplementation. (Adapted from Lawless *et al.*, 1994.)

	Placebo group		Iron treatment group	
	Before	After	Before	After
Porridge consumed				
In ml	623	699	621	876*
In energy (kJ)	1688	1894	1684	2373*
Appetite score	3.71	3.74	3.59	3.86*

*Statistically significant difference compared with the placebo group.

Case Study 7.3: Adverse effects of iron supplementation of children in high malaria transmission areas.

International guidelines have favoured the recommendation to supplement iron and folate to children younger than 2 years in areas with a high prevalence of anaemia to reduce the impact of iron deficiency on the growth and development of young children. Reports in the literature with regard to adverse outcomes of iron supplementation to children in areas with high endemicity of malaria prompted the investigation reported in this case study. The objective of the investigation was to assess the effect of iron and folate supplementation on morbidity and mortality in a malaria-endemic area in Zanzibar.

A randomized, double-masked, placebo-controlled trial was carried out on pre-school children with routine supplementation of iron and folate, iron, folate and zinc, or placebo. Overall there was a higher risk (12% higher) of serious adverse events, i.e. death or severe morbidity leading to hospital admission, in the groups that received iron and folate with or without zinc compared with the placebo control group. Table 7.6 presents the relative risk of adverse events, hospital admissions and mortality in this group compared with the control group.

The relative risk was significantly higher among 12- to 23-month-old children and among those who had the supplement for more than 3 months. The authors concluded that the routine supplementation of iron and folate in pre-school children of a population with high rates of malaria increases risk of severe illness and death in these children.

Table 7.6. Relative risk of adverse events, hospital admissions and mortality among groups supplemented with iron and folate with or without zinc, compared with placebo. (Adapted from Sazawal *et al.*, 2006.)

	Relative risk		
	Adverse events	Hospital admissions	Mortality
Overall	1.12*	1.11*	1.15
Age group			
1–5 months	1.10	1.01	1.71
6–11 months	1.04	1.04	1.03
12–23 months	1.19*	1.17*	1.29
>24 months	0.99	1.0	0.98
Duration of supplementation			
<3 months	1.07	1.08	1.03
>3 months	1.13*	1.12*	1.21

*Statistically significant.

Reference

Sazawal, S., Black, R.E., Ramsan, M., Chwaya, H.M., Stoltzfus, R.J., Dutta, A., Dhingra, U., Kabole, I., Deb, S., Othman, M.K. and Kabole, F.M. (2006) Effects of routine prophylactic supplementation with iron and folic acid on the admission to hospital and mortality in preschool children in a high malaria transmission setting: a community-based, randomised, placebo controlled trial. *Lancet* 367, 133–143.

8 Zinc Deficiency and Infections

- Zinc deficiency compromises several aspects of the immune response and increases the risk of infection.
- Zinc deficiency in children increases the risk of diarrhoeal disease and respiratory illness.
- Zinc supplementation in children reduces the incidence and duration of diarrhoeal disease episodes and respiratory disease.
- Zinc has a potential role in a number of other infectious diseases associated with impaired cellular immunity like tuberculosis, leprosy and leishmaniasis.
- Zinc has been used in the treatment of a wide range of infections like influenza, hepatitis C and common cold.
- Zinc plays an important antioxidant role in the body and hence provides some benefit in autoimmune diseases like rheumatoid arthritis.
- Zinc supplements have beneficial effects even during an acute episode of infection and have been used as an adjunct to therapy.

8.1 Introduction

Zinc is an important micronutrient. It is found in every cell of the body and in all organs and tissues. After iron it is the second most abundant metal in the body and is involved in a wide range of physiological functions (Box 8.1). Zinc is required for DNA synthesis and replication, for cell division and for cell growth and differentiation. It also plays an important role in the defence mechanism of the body and in the normal functioning of the immune mechanisms. Zinc also serves as an important antioxidant in the body. The body does not store zinc and hence the diet is an important source to meet the body's zinc requirements. Zinc is abundant in food and is provided by animal proteins such as meat, seafood and dairy products, as well as cereals and nuts.

Although the essential role of zinc for growth and survival in animals is well known, its role in man was recognized only more recently. It was the discovery, based on studies in the Middle East, that forms of dwarfism and hypogonadism can be attributed to zinc-deficient states that initiated much of the interest in zinc as an important nutrient in man (see Box 8.2). The observations that these zinc-deficient dwarfs were susceptible to fre-

quent infections and that they succumbed to these infections at an early age, suggested an important role for zinc in the host's immune function. It is now well recognized that zinc exerts a ubiquitous effect on the body's immune mechanisms and its ability to resist infections and fight disease.

Zinc deficiency is widespread in developing countries, particularly among children, women and the elderly. In infants and children zinc deficiency is associated with increased risk of infections. There is clinical and epidemiological evidence that zinc deficiency is associated with diarrhoeal disease and respiratory illness. Low plasma zinc level increases the risk of diarrhoeal disease and respiratory illness in children, and several studies have demonstrated the benefits of zinc supplementation in children. Zinc supplementation may also reduce clinical disease due to malaria and can reduce attendance at health centres for treatment of malaria.

Zinc supplementation is known to reduce the risk of infection as well as the duration and severity of illness during an acute infectious episode. Zinc supplements elicit beneficial responses even during an acute episode of illness; for instance, they decrease the duration of the common cold. Zinc is also effective in promoting recovery from acute watery diarrhoea and in reducing the associated flattening of the growth curve that accompanies severe diarrhoeal disease.

There is evidence that zinc supplementation reduces morbidity and promotes growth in small-for-gestational-age babies in Brazil.

Box 8.1. Physiological and Nutritional Aspects of Zinc.

Zinc is a catalytic metal ion present in the cytoplasm of the cells of the body. Zinc is present in all cells, although about 80% of it is present in muscle and bone alone. It is present both in the plasma and the red cells of blood; a third of the zinc in circulating plasma is bound to a macroglobulin and to albumin. Seminal fluid has a concentration of zinc 100-fold higher than plasma and is a contribution from the prostate gland, which is one of the organs in the body with the highest concentration of zinc. There is no readily mobilizable store of zinc in the body, unlike iron. Zinc is a constituent of numerous enzymes of the body such as carbonic anhydrase, carboxyopeptidase, alkaline phosphatase, DNA and RNA polymerases, reverse transcriptase and superoxide dismutase, among others. Zinc is also essential for both the synthesis and action of the hormone insulin. The presence of zinc in many enzymes and in hormones like insulin enhances the role zinc plays in major metabolic processes, including protein and nucleic acid synthesis. Zinc regulates the actions of a number of genes – some positively and others negatively; and since many of these genes are involved in signal transduction, fatty acid synthesis and degradation, platelet activation, etc., zinc status affects normal physiological functions in innumerable and complex ways.

Sources of zinc in the diet

Zinc is present in a wide variety of foods of animal and plant origin although its bioavailability from different foods is highly variable. Zinc from animal and marine sources of food is readily absorbed compared with zinc from plants. Poultry, beef, pork and lamb meats, fish and cheese are good sources of zinc. Red meat and liver have more zinc than white meat; shellfish are rich in zinc and oysters are one of the richest sources. While wholegrain cereals, nuts and legumes are important sources of zinc in the diet, roots and tubers and fruits and vegetables are poor sources of dietary zinc.

Zinc absorption and bioavailability

The absorption of zinc in the gut probably occurs throughout the small intestine. Zinc absorption from the jejunum is highest, with the duodenum and ileum absorbing much less zinc. Several zinc transporter and binding proteins have been identified in intestinal epithelial cells; although the exact mechanism of absorption has not been fully worked out, it is known that the absorbed zinc is bound to albumin and then transported to the liver. Zinc homeostasis is regulated largely by its uptake and loss through the shedding and constant replacement of intestinal epithelial cells.

Zinc in cereal grains and legumes is less bioavailable as these foods are also rich in phytate, which impairs absorption by forming insoluble complexes of zinc. Milling of cereals removes the bran which contains much of the phytate and results in more zinc becoming bioavailable. Fermentation of cereal flour hydrolyses phytic acid and increases zinc availability, as does soaking unrefined cereal flours which lose water-soluble phytates. The amount of zinc in cereals and staples also depends on the zinc content of the soil in which they have grown.

The presence of other nutrients may also influence zinc availability. Increasing the protein content of the meal increases zinc absorption; the presence of animal protein further enhances this positive effect. Calcium has no effect on zinc absorption except in situations where the phytate content of the diet is also high. The presence of iron results in competitive interaction with zinc, the extent of which in turn may depend on the form and amount of iron.

The World Health Organization has categorized diets into three categories based on the phytate/zinc molar ratio as: (i) low zinc bioavailable diets, high in unrefined cereals with phytate/zinc molar ratios exceeding 15; (ii) moderate zinc bioavailable diets, which are mostly mixed diets with animal or fish protein and phytate/zinc molar ratios less than 10; and (iii) high zinc bioavailable diets, which are low in cereal fibre and high in animal protein with phytate/zinc molar ratios less than 5.

Zinc homeostasis, like that for iron, is regulated – although the mechanisms involved have not been as clearly worked out as for iron. It has been postulated that zinc homeostasis may be mediated by metallothioneins, which are low-molecular-weight proteins with high sulfur content and containing zinc. The amounts of zinc in these proteins are greater than in other metalloproteins, and in addition contain other trace metals like copper, mercury and cadmium. The regulation of zinc status of the body is by alterations in zinc absorption in the gut and its excretion, mainly in the faeces, but also in urine. Pancreatic and intestinal secretions contain zinc (endogenous zinc) and when

---

dietary zinc intakes are low, absorption is enhanced and endogenous zinc secretion is suppressed. When intakes are high enhanced secretion of endogenous zinc helps rid the body of the excess.

Physiological functions of zinc

Zinc has many physiological functions largely because it is an important constituent of innumerable enzymes (zinc metalloenzymes) in the body, especially those involved with the metabolism of proteins, carbohydrates and fats. Zinc metalloenzymes are both catalytic and non-catalytic. Zinc is required for protein synthesis, for the integrity of cell membranes, for tissue growth and repair, and for wound healing. It is required for the maintenance of DNA and RNA in the cells. It is essential for the production of prostaglandins, bone minerali-

zation and for blood clotting. Zinc affects the activity of hormones, specifically that of glucagon, insulin, growth hormone and sex hormones. Zinc-depleted states may manifest with reduced glucose tolerance. Zinc also influences vitamin A metabolism.

Zinc is an important nutrient for normal growth and development; it plays a role in male reproductive function and is essential for the normal functioning of the immune system. Zinc is an essential constituent of seminal fluid derived largely from the secretions of the prostate gland and hence plays an important role in sperm production and maturation. Even in zinc deficiency the amount of zinc in the ejaculate remains high. In men zinc is thus lost as part of normal sexual and reproductive function, a role that iron fulfils in women. Zinc is also required for normal vision and taste sensation.

Box 8.2. Zinc Deficiency States.

Mild zinc deficiency manifests with growth retardation and stunting in children, while severe deficiency manifests with severe growth retardation and dwarfism associated with hypogonadism and delayed sexual maturation. Mildly zinc-deficient males show decreased serum testosterone levels and oligospermia. Other manifestations of zinc deficiency include skin lesions, impaired wound healing and loss of taste. Behavioural changes, night blindness and hypopigmentation of hair have also been observed.

The manifestations of zinc deficiency depend on the situation or clinical setting. In patients on total parenteral nutrition, zinc deficiency manifests with symptoms suggestive of mental changes like confusion and depression as well as skin lesions (eczema) and loss of hair (alopecia). In young children, on the other hand, it manifests as growth retardation associated with poor appetite and poor taste acuity. Night blindness, which is a symptom of vitamin A deficiency, is also seen in zinc-deficient states. The mechanism in this case is different and is due to zinc deficiency affecting the coenzymes for the conversion of retinol.

Acrodermatitis enteropathica is a rare genetic disorder resulting in malabsorption of zinc by the intestinal cells and is characterized by intermittent diarrhoea, dermatitis characterized by an inflammatory rash (red inflamed patches of dry scaly skin around body openings like the mouth and anus, and on the skin of elbows, knees, hands and feet) with glossitis (inflamed tongue) and hair loss. It is also associated with recurrent infections and growth retardation. A similar pic-

ture may be seen in severe malnutrition, with zinc deficiency manifesting with alopecia, diarrhoea, glossitis and peri-orofacial skin rash.

Sickle cell disease is a more common genetic disorder where the haemoglobin is abnormal and leads to abnormalities in the shape of red blood cells, which are hence increasingly destroyed at a high rate causing anaemia. Children with sickle cell disease often show growth retardation and slow maturation and there is some evidence that people with this disease may be more likely to be zinc deficient. Although it is not clear why these children are zinc deficient, there is good evidence to show that they benefit from zinc supplementation in terms of growth in height. Individuals with sickle cell disease also show evidence of impaired immune function such as decreased peripheral T-lymphocyte numbers, decreased CD4+/CD8+ ratios, decreased natural killer-cell activity and decreased production of interleukin-2. They also have reduced delayed cutaneous hypersensitivity responses. All these immunological functions are restored to near normality when people with sickle cell disease are supplemented with zinc.

Secondary zinc deficiency occurs in gastrointestinal disorders with malabsorption like Crohn's disease, short bowel syndrome and cystic fibrosis. Secondary zinc deficiency may also accompany other disease states including renal and liver diseases, diabetes and alcoholism. The elderly as a group are generally more vulnerable to zinc deficiency states.

8.2 Zinc and Immune Function

Zinc has an important role in ensuring the normal functioning of the host's defence mechanisms and immune systems. Zinc deficiency damages epidermal cells (which manifests as an inflammatory skin rash) and thus breaks down the integrity of the physical barrier that normally prevents the entry of a pathogen. Damage to the epithelial linings of the gastrointestinal and respiratory tracts also occurs in zinc-deficient states.

In severely zinc-deficient children substantial reductions in the size of the thymus occurs, thus affecting cell-mediated immunity and T-cell functions. Mild zinc deficiency induced in human volunteers also depresses cell-mediated immune responses. It reduces serum thymulin (a thymus-specific hormone) and although inactive thymulin peptides are present in these zinc-deficient individuals, zinc is required for activation of this hormone. Zinc is also required for the biological actions of thymulin. Thymulin binds to receptors on T lymphocytes, induces several T-cell markers and promotes T-cell function which includes allogenic cytotoxicity, suppressor functions and IL-2 production.

Zinc deficiency results in lymphopaenia and a reduction in T-lymphocyte numbers. There is a decrease in the ratio of CD4+/CD8+ cells, an imbalance in Th1 and Th2 function, and reduced NK-cell activity. Zinc is required for the regeneration of CD4+ T cells. Since zinc is also required for the maturation of Th cells mediated by thymulin, zinc deficiency affects Th1-cell numbers and the resulting shift from Th1 to Th2 function leads to cell-mediated immune dysfunction.

Precursors of CTLs are decreased and T-cell responses like the proliferation in response to mitogens and cytotoxicity are also suppressed during zinc deficiency. Production of IL-2 and INF-γ is decreased while the production of IL-4, IL-6 and IL-10 is not affected. IL-2 production appears to be very sensitive to zinc status, and the changes in IL-2 production result in decreased activities of NK cells and T cytolytic cells which are involved in killing pathogens like viruses and bacteria. DCH responses are suppressed in children with zinc deficiency. All observed changes in cell-mediated immune function and T-cell responses including DCH test are reversed following zinc replacement or supplementation. The role of zinc in T-lymphocyte production and their functions is summarized in Fig. 8.1.

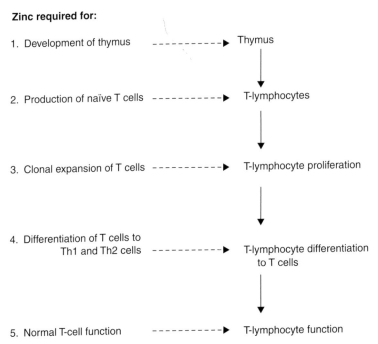

Zinc required for:

1. Development of thymus ----------► Thymus

2. Production of naïve T cells ---------► T-lymphocytes

3. Clonal expansion of T cells ---------► T-lymphocyte proliferation

4. Differentiation of T cells to Th1 and Th2 cells ---------► T-lymphocyte differentiation to T cells

5. Normal T-cell function ---------► T-lymphocyte function

Fig. 8.1. Schematic diagram illustrating the various levels at which zinc ions play an important role in T-lymphocyte generation, proliferation and function. (Adapted from Overbeck *et al.*, 2008.)

B-lymphocyte development in the bone marrow is adversely affected in zinc deficiency, resulting in lowering of the number of B cells in the circulation and in the spleen. B-cell proliferation and antibody responses are inhibited by zinc deficiency and the T-dependent antibody responses seem to be affected more.

Neutrophil chemotaxis and function are impaired in zinc-deficient patients. Monocyte and macrophage functions are also compromised. This is demonstrated by the suppression of the chemotactic response of monocytes and impaired killing of intracellular parasites in zinc deficiency. Increased concentrations of zinc also seem to show similar inhibition of macrophage activation, mobility and phagocytosis and would account for the findings in marasmic children upon rehabilitation with a zinc-supplemented regimen who demonstrate suppression of monocyte phagocytic and intracellular killing activity. It is postulated that this effect of elevated zinc may be mediated through its effects on the complement. Elevated zinc levels inhibit complement activation, which may in turn influence complement-mediated phagocytosis. Table 8.1 summarizes the important features of zinc deficiency on immune function in man.

Zinc deficiency on the other hand increases the level of TNF-α and other related pro-inflammatory cytokines while zinc supplementation reduces not only the synthesis and levels of these harmful cytokines, but also decreases the levels of lipid peroxidation products, DNA adducts and other markers of oxidative stress. Zinc in addition to its effects on immune function also exhibits both anti-inflammatory and antioxidant effects in the body. Oxidative stress is an important contributing factor in several chronic diseases such as atherosclerosis, cardiovascular disease, cancer and in the ageing process. Reactive oxygen species (ROS) are synthesized continuously in the body and are responsible for this oxidative stress. Zinc is an inhibitor of the plasma membrane enzymes (oxidases) that release reactive oxygen from the oxygen molecule. Zinc induces the production of metallothionein which is an excellent scavenger of free hydroxyl ions. Zinc also competes with other metals like iron and copper to bind to cell membranes and reduces the production of hydroxyl ions. The antioxidant effects of zinc are now well established and it has been demonstrated that zinc not only protects cells in the body against oxidative stress, but also negatively regulates gene expression of inflammatory cytokines such as TNF-α and IL-1β which are known to gener-

Table 8.1. Zinc deficiency states and immune function.

Cell-mediated immune function	Impaired
Thymus weight	↓↓
Thymulin activity	↓↓
Total T lymphocytes	↓
CD4+/CD8+ ratio	↓
Cytotoxicity	↓
Interleukin (IL-2) secretion	↓
INF-γ secretion	↓
DCH response	↓↓
Humoral immunity	Some B-cell functions impaired
B lymphocytes	↓
Immunoglobulin levels	↓ or ↔
Antibody response to tetanus toxoid	↓ (↑ with zinc supplements)
B-cell proliferation	↓
Other immune functions	
Macrophage phagocytosis	↓
Macrophage killing capacity	↓
Neutrophil migration	↓
Neutrophil phagocytosis	↓
Neutrophil bactericidal activity	↓
NK-cell activity	↓
TNF-α secretion	↑
Complement	Affected?

↓, decreased; ↓↓, moderately decreased; ↔, no significant change; ↑, increased.

ate ROS. Elderly individuals tend to have lower plasma zinc levels, increased oxidative markers and increased generation of inflammatory cytokines, all of which are reversed with zinc supplementation.

Antibody production during both the primary and the immunologic memory (secondary) response appears to be disturbed by zinc deficiency. Experimental studies show that antibody production in response to TD antigens is more sensitive to zinc deficiency than that in response to Ti antigens. This raises an important question of whether zinc supplementation can influence the outcomes of vaccination. Zinc supplementation appears to have no effect on the influenza vaccination response. The response to bacterial antigens seems to be different from that seen with viral vaccination. With tetanus toxoid zinc supplementation increased the anti-tetanus toxin IgG titre and with cholera vaccination zinc supplementation increased vibriocidal antibody titre and faecal antibody titre. This is potentially an area where the benefits of zinc sup-plementation are likely to be investigated further.

Whether zinc excess can alter immune function is a question worth investigating. One study showed reduced proliferative responses of lymphocytes to mitogens and reduced chemotactic and phagocytic activity of neutrophils with very high doses (nearly 20 times the recommended requirement) of zinc daily; this was attributed to the copper deficiency noticed with high intakes of zinc as the probable cause. However, other studies of daily zinc admin-istration, but not at such high doses, were not found to be deleterious to immune function in either children or elderly subjects.

8.3   Zinc Deficiency and Risk of Infection

The important role of zinc in human body defence mechanisms and immune function naturally raises the question of the relationship between zinc status and susceptibility to infectious disease. Observational studies have implicated poor zinc status with increased risk of infections. Children up to 10 years of age who were more susceptible to repeated infec-tions have been shown to have low serum zinc (and also low iron) levels compared with healthy con-trols. The low zinc status in these children was also linked to a shorter duration of breastfeeding.

Zinc and diarrhoeal disease

Children who present with acute and persistent diarrhoea often have low serum zinc levels which also correlate with the duration of the diarrhoeal episode. Whether this is the result of the body redistributing this important metal during an acute infective episode, or the result of increased loss accompanying the water and other electrolyte losses during a diarrhoeal episode, is not certain. Studies on apparently healthy as well as malnour-ished children in urban slums in India showed a higher incidence and severity of diarrhoea in those children who had low zinc levels during follow-up and when asymptomatic for several months. These findings of an increased risk of diarrhoeal disease in low zinc status have led to several clinical trials with zinc supplementation, almost all of which have reported a reduction in the incidence and severity of diarrhoeal disease in children (see sec-tion 8.4). This important relationship between zinc and risk of diarrhoea may be related to the role

that zinc plays in a wide array of enzymes present in cells. These include intestinal cells (enterocytes) involved in water and electrolyte transport and intestinal permeability. Zinc also plays a role in the repair and healing of pathogen-induced damage to enterocytes. Zinc may in addition play a role in enhancing local immune responses, thus restricting pathogen growth and enabling their early clearance from the gut. Diarrhoeal disease also contributes to the loss of zinc as it increases the loss of endog-enous zinc which is normally reabsorbed.

Zinc and acute respiratory infections and pneumonia

The study referred to above in India which observed the relationship between low zinc status and risk of diarrhoeal disease also showed that the children with low zinc status on follow-up had a higher incidence of ARI than those with normal zinc lev-els. Studies where children were followed up after an acute episode of diarrhoea with zinc being administered for 2 weeks after the diarrhoeal epi-sode showed a small decrease in hospitalization rates from ARI on follow-up for several months. The generally beneficial results of zinc supplemen-tation trials seem to support the association between poor zinc status and increased risk of ARI and pneumonia.

Table 8.2 summarizes the percentage higher risk of diarrhoeal diseases of different types and ALRTI in zinc-deficient children.

Zinc status and other infectious disease risk

Children with malaria generally tend to have low zinc levels. It has been observed that the zinc levels of children rise shortly after recovery from malaria, probably reflecting the redistribution of zinc along with other minerals during the acute phase of the

Table 8.2. Percentage higher risk of several morbidities in zinc-deficient children.

Morbidity	Higher risk (%)
Diarrhoea	+47
Watery diarrhoea	+37.5
Severe diarrhoea	+70
Diarrhoea with fever	+75
ALRTI	Not significant

infection. A cross-sectional study in Malawi appears to suggest a relationship between low zinc status and increased incidence of malaria in women. The relationship was shown only between hair zinc content and not with plasma zinc levels. Hence it may not be incorrect to conclude that no studies have shown an association between low plasma zinc status and increased risk of malaria.

It has also been postulated that zinc deficiency may increase the susceptibility to TB and leishmaniasis, both of which are caused by intracellular pathogens, although there is no epidemiological study to support this. Patients with TB are often observed to have low zinc levels, which appear to be related to raised CRP levels in these patients. Similar findings of low zinc status are also seen in patients with leprosy, another intracellular pathogen. The severity of the zinc deficiency seems to vary with the severity of the condition (tuberculoid leprosy compared with the more severe lepromatous leprosy) with the lowest levels seen in those who have reactions (*erythema nodosum leprosum*), suggesting that the low zinc status is a reflection of the acuteness of the phase of the infection. Clinical trials of zinc supplementation resulted in better control of leprosy reactions in patients and probably better clinical outcomes.

HIV/AIDS is an infection which is associated with multiple micronutrient deficiencies including that of zinc. Zinc deficiency may hence influence the progression of the disease. HIV/AIDS and the role of nutrients including zinc in this infectious disease are discussed in detail in a separate chapter (Chapter 9).

8.4 Zinc Supplementation and Its Effects on Infectious Disease Risk

A deliberate attempt has been made here to separate the discussion based on supplementation trials and their impact on infectious disease risk. While these generally support the observation that poor zinc status increases risk of some infections like diarrhoeal disease and ARI, it is useful to distinguish the indirect evidence supporting this view from the direct observations recorded of a linkage between poor nutrient status and the risk.

Zinc supplementation and diarrhoeal disease

Pooled data from several randomized controlled trials of zinc supplementation (Table 8.3) have shown that the incidence of diarrhoea is significantly lowered by 18% among those receiving zinc

Table 8.3. Randomized trials[a] of zinc supplementation and diarrhoeal disease (prevention and treatment) in children compared with controls. (Adapted from Cuevas and Koyanagi, 2005.)

Country	Age (months)	Effect of zinc supplementation	Specific objective(s) of the study
Ethiopia	6–12	Lowered incidence of diarrhoeas	Growth in stunted children and morbidity
Burkina Faso	6–31	Reduced prevalence of diarrhoea	Morbidity
India	6–30	Lower incidence of diarrhoea; prevention of prolonged episodes and high stool outputs	Diarrhoeal disease incidence
Bangladesh	1–4	No effect on diarrhoeal morbidity	Growth and morbidity
India	3–4	Fewer liquid stools; lower ORS requirements	Treatment of malnourished children with diarrhoea
Nepal	6–35	Reduced risk of prolonged diarrhoea	Treatment of acute diarrhoea
Bangladesh	3–59	Better outcomes of diarrhoea; reduction in mortality	Treatment of acute diarrhoea
Brazil	<60	Shorter duration of diarrhoea; fewer watery stools	Treatment of acute diarrhoea
India	6–35	Better outcome of diarrhoea and reduced number of stools; zinc alone better than zinc in ORS	Treatment of acute diarrhoea; also comparison of zinc alone and ORS versus ORS containing zinc

ORS, oral rehydration salts.
[a]The first four studies examined the role of zinc in prevention of diarrhoeal disease morbidity, while the rest evaluated the therapeutic role for zinc during a diarrhoeal episode.

supplements. These clinical trials have been of two types: either (i) a short-term supplementation, usually as a 14-day supplement after a diarrhoeal episode in a child which was treated; or (ii) a trial with zinc given for several months and follow-up to evaluate the incidence and severity of episodes of diarrhoea. Pooled data from the short-term studies indicate that there was a 34% decrease in diarrhoea prevalence in the supplemented group. In the long-term continuous supplementation trials a decrease of 27% in the incidence of persistent diarrhoea was noted. A more recent study in Bangladesh corroborates the conclusion that zinc supplementation reduces the risk of diarrhoeal disease in children. Moreover, studies comparing daily with weekly supplements show that both regimens are effective in lowering rates of diarrhoea during the supplementation when compared with a non-supplemented group. These supplementation trials support the hypothesis that poor zinc status increases risk of infection by pathogens that cause diarrhoeal disease.

Zinc supplementation and acute respiratory infections and pneumonia

Pooled analysis of randomized controlled trials was carried out to evaluate the risk of ARI and pneumonia following zinc supplementation. It showed that the zinc-supplemented group had a significant reduction in the incidence of pneumonia. This is supported by a more recent study in India showing a similar effect in slum children, where the zinc-supplemented group had a lower incidence of pneumonia (2.5% absolute risk reduction). Zinc supplementation lowered the relative risk of pneumonia in children. An analysis of all the studies done so far provided a pooled reduction of 34% in the incidence of episodes of pneumonia in zinc-supplemented children. Table 8.4 summarizes studies on zinc supplementation and respiratory infections.

Zinc supplementation and other infections

The effects of zinc supplementation on risk of malaria in children appear to be inconsistent. While two studies (one in Papua New Guinea and the other in Gambia) reported a decrease in febrile illness with confirmation of malarial parasitaemia in those on zinc supplements, another study in West Africa showed no difference in the incidence of malaria between zinc-supplemented children and a placebo group. Zinc supplementation has also been shown to reduce the discharge of eggs of *Schistosoma mansoni* in infected children when compared with un-supplemented children. Zinc provided as a prophylactic against common cold resulted in lower mean number of episodes of common cold.

Table 8.4. Randomized controlled trials of zinc supplementation and respiratory infections. (Adapted from Cuevas and Koyanagi, 2005.)

Country	Age (months)	Effect of zinc supplementation	Principal objective(s) of the study
Bangladesh	3–24	Lower respiratory morbidity	Treatment of malnourished children with diarrhoea
Bangladesh	3–59	Lowered incidence of subsequent lower respiratory tract infection	Treatment of diarrhoea
Ecuador	12–59	Less fever and cough in supplemented group	Respiratory infections in malnourished children
India	6–30	Lower incidence of pneumonia	Respiratory illness prevention in normal children
Bangladesh	1–6	Lowered risk of lower respiratory tract infections	Respiratory infections, growth and morbidity in normal children
India	>9	No beneficial effect seen	Measles-related pneumonia
India	2–24	Early resolution of fever only in boys	Recovery from lower respiratory tract infections
Guatemala	6–9	Higher but not significant incidence of respiratory illness in supplemented group	Diarrhoea and respiratory morbidity in normal children

8.5 Zinc as an Adjunct in the Treatment of Infections

Diarrhoeal disease

The administration of zinc along with oral rehydration salts during an episode of diarrhoea resulted in a reduction of the duration of the acute diarrhoea, i.e. fewer days of diarrhoea. It also lowered stool output and hence lowered the requirement for oral rehydration. There were fewer watery stools with zinc. It also reduced the risk of prolonging the diarrhoeal illness. These effects are not influenced by either the nutritional status of the child or the excretion of the pathogen in the stool. However, incorporation of zinc in the oral rehydration solution is not as effective as the administration of zinc as an adjunct to the oral rehydration fluids.

Zinc administration during the acute episode reduces the risk of developing persistent diarrhoea which is often beset with treatment failure, contributing to the high mortality from diarrhoeal disease in developing countries. Zinc is beneficial also because it reduces the problem of treatment failure in those with persistent diarrhoea. Children with persistent diarrhoea treated with zinc had a 42% lower treatment failure. Thus zinc contributes both to the treatment and the prevention of diarrhoeal disease in children.

Acute respiratory infections and pneumonia

Whether administration of zinc improves the outcome of treatment of acute pneumonia as with acute episodes of diarrhoea remains unresolved. In Bangladesh, children with severe pneumonia on antibiotic therapy had reduced symptoms of severity (duration of chest in-drawing, respiratory rate and hypoxia) if they received zinc in addition. The overall duration of the pneumonia and the number of days of hospitalization were also reduced in the zinc group compared with the placebo group. In a study in India, when zinc was provided as an adjunct during the management of measles-associated pneumonia, no additional beneficial effect was noticed with zinc. Neither the time to recovery nor the number of children considered to be cured was different in the two groups, i.e. zinc and placebo. However, when the same investigators compared the outcomes in a larger sample of children admitted with severe lower respiratory infections, they reported that zinc administered as an adjunct to the treatment resulted in a shorter duration of fever and reduced duration of severity of illness in boys who received zinc, but not in girls.

Treatment of other infections

Zinc administration has apparently no role in the treatment of malaria. When children with malaria were given either zinc or a placebo along with chloroquine to treat the malaria, no differences were observed between the length of time for fever reduction or in the proportion of children who had significant reductions in the parasitaemia.

The supplementation of zinc along with chemotherapy for the treatment of TB demonstrates positive benefits. Zinc in combination with vitamin A supplementation resulted in earlier sputum conversion, i.e. clearance of TB bacilli in sputum, as well as resolution of cavities in the chest X-ray in Indonesian adults. A similar outcome of early sputum conversion was reported from a smaller study in adults in India with zinc supplementation alone. Zinc supplementation of children who were exposed to adults with pulmonary TB in their homes showed a better response (such as increased induration diameter) to DCH tests with tuberculin.

Zinc has been used in the treatment of chronic hepatitis C infections. Zinc supplementation increases serum zinc levels and improves the response to interferon therapy for hepatitis C. It also seems to decrease gastrointestinal disturbances and body weight loss associated with chronic hepatitis C infection.

Zinc has been used as an adjunct to antimicrobial treatment of *Helicobacter pylori* infection, where it was found to increase cure rates compared with antimicrobials alone.

Treatment of common cold

Zinc has been used to treat common cold. Several clinical trials indicate inconsistent results with regard to the severity and duration of the illness. Some trials show benefit while others show none using zinc lozenges. More recent trials also support the inconsistent outcomes when zinc was compared with placebo in the treatment of natural cold infection. Thus zinc is unlikely to be efficacious in the treatment of cold, although it is not likely to cause any adverse effects if used during a viral common cold infection.

Wound infections

Zinc deficiency has adverse effects on wound healing and will probably increase the time for tissue repair. Wounds heal faster with both oral zinc supplementation and topical application. A randomized comparison of the duration of wound healing in surgical patients with oral zinc showed that the time for healing was almost halved in the zinc-supplemented group. The topical application of zinc to incision wounds demonstrated a decrease in wound size in the group with the zinc treatment. Oral zinc treatment also decreased the mean healing time in patients with burns.

Autoimmune disease

Zinc supplementation seems to provide some benefit to patients with autoimmune diseases like type 1 diabetes mellitus and rheumatoid arthritis. Zinc deficiency increases the risk of oxidative stress since zinc is a good antioxidant. In both these autoimmune diseases, ROS are implicated in the pathogenesis. Hence it is logical to assume that zinc provided as an adjuvant may benefit patients with type 1 diabetes and rheumatoid arthritis. The results do not appear to be always favourable, although in the case of rheumatoid arthritis patients some studies have shown that zinc supplementation reduces joint swelling, morning stiffness and the time to walk a given distance.

8.6 Zinc Toxicity

While zinc supplementation within physiological levels is considered safe, supplementation or therapeutic trials have been carried out using a wide range of doses of zinc. Moderately high doses of zinc give a metallic flavour and cause nausea and vomiting. Large doses of zinc may interfere with the absorption and metabolism of other metals like copper. There have been reports of higher mortality among malnourished children who received high doses of zinc compared with those on lower doses. In adult men high intakes of zinc had an increased risk of prostate cancer.

Further Reading

Cuevas, L.E. and Koyanagi, A.I. (2005) Zinc and infection: a review. *Annals of Tropical Paediatrics* 25, 149–160. *This review summarizes current knowledge on the role of zinc in childhood diarrhoea, respiratory infections and malaria, and its potential role in diseases associated with impaired immunity like TB, leprosy and leishmaniasis.*

Fischer-Walker, C. and Black, R.E. (2004) Zinc and the risk of infectious disease. *Annual Review of Nutrition* 24, 255–275. *A review that summarizes the results of all studies that have assessed the efficacy of zinc for the prevention or treatment of infectious diseases.*

Prasad, A.S. (2002) Zinc, infection and immune function. In: Calder, P.C., Field, C.J. and Gill, H.S. (eds) *Nutrition and Immune Function*. CAB International and The Nutrition Society, Wallingford, UK, pp. 193–207. *Provides an excellent summary of the current knowledge of the ubiquitous effects of zinc on immune function and disease resistance.*

Case Studies

Case Study 8.1: Zinc supplementation in the management of diarrhoea due to cholera.

Zinc supplementation has been shown to be beneficial in children with diarrhoeal disease even in community settings. This case study evaluates the role for zinc in the management of severe diarrhoea associated with cholera. Cholera, a bacterial infection caused by the pathogenic agent *Vibrio cholerae*, manifests with severe and frequent watery diarrhoea that rapidly causes severe dehydration in the host, which can be life threatening.

This study from Bangladesh investigated the impact of zinc supplementation in addition to the standard management with antibiotic and oral rehydration therapy (ORT) in children with cholera. A double-blind, randomized, placebo-controlled trial was conducted in children aged 3 to 14 years who were admitted with watery diarrhoea confirmed to be due to cholera by both stool examination and stool culture. Children admitted were randomized to receive zinc or a placebo along with antibiotics (erythromycin) and ORT until recovery. The mean data from this study are presented in Table 8.5.

Table 8.5. Data showing effect of zinc supplementation on cholera-induced diarrhoea. (Adapted from Roy *et al.*, 2008.)

	Zinc supplement group	Placebo group
Duration of diarrhoea (h)	64.1*	72.8
Total stool weight (kg/day)	1.6*	1.8
Total vomitus weight (g)	789.9	565.1
Total ORS intake (ml)	706.9	693.9
Percentage recovered in 2 days	49*	32
Percentage recovered in 3 days	81*	68

ORS, oral rehydration salts.
*Statistically significant difference compared with the placebo group.

The study demonstrated that zinc supplement as an adjunct to the standard treatment is effective even in the severe watery diarrhoea seen in cholera infections in children in developing countries, as it speeds up recovery and reduces duration of diarrhoea and stool output. By reducing hospitalization time it contributes to save treatment and other costs to the family. Hence zinc is an effective adjunct to be used in the management of diarrhoea due to cholera.

Reference

Roy, S.K., Hossain, M.J., Khatun, W., Chakraborty, B., Chowdhury, S., Begum, A., Mah-E-Muneer, S., Shafique, S., Khanam, M. and Chodury, R. (2008) Zinc supplementation in children with cholera in Bangladesh: randomised control trial. *British Medical Journal* 336, 266–268.

Case Study 8.2: Comparison of the efficacy of treatment of acute lower respiratory tract infection in children with zinc and vitamin A.

The objective of this study was to evaluate the effect of the addition of zinc or vitamin A on clinical recovery following the standard treatment for severe acute lower respiratory tract infection (ALRTI) in children. The study was based on ear-lier reports of intervention studies that demonstrated a 42% reduction in the mortality associated with ALRTI in children.

Children aged 2–24 months admitted to hospital with a diagnosis of severe ALRTI were randomly assigned to one of four groups, receiving (i) zinc alone, (ii) vitamin A alone, (iii) zinc and vitamin A or (iv) neither zinc nor vitamin A, along with the standard treatment including antibiotics. All groups had about equal numbers (34–37%) who were breastfed, or had low weight-for-age scores, or were considered to be very ill.

The study reported differences in the response to the supplementation of zinc between genders which are not easily explained, and hence only the data from boys with ALRTI are provided here. Boys who were zinc supplemented had significantly shorter duration of some of the illness indicators evaluated compared with the placebo group, as shown in Table 8.6.

Only the differences in duration for the changes in very ill status and fever resolution were statistically significant; and only in boys. The comparison in girls was not significant for any of the illness indicators. In the boys of the zinc-supplemented group the rate of recovery for the composite illness indicator, i.e. very ill status at any given point, was 2.6 times and for the resolution of fever was 3.1 times that seen in children not supplemented with zinc.

Figure 8.2 reproduced from this study shows survival curves of boys determined by Kaplan–Meier estimates and compares those who received only zinc (Z) with those who received the placebo (P) for the indicators very ill status (A) and fever (B).

Kaplan–Meier estimates (also known as product limit estimates) are estimates of survival function from lifetime data. The Kaplan–Meier plot of survival function is a series of steps of declining magnitude plotted against time. It measures the fraction

Table 8.6. Effect of zinc supplementation on illness indicators of ALRTI in boys. (Adapted from Mahalanabis *et al.*, 2004.)

	Very ill status (h)	Feeding difficulty (h)	Fever (h)	Tachypnea (h)
Placebo group	97	73	56.5	79
Zinc group	60*	54.5	23*	70.5

*h = hours.
*Statistically significant difference compared with the placebo group.

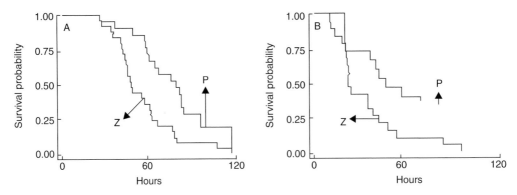

Fig. 8.2. Survival curves for two illness indicators, 'very ill status' (A) and 'fever' (B), in boys who received zinc (Z) compared with boys who received a placebo (P). (Reproduced with permission from Mahalanabis *et al.*, 2004.)

of patients surviving or living for a certain amount of time after treatment (in the current case, hours after treatment).

The study clearly demonstrates a benefit to the (male) child with ALRTI of zinc supplementation as an adjunct to standard treatment. This probably suggests a role for zinc in treatment, although more studies are needed to show that this effect and efficacy of zinc are universal to all children irrespective of gender. The arm of this study that looked at the effect of supplementation with vitamin A demonstrated no benefit in the illness parameters studied compared with the group. The vitamin A supplementation arm seems to corroborate the lack of clear benefit of vitamin A administration on acute respiratory infections in children.

Reference

Mahalanabis, D., Lahiri, M., Paul, D., Gupta, S., Gupta, A., Wahed, M.A. and Khaled, M.A. (2004) Randomized double-blind, placebo-controlled clinical trial of the efficacy of treatment with zinc or vitamin A in infants and young children with severe acute lower respiratory infection. *American Journal of Clinical Nutrition* 79, 430–436.

Case Study 8.3: Use of zinc along with oral rehydration salts by caregivers in the community and its impact on infectious disease morbidity.

The role of zinc in the management of diarrhoea, and its effect on infectious disease morbidity related to both diarrhoeal and respiratory illness and hospitalization associated with illness, were evaluated at the community level in India. The study involved six clusters were of approximately 30,000 people each near Delhi; three clusters were each randomly assigned to either an intervention group or a control group. Both groups were served by community health workers who, in addition to growth monitoring of children and providing nutritional supplements, were also expected as caregivers to provide oral rehydration salts (ORS) for the management of diarrhoeal disease. The caregivers in the intervention group only were provided with education about zinc and were supplied with a provision of dispersible zinc tablets along with ORS. The objectives of the study were to evaluate whether education about zinc and the provision of zinc supplements to caregivers is effective in the treatment of acute diarrhoeas, and also to examine the impact of this intervention on disease morbidity in the intervention group compared with the control group.

Surveys were conducted at 3 and 6 months after the intervention. Table 8.7 summarizes the data collected at the end of 6 months only, although similar trends were evident even after 3 months of the intervention.

This large community intervention, cluster-randomized trial showed that care seeking for diarrhoeal disease was reduced by 34% in the intervention group and also reductions in the 24-hour and 14-day prevalence of diarrhoea and acute lower respiratory tract infection, all of which were statistically significant (all odds ratios in Table 8.7 were significant in comparison with the control group). Hospital admissions in the preceding 3 months were also reduced in the intervention

Table 8.7. Data showing the effect of zinc supplement use along with ORS on acute diarrhoea, disease morbidity and hospital admissions. (Adapted from Bhandari *et al.*, 2008.)

	Intervention group (%)	Control group (%)	Odds ratio[a]
Morbidity in past 24 h			
Diarrhoea	6.1	8.0	0.75
Pneumonia	0.4	1.0	0.37
ALRTI	0.3	0.9	0.28
Morbidity in past 14 days			
Diarrhoea	14.3	22.9	0.56
Pneumonia	2.4	4.2	0.55
ALRTI	1.8	3.8	0.47
Hospital admissions			
All causes	2.8	6.5	0.41
Diarrhoea	1.1	1.6	0.69
Pneumonia	1.4	4.5	0.29

ALRTI, acute lower respiratory tract infection.
[a]Odds ratio is the ratio of the odds of an event occurring in one group (intervention) to the odds of it occurring in another group (control).

groups – for all causes as well as those specific to diarrhoea and pneumonia – again showing a statistically significant reduction.

The information provided by this study supports the fact that diarrhoeas are effectively treated when caregivers receive education on zinc supplementation and have ready access to supplies of ORS and zinc. The study data also support the fact that fewer children were hospitalized from the intervention group and that their use of ORS for the management of diarrhoeas increased compared with the control group. Satisfactory explanations for the reduction in morbidity related to both diarrhoea and respiratory illness in the intervention community are not readily forthcoming, as zinc was provided only as an adjunct to ORS therapy to children with diarrhoeal disease by the caregivers.

The study is also supported by other reports from Bangladesh, that zinc along with ORS and with appropriate education is associated with a higher use of ORT and lower use of antibiotics. This is an important observation, since excessive use of antibiotics contributes to increase in antimicrobial resistance in developing countries.

Reference

Bhandari, N., Mazumder, S., Taneja, S., Dube, B., Agarwal, R.C., Mahalanabis, D., Fontaine, O., Black, R.E. and Bhan, M.K. (2008) Effectiveness of zinc supplementation plus oral rehydration salts compared with oral rehydration salts alone as treatment for acute diarrhoeal diseases in a primary care setting: a cluster randomized trial. *Pediatrics* 121, e1279–e1285

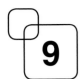

9 Nutrition, HIV/AIDS and Tuberculosis

- Infection with HIV results in compromising the body's immunological mechanisms.
- The presence of other infections in the host such as sexually transmitted infections and tuberculosis can increase susceptibility to HIV infection.
- HIV infection has a dramatic impact on the body's immune system, and HIV infection and AIDS increase susceptibility to concurrent, opportunistic infections.
- Several nutrients play an important role in immune function and may influence infection with HIV. Poor nutrition and micronutrient deficiencies of the host increase both the transmission and the progression of HIV/AIDS.
- HIV may be transmitted vertically from mother to child through breast milk. Micronutrients play a role in the transmission of HIV from mother to child. Infant feeding practices are important during HIV infection.
- HIV/AIDS severely compromises the nutritional status of the host and leads to progressive wasting.
- A range of factors are altered by undernutrition in the human host, increasing susceptibility to and progression of infection with tuberculosis. Poor nutritional status increases susceptibility to tuberculosis infection.
- Poor nutritional status is often a sequela of tuberculosis in man and may be mediated by poor appetite, the repeated febrile episodes that increase energy output, and increased protein breakdown.
- Tuberculosis may compromise the nutritional status of an individual.

9.1 Introduction

HIV infection, which may result in AIDS, and TB are major global public health problems. UNAIDS estimates that 33.2 million people in the world were living with HIV infection in 2007 and over 2.5 million were newly infected that year, while another 2.1 million died of the disease of whom 270,000 were children. Two-thirds of those infected with HIV were in sub-Saharan Africa.

The WHO estimates the incidence (new cases arising in a year) of TB at 9.2 million in 2006, with 95% of those infected likely to have occurred in developing countries. TB is a major killer and was responsible for over 1.7 million TB-related deaths in 2006, 25% of which were co-infected with HIV. Both these infections impose a major health burden on developing countries, and are associated with poor socio-economic circumstances and poor nutrition.

Poor nutritional status and micronutrient deficiencies are commonly associated with HIV and TB infections and probably increase the suscepti-

bility to these infectious diseases. Both HIV/AIDS and TB in turn increase the risk of deterioration of the nutritional status of the infected individual. HIV infection attacks the immune system directly and complicates the scenario by increasing risk of other infections in the host. Increasing evidence supports an important role for nutritional supplementation in improving therapeutic response and clinical outcomes to drug treatment for these infections. Many of these issues are discussed in this chapter.

9.2 HIV Infection and the Immune System

Infection with HIV eventually causes a dramatic impact on the body's immune system (see Box 9.1). The virus infects and kills the CD4+ Th lymphocytes which play a crucial role in the immune response. When an individual is infected with HIV, his or her immune system responds vigorously. HIV-specific cytotoxic T cells are generated, which kill the infected cells while the neutralizing antibodies that are produced limit the spread of the cell-free virus. However, even these vigorous responses of the immune system appear to be inadequate since the virus escapes, leaving the host's immune system chronically over-activated and exhausted. The immune system finally collapses and the host is left in a state of severe acquired immune deficiency.

Lymph nodes are the main reservoir for HIV, and billions of virus particles are produced. Millions of CD4+ T cells are destroyed every day during the asymptomatic phase. CD8+ T cells play an important role in the immune defence against HIV. Large numbers of cytotoxic (CD8+) T lymphocytes (CTLs) are generated during the early phases of the infection and may help slow down the progression of the disease. CTLs may help control HIV replication either by killing infected cells or by the mediation of soluble factors such as chemokines and antiviral factors. The persistent replication of HIV renders the CTLs unable to eradicate the viral infection. The virus in turn generates a large number of viral variants that are not readily recognized by CTLs and this ultimately results in the progression of the disease.

Other infections and susceptibility to HIV infection

The success of the replication of HIV in CD4+ T cells is influenced by the state of activation of these cells. Concurrent infections that stimulate the immune system may enhance HIV replication in infected T cells and accelerate the disease's progression. Individuals with other infections that have activated the body's immune system may also be more susceptible to infection with HIV. This may explain why the spread of HIV/AIDS is more rapid in developing countries, where both poor nutrition and an environment prone to infectious disease may promote susceptibility to HIV.

Tuberculosis

TB is an infection that chronically activates the immune system and increases an individual's susceptibility to HIV infection. Experimental studies have demonstrated that HIV replication occurs more readily in monocytes of TB patients than in those of controls. The infective agent of TB, *Mycobacterium tuberculosis*, increases HIV replication in peripheral blood mononuclear cells and this is correlated with

the level of cellular activities seen. During the acute phase of infection with *M. tuberculosis*, HIV replication has been known to be increased by five- to 160-fold. These observations support the clinical finding of an accelerated course of HIV infection when concurrently infected with TB.

Sexually transmitted diseases

Sexually transmitted diseases (STDs) also increase susceptibility to HIV infection. Ulcerative STDs probably facilitate the entry of the virus through mucosal lesions. Whether or not STDs (particularly non-ulcerative types like gonorrhoea and chlamydia) also have a direct effect on the immune system is not clear. However, it is reasonable to assume that infections with agents responsible for STDs are likely to result in activation of the immune system of the host and thus influence susceptibility to HIV infection.

Helminthic infections

Helminthic infections, such as that due to *Schistosoma mansonii*, may increase the susceptibility to HIV infection. Helminthic infections are known to influence immune responses to concurrent viral infections and the immune dysregulation that occurs with helminthic infections, such as schistosomiasis, may increase susceptibility to HIV.

HIV infection and susceptibility to other infections

Infection with HIV induces a selective and progressive immune deficiency and thus seriously compromises the host's immune system. Cell-mediated immunity, which is required to confer protective immunity against infectious agents, is specifically compromised. The resurgence of TB worldwide is partly attributable to the increasing spread of HIV and AIDS. HIV infections not only affect the incidence of TB, but also its clinical presentation. Reactivation of pulmonary TB may occur in the presence of HIV infection, whereas HIV-induced immunodeficiency may result in atypical, extra-pulmonary or even disseminated forms of TB. Visceral leishmaniasis is another infection increasingly seen in patients with HIV in areas endemic for leishmaniasis.

Opportunistic infections are a characteristic feature of the severe immunodeficiency of the

Box 9.1. HIV and AIDS.

HIV, a retrovirus, is the causative agent of AIDS. Two strains of HIV have been identified.

- HIV-1, the predominant isolate in clinical AIDS, found in Central Africa and other regions of the world including East Africa, North America, Europe and Asia. HIV-1 is believed to have jumped species from chimpanzees to bush-meat hunters in West Africa (likely to be Cameroon).
- HIV-2, which has not demonstrated the virulence of HIV-1 and is mostly confined and limited to West Africa. HIV-2 is believed to have jumped species from the sooty mangabey to man.

There are four modes of transmission of HIV infection: (i) person-to-person from sexual contact; (ii) following transfusion of infected blood or blood products; (iii) from mother to child *in utero*, intrapartum or during breastfeeding; and (iv) by percutaneous injection with contaminated needles or other devices. The highest risk is with direct blood-to-blood contact such as with blood transfusion, needle puncture or following significant mucosal disruption during sexual activities. The size of the infectious inoculum, the viral load of the infected person, and the presence of genital ulcers and mucosal abrasions are other factors that are associated with risk of transmission. Although the virus has been isolated from blood, semen, cerebrospinal fluid, saliva and breast milk, it has only been known to transmit through blood, semen and breast milk. The transmission of HIV is thought to be cell-mediated since HIV specifically replicates in T lymphocytes carrying the CD4$^+$ antigen on their surface. HIV has a long latent or incubation period (5–65 months).

HIV primarily infects cells of the human immune system, and specifically the T helper (Th) cells (CD4$^+$ cells), macrophages and dendritic cells. The first step in the infection is the attachment of the virus particle to the surface receptors on these target cells, followed by fusion of the viral envelope with the cell membrane of the target cell and the entry of the virus into the cell. The enzyme reverse transcriptase enables the synthesis from the viral RNA of a complementary DNA molecule which by the action of another viral enzyme, integrase, helps integrate the viral DNA into the cell genome. The integrated viral DNA in the genome remains dormant during the latent phase of the infection. In the final stage of the infection, the replicated viral RNAs

leave the nucleus and new HIV virons are packaged and then transmitted by release outside the cell by a process of budding from the host cell. The mature HIV virons are then capable of infecting new cells in the immune system. The reverse transcription process is error prone and thus causes frequent mutations in the virus.

HIV specifically infects the CD4$^+$ Th cells of the immune system, and progressive reduction leading to low levels of CD4$^+$ T cells with increasing viral load is a characteristic feature of this disease. The decrease in CD4$^+$ T cells occurs as a result of direct viral killing, killing of the infected cells by CD8$^+$ cytotoxic T cells and an increase in apoptosis (programmed cell death) of infected cells.

An infection due to the HIV virus occurs in four clinical stages. The first phase, i.e. the *incubation period*, is an asymptomatic phase and lasts from 2 to 4 weeks. During the next phase of *acute infection*, which may last for about 4 weeks, the clinical infection is characterized by fever, lymphadenopathy (swelling of the lymph nodes), sore throat, rash, myalgia (muscle pain), and mouth and oesophageal ulcers. The next phase of the HIV infection is a *latent stage* with few or no symptoms and may last from 2 weeks to even up to 20 years. *Clinical AIDS* is the final phase with symptoms due to various opportunistic infections and or malignancies.

Eventually most HIV-infected individuals develop AIDS with progressive failure of the immune system and death may occur from opportunistic infections or from malignancies. A compromised immune system presents opportunities for pathogens to infect the host; these infections caused by pathogens that do not usually cause diseases in individuals with a healthy immune system are referred to as 'opportunistic' infections.

The clinical entity of AIDS is characterized by opportunistic infections and malignancies in the absence of any other known cause for immune deficiency. The most frequent opportunistic infections are:

- *Pneumocystis jiroveci* (*carinii*) pneumonia;
- disseminated cytomegalovirus pneumonia;
- disseminated atypical mycobacterial infections.

The most common malignancy is Kaposi's sarcoma. The AIDS-related complex is seen in many individuals who are HIV-positive and may eventually develop into full-blown clinical AIDS.

AIDS-related complex. Opportunistic infections are those caused by agents or pathogens that do not normally cause disease or death in normal people, but do so in immunocompromised individuals such as those with HIV/AIDS. These opportunistic infections include infections with toxoplasmosis, *Pneumocystis carinii* and *Herpes simplex*. Very often, latent infections due to *Toxoplasma*, *Pneumocystis* and herpes virus may be reactivated by HIV infections. For some unknown reason, infections such as amoebiasis and malaria do not seem to be affected by the HIV status of the host.

Table 9.1 summarizes many of the HIV/AIDS-related opportunistic infections in the human host.

9.3 Nutrition and HIV Infections and AIDS

The interrelationship between nutritional status and infection with HIV is largely the result of the fact that both compromise immune function and also that they interact with each other to worsen the disease and the nutritional status of the host. HIV infection has a serious effect on the normal functioning of the immune system. HIV infection and the associated co-morbidities due to opportunistic infections can compromise the nutritional status of the individual. Recent evidence seems to support a specific role for micronutrients in the transmission and progression of HIV/AIDS.

The nutritional status of the host can alter the immune response. Poor nutritional status can increase susceptibility to infection with HIV; it is also likely to influence the immune system, which may be further compromised by the HIV infection, to increase the host's susceptibility to other infections. Poor nutrition affects the host's immune system in many ways depending on whether it is a generalized nutritional deficiency or a more specific micronutrient deficiency.

Generalized undernutrition such as PEM causes a profound reduction of CD4+ Th cells, while humoral responses are less affected. Mucosal responses may be severely depressed, enhancing the risk of mucosal infections such as infection with diarrhoeal disease agents, which in turn may further compromise nutritional status and immunocompetence of the host. This explains to a large extent the close association between

Table 9.1. Some common HIV/AIDS-related opportunistic infections in the human host.

Infecting organism	Types of infection
Viruses	
Cytomegalovirus	Pneumonia
	Disseminated infection
	Retinitis
	Encephalitis
Epstein–Barr virus	Lymphoproliferative disorders
	Burkitt's lymphoma
	Oral hairy leucoplakia
Herpes viruses	Localized and disseminated infection
	Oral ulcers and genital herpes
	Kaposi's sarcoma
Fungi	
Candida albicans	Mucocutaneous infection
	Oesophagitis
	Disseminated candidiasis
Cryptococcus neoformans	Meningitis
	Disseminated infection
Histoplasma and *Coccidioides*	Disseminated infections
Aspergillus	Invasive pulmonary infection
Protozoa	
Pneumocystis carinii	Pneumonia
	Retinal infection
Toxoplasma gondii	Encephalitis
Cryptosporidium	Enteritis
Bacteria	
Mycobacterium	TB
	Disseminated infections both TB and non-TB
Nocardia	Pneumonia
	Disseminated infection
Legionella	Pneumonia
Campylobacter	Enteritis

undernutrition and infection with HIV/AIDS. Issues related to HIV-associated weight loss, wasting and undernutrition are discussed separately below.

Micronutrients and HIV transmission and progression

Micronutrient deficiencies of vitamins and minerals may also increase susceptibility to HIV infection. Iron deficiency, for instance, is characterized by reduced intracellular killing of bacteria by phagocytes, decreased T-cell numbers, reduced lymphocyte transformation and a lowered lymphokine production. Zinc deficiency is associated with depressed antibody production, reduced lymphocyte proliferative responses to mitogens, depressed polymorphonuclear leucocyte function, and depressed NK-cell and cytotoxic T-cell function. Selenium is essential to mount protective immune responses to viruses, and selenium deficiency impairs T-cell functions and decreases NK-cell activity. Vitamin deficiencies also affect the host's immune functions. Vitamin A deficiency depresses cell-mediated immunity and T-cell-dependent antibody production. Vitamins E and C are antioxidant nutrients that enhance immunity by maintaining the functional and structural integrity of immune cells. Thus, micronutrient deficiencies – both mineral and vitamin – can seriously compromise immune function and increase susceptibility to HIV and promote progression of the disease. They may also compromise the host's immunity in other ways and complement the immune deficiency imposed by HIV to increase susceptibility to opportunistic infections that are associated with HIV status.

In the USA, HIV-infected men with high intakes of vitamin A, thiamin, riboflavin, niacin, B_6 and possibly vitamin C showed reduced disease progression and/or mortality. A similar study also associated reduced disease progression with high intakes of riboflavin, vitamin E, iron, and possibly vitamin A, vitamin C and thiamin. Low serum selenium was shown to increase the risk of mortality tenfold among HIV-infected subjects. The beneficial responses have been observed in populations with high dietary intakes and high supplemental intakes of micronutrients in developed countries. They neither provide evidence of the role of micronutrient deficiencies in increasing the risk of HIV infections in developing countries nor throw light on the impact such deficiencies may have on the progression of HIV infections. They also do not provide support for a therapeutic role for micronutrient supplementation in the management of the infection.

Tables 9.2 and 9.3 summarize the data on the association between micronutrient status and transmission of HIV (including vertical transmission discussed below) and HIV/AIDS disease progression, respectively.

Micronutrient deficiencies in HIV/AIDS

Deficiencies of micronutrients are common in HIV-infected individuals and may be the result of pre-existing poor micronutrient status as seen in populations from poor countries with a consequent increased susceptibility to infections. They may also occur as a result of the HIV infection due to gut infection with opportunistic pathogens, compromised gut barrier function and malabsorption. In addition to studies that have looked at specific micronutrient deficiencies, the relationship between HIV infection and multiple micronutrient deficiencies has also been reported.

Multiple micronutrient deficiencies

Multiple micronutrient deficiencies are just as common as single micronutrient deficiencies in HIV infection and are evident in all phases of the disease including during the symptomatic phase. Most common are those of fat-soluble vitamins and of selenium, while serum carotene levels are the most affected compared with any other micronutrient. There also appears to be an association between disease progression and mortality with micronutrient deficiencies.

Table 9.2. The association between micronutrient status and supplementation on the transmission of HIV. (Adapted from Kiure and Fawzie, 2004.)

Nutrient	Findings and clinical outcomes
Vitamin A	Low vitamin A status associated with: • increased HIV shedding in lower genital tract • subclinical mastitis and increased viral load in blood and breast milk • increased heterosexual and vertical transmission Vitamin A supplementation: • has no increase in reducing viral shedding in lower genital tract • does not reduce postpartum subclinical mastitis • increases transmission if given both prenatally and during lactation
Vitamins B, C & E	Daily supplementation during lactation has no overall effect on the risk of vertical transmission of HIV

Table 9.3. The association between micronutrient status and supplementation on HIV/AIDS disease progression. (Adapted from Kiure and Fawzie, 2004.)

Nutrient	Effect on markers of disease	Clinical outcomes
Vitamin A	Deficiency of vitamin A associated with: • low CD4+ cell counts • high viral loads Supplementation has: • no effect on CD4+ cell counts or on viral load in adults	Deficiency of vitamin A associated with: • increased mortality Supplementation: • efficacy on clinical outcomes not known • of mothers/children reduced risk of diarrhoea, pneumonia and overall mortality • reduces risk of LBW • of HIV-positive mothers (antenatal) reduces anaemia in children
Vitamin B complex, vitamins C and E	High intakes and plasma levels associated with: • reduced risk of low CD4+ cells Supplementation trials report: • protective effect on CD4+ cells • marginal effects on viral load • mothers (pregnant/lactating) increase CD4+ cell counts	High dietary intakes of vitamin C or E; high serum levels of vitamin E; high intakes and high levels of B vitamins associated with: • reduced disease progression Supplementation of mothers (pregnant/lactating): • reduced adverse birth outcomes (fetal loss, LBW, preterm birth) • lowered risk of diarrhoea in children
Selenium	Low selenium status associated with: • low CD4+ cell counts Supplementation trials of short duration: • no effect on viral load • non-significant increase in CD4+ cell counts	Low plasma levels associated with: • increased risk of mortality in adults • increased risk of vertical transmission
Zinc	Normalization of zinc levels and high dietary intakes increased CD4+ cell counts	High dietary zinc intakes had harmful effects on disease progression Low biochemical levels associated with increased disease progression

Vitamin A and β-carotene deficiencies

Vitamin A deficiency is common in patients with HIV irrespective of the stage of the clinical infection, including during the asymptomatic phase, and the prevalence of deficiency is higher in women than men. Vitamin A levels in the blood deteriorate as the infection progresses even if nutritional intakes are adequate and an association between the development of vitamin A deficiency and the decrease in CD4+ cell counts has been shown. Vitamin A deficiency was observed in 20% of those who died from AIDS compared with only 7% in matched HIV-positive controls.

Sixty-three per cent of HIV-positive pregnant mothers in Malawi had vitamin A deficiency and so did 70% of their infants, irrespective of whether they were HIV-positive or not. Serum levels of vitamin A, i.e. retinol, in HIV-infected women in Malawi were inversely related to mortality, as also was the case in HIV-infected intravenous drug users. Mortality of infants (up to 1 year of age) was 93% among women with low serum retinol levels compared with 14% among infants whose mothers were vitamin A replete. Low vitamin A levels have been associated with advanced HIV infection in the mother and increased vertical transmission to the infant.

Deficiencies of the vitamin A precursor carotene and carotenoids are also common in HIV infection. In adults the prevalence of carotene deficiency varies from 30 to over 70%. Like retinol, there appears to be a close association between serum carotene levels and CD4$^+$ T-cell counts and CD4$^+$/CD8$^+$ ratios irrespective of the clinical stage of the disease. However, the severely lowered levels often seen in the early phase of the disease have been attributed to the higher antioxidant requirement during the early stages of the infection. Even during pregnancy similar relationships between serum carotene and vitamin A levels and CD4$^+$ counts and CD4$^+$/CD8$^+$ ratios have been reported. A similar correlation with levels of carotene and the severity of the infection was also reported in children, with a 13-fold decrease in AIDS compared with a 6.5-fold decrease in HIV infection.

Deficiencies of fat-soluble vitamins like A occur in HIV-infected individuals because of diarrhoea and fat malabsorption. The latter seems to occur even in the absence of diarrhoea and may be due to the villous atrophy and impaired enterocyte function in HIV-infected individuals.

Vitamin E deficiency

Low serum levels of vitamin E are seen in HIV-infected individuals as well as those with frank AIDS. The low levels seem to be related to low intakes in the diet consequent to the infection, the oxidative stress of HIV infection and the associated opportunistic infections associated with HIV infections.

Vitamin B-complex deficiencies

Deficiencies of B-group vitamins, in particular those of B_6, B_{12} and riboflavin, are common in HIV

infection even in the absence of symptoms. Patients with B_6 deficiency show altered immune function like reduced NK-cell cytotoxicity and decreased mitogen responsiveness.

Vitamin B_{12} deficiency is much more common in HIV-infected individuals and is seen even in the early asymptomatic phase. Since B_{12} and folate are essential for cell proliferation, the B_{12} deficiency may be caused by the increase in lymphocyte proliferation and turnover in an HIV-infected individual. Reduction in the levels of B_{12} may also result from the direct effects of HIV infection on the gut, which results in the production of antibodies to the acid-secreting cells and manifests with a reduction in gastric acid secretion. These acid-secreting cells also produce intrinsic factor, needed for the absorption of B_{12}, which along with the inflammation of parts of the intestine where B_{12} absorption takes place contributes to the B_{12} deficiency. Low serum B_{12} levels are associated with anaemia, low CD4$^+$ counts and low CD4$^+$/CD8$^+$ ratios. The development of vitamin B_{12} deficiency and the fall in CD4$^+$ count also seems to be correlated well. Low serum B_{12} levels are good predictors of the increased risk of progression of the disease to frank AIDS. There is a possibility of an association between low serum B_{12} and the altered cognitive function and other neurological impairments seen in HIV-positive individuals.

Deficiency of zinc and selenium

Deficiency of zinc is common in HIV infection; low or marginal zinc levels are often seen both in the early asymptomatic phase of the disease and in AIDS patients. Serum zinc levels may be lowered during the acute phase of the infection as zinc uptake by the liver increases. Anorexia, diarrhoea and malabsorption may further contribute to the zinc deficiency. An association is seen between intakes of zinc from the diet and CD4$^+$ cell counts and the progression to AIDS from the HIV-positive state. An increase in AIDS mortality seems to be associated with low baseline levels of zinc. Since the thymic hormone thymulin is activated by zinc, thymulin levels may be more sensitive markers of these changes.

HIV infections are associated with selenium deficiency. Low levels of selenium have been reported in HIV and AIDS patients, often well before malabsorption manifests in them. An association of low selenium levels with progression of the disease has been seen in several studies, and a correlation has been shown between selenium levels and CD4[+] counts with mortality. HIV patients with low selenium levels have a 20-fold greater risk of death from HIV-related causes, a risk greater than that associated with CD4[+] counts and greater than that seen with any other micronutrient deficiency. It appears that low plasma selenium levels are independent predictors of rapid disease progression and mortality.

Micronutrient supplementation and HIV/AIDS

There is increasing evidence in the literature to suggest that vitamin and mineral supplementation may improve the survival of HIV-positive patients. Vitamin and mineral supplements are cheap compared with HIV antiviral therapy, and may have an important place in the management of HIV/AIDS in developing countries where even the traditional single antiretroviral drug is too expensive. Micronutrient supplements may delay the onset of AIDS, reduce opportunistic infections, reduce morbidity and delay mortality in developing countries. Evidence is accumulating on the role of nutrition in decreasing the wasting that accompanies advanced HIV infection and in preventing the progression of the disease. The possibility also exists that specific micronutrients may affect the transmission and progression of HIV. Since several key micronutrients play an important role in maintaining health in immunodeficiency states like HIV infection, this section reviews the evidence for a role for micronutrient supplementation (multiple or single nutrients) in the treatment and care of HIV/AIDS.

Multiple micronutrient supplementation

In developed countries intake of micronutrient supplements is common among HIV-infected individuals and it is estimated that, in North America alone, between two-thirds to three-quarters of HIV-infected people take multivitamin and mineral supplements. However, the levels of micronutrients appear to be lower in HIV-positive individuals compared with HIV-negative controls even with supplementation. Micronutrient supplementation seems to be associated with slower disease progression and a reduced risk of mortality. Excessive intake of micronutrients does not confer better outcomes than moderate increase in intakes of vitamins and minerals.

Supplementation of vitamin A and β-carotene in HIV infection

Several studies including one in HIV-infected pregnant women showed no effect of supplementation with vitamin A or β-carotene or both on viral load. A randomized placebo-controlled study with vitamin A supplementation of children of HIV-positive mothers in South Africa showed that supplemented children had reduced incidence, shorter durations of and reduced hospitalization due to diarrhoeal diseases. A trial in Tanzania demonstrated a significant increase in height of children with HIV infection supplemented with vitamin A. Studies in Tanzania have also shown that life expectancy of HIV-infected children may be prolonged by vitamin A supplementation, suggesting that vitamin A may play a role in slowing the course of HIV infection in children. The general conclusion is that vitamin A supplementation benefits most those HIV-infected individuals who are deficient, compared with those who are replete.

Carotenoids, the precursors of vitamin A, are increasingly used in clinical trials in preference to supplementing with vitamin A during the treatment of the infection. Supplementation with β-carotene appears to improve CD4[+] cell counts, CD4[+]/CD8[+] ratios and NK cells; however there are reports of no significant impact of carotene supplementation on lymphocyte function too. There are studies that seem to show that carotenoids help alleviate symptoms of the disease, and influence the progress of the disease and risk of mortality. However, the jury is still out on the benefits – if any – of carotene supplementation in the HIV-positive population.

Vitamin E supplementation in HIV infection

Supplementation with large doses of vitamin E along with vitamin C seems to reduce oxidative stress and viral load in HIV-infected individuals. Increased intake of vitamin E seems to decrease the risk of progression of the disease, with subjects having the highest levels of vitamin E having significantly lower risk. Vitamin E supplementation studies in HIV patients seem to support its immunostimulatory and antioxidant function.

Vitamin B complex in HIV infection

The absence of well-designed randomized trials with B-complex vitamins, and B_{12} in particular, has confined reports of benefits of supplementation to be based entirely on anecdotal evidence or case reports. The B complex group investigated include thiamin (B_1), riboflavin (B_2), niacin (B_3), pyridoxine (B_6) and cobalamine (B_{12}). It may be important to mention that antiretroviral drugs like zidovudine show increased toxicity in the presence of B_{12} deficiency which justifies the administration of B-complex vitamins along with antiretroviral therapy.

Zinc and selenium supplementation in HIV infection

A few studies have shown that zinc supplementation improves both lymphocyte counts (CD4+ counts and CD4+/CD8+ ratios) and clinical outcomes in HIV-infected adults and children. There also appears to be an association with zinc supplementation and antiretroviral therapy. Zinc supplementation seems to confer clinical benefit and reduced incidence of opportunistic infections during antiretroviral therapy.

Studies using selenium supplementation in HIV infection provide variable results, some showing benefit, others none. Since the reports are based on small observational studies it is difficult to draw useful conclusions despite the importance of selenium deficiency in HIV infection.

Tables 9.2 and 9.3 summarize some of the data on the impact of supplementation of several micronutrients on the transmission of HIV and HIV/AIDS disease progression, respectively.

Micronutrients and the vertical transmission of HIV

Mother-to-infant transmission of HIV can occur prenatally during pregnancy, at the time of delivery of the infant and postnatally through breast milk in HIV-positive mothers. This transmission from HIV-positive mothers to their infants is referred to as *vertical transmission*. The rate of vertical transmission is higher in developing countries (25–35%) than in developed, industrialized countries (15–25%).

The higher rates of vertical transmission of HIV in developing countries may be attributable to micronutrient deficiencies in women of reproductive age, exacerbated by the nutritional stress of pregnancy and lactation. Maternal micronutrient deficiencies increase the risk of poor micronutrient status of the infant, and thereby affect the infant's immune status and susceptibility to HIV infection.

Table 9.4 summarizes some of the maternal and fetal factors that relate micronutrient supplementation to the vertical transmission of HIV. Among micronutrients only vitamin A deficiency and supplementation studies have been carried out extensively and are reviewed here. See also Table 9.2 for associations between micronutrients and vertical transmission of HIV.

Vitamin A deficiency and vertical transmission of HIV

In Kenya, HIV-infected women with low serum vitamin A levels were more likely to shed the virus

Table 9.4. Maternal and fetal factors that relate micronutrient deficiencies to vertical transmission of HIV. (Adapted from Dreyfuss and Fawzie, 2002.)

	Increases with micronutrient supplementation	Decreases with micronutrient supplementation
Maternal factors		
Placenta	Epithelial integrity	
Lower genital tract	Mucosal immunity Epithelial integrity	Systemic viral load
Breast	Mucosal immunity Epithelial integrity	Systemic viral load
Progression of HIV disease	Cellular immunity Humoral immunity	Clinical progression and opportunistic infections Systemic viral load
Fetal or child factors	Gastrointestinal epithelial integrity Cellular and humoral immunity	LBW Preterm birth

in vaginal secretions and breast milk. This implies that maternal vitamin A deficiency increases the HIV exposure of the infant as it passes through the birth canal and during breastfeeding. Low serum vitamin A levels among HIV-infected pregnant women increased the risk of vertical transmission. Women with low vitamin A status in Malawi showed a fourfold increase in the risk of having an HIV-infected child, while mothers with high serum vitamin A levels had significantly lower risk of vertical transmission.

The mortality rates of infants were approximately two to four times higher if they were born to HIV-infected mothers with moderate to severe vitamin A deficiency. A Rwandan study of HIV-infected mothers confirmed that low serum vitamin A levels during pregnancy meant they were increasingly likely to have an infant who died soon after or was HIV-positive. Several subsequent studies on HIV-infected pregnant women in the USA were not conclusive that vitamin A deficiency was associated with an increased risk of vertical transmission of the infection. While a large study showed an association between severe deficiency of vitamin A and a fivefold increase in relative odds of vertical transmission, other studies did not confirm this although they provided evidence suggestive of a protective effect of vitamin A.

Vitamin A supplementation and vertical transmission of HIV

Randomized supplementation trials have been carried out based on the evidence of vitamin A deficiency states on the vertical transmission of HIV from mother to infant. A randomized control trial in HIV-infected pregnant mothers who were supplemented with retinol showed no significant difference in vertical transmission assessed 6 weeks and 12 months after birth. A similar result, i.e. no impact on vertical transmission, was observed in a supplementation trial with vitamin A and carotene in South Africa when assessed in infants at 3 months of age.

A placebo-controlled trial of vitamin A and carotene was compared with multivitamin supplementation in HIV-positive mothers in Tanzania. While neither vitamin A with carotene nor multivitamin supplements altered the incidence of vertical transmission, multivitamins unlike vitamin A and carotene were effective in reducing fetal death by approximately 39% and LBW by 40%. The summary of the results of four trials with a total of over 3000 HIV-infected pregnant mothers does not support the use of vitamin A supplementation for the prevention of mother-to-infant transmission of the infection. Effects on birth weight were however evident in the supplemented group, as was reduced maternal mortality, in another study in HIV-infected and uninfected mothers in Nepal.

HIV and breastfeeding

Prevention of vertical transmission of HIV means improving maternal health, evaluating the role of breastfeeding in postnatal transmission and devising economically viable interventions to reduce mother-to infant transmission. Breastfeeding is preeminent for infant nutrition because of its nutritional, immunological, social and nurturing benefits. However, mother-to-child transmission of HIV infection is likely to occur by breastfeeding an infant and hence mothers need to be counselled about the various options available to them. Early cessation of breastfeeding appears to reduce the risk of HIV transmission by reducing the length of time during which an infant is exposed to HIV through breast milk. The option of recommending infant formula feeding should be considered for HIV-positive mothers when the family has reliable access to sufficient formula for at least 6 months and has access to other essential resources such as clean water, fuel, utensils, skills and time to prepare the infant formula milk hygienically and accurately. Heat treatment of expressed breast milk is another option since heat treatment kills the virus in breast milk. Wet-nursing may be another option available to the family.

More recent data from trials show that the problem of HIV transmission through breast milk is related to other infant feeding practices associated with breastfeeding. Summary of data collected from over 14,000 mother–infant pairs showed that postnatal transmission of HIV occurred in 12% of infants who were breastfed but two-thirds of infection occurred after 6 months. Comparison of those infants who were exclusively breastfed with others who had early mixed feeding along with breast milk showed the latter to have nearly a fourfold greater risk at 6 and 12 months than those who were exclusively breastfed. Thus it would appear that exclusively breastfed infants are at significantly reduced risk than those who receive other foods and fluids along with the breast milk.

HIV-positive mothers in developing countries have to balance the risk of transmitting HIV infection to their infant through breast milk with the other health benefits of breastfeeding. However, studies in South Africa do not support the view that exclusive breastfeeding protects these infants from common childhood illnesses nor does it delay the progression to AIDS. One can only conclude that, when and where possible, alternative strategies need to be adopted to reduce vertical transmission of HIV.

HIV-associated weight loss, wasting and undernutrition

HIV infection in adults is associated with severe wasting and unintentional weight loss which can occur even in the absence of fever or diarrhoea. Prior to the availability of antiretroviral therapy, wasting and weight loss characteristic of severe malnutrition was the most frequent AIDS-defining condition. It was assumed that unintentional weight loss in HIV-infected individuals would be eliminated with the advent of highly effective antiretroviral therapy – just as significant reductions were observed in morbidity and mortality.

The cause of HIV-associated wasting is multifactorial and includes both decreased nutrient intake (due to oral and upper gut lesions, anorexia and malabsorption) and altered nutrient metabolism (resulting from uncontrolled HIV infection, metabolic demands imposed by antiretroviral therapy, opportunistic infections, cytokine dysregulation and hormonal deficiencies of thyroid and testosterone) (see Table 9.5). Socioeconomic factors, access to care and psychological factors also play a part. Weight loss in HIV-infected individuals seems to occur early in the disease before significant compromise in immune function is evident. The loss of lean body mass seems to be related to the quality of life of the individual and strategies are hence focused on increasing lean tissues of the body. While nutritional support and advice seems to have some effect on increasing lean body mass, the best results both in terms of gain in body weight and lean body mass seem to occur with anabolic steroids and testosterone.

The progression of HIV infection to frank AIDS is linked closely to nutritional status. Good nutrition strengthens and protects the host's immune system and other aspects of host defence. During

Table 9.5. Causes of weight loss in HIV/AIDS-infected individuals. (Adapted from Mangili *et al.*, 2006.)

Inadequate and poor nutrient intakes	Oral and upper gastrointestinal lesions Anorexia Malabsorption Diarrhoeal disease due to opportunistic infections Psychosocial conditions and economic circumstances
Altered metabolism and changes in energy expenditure	Uncontrolled HIV infection and viral load Metabolic demands of highly active antiretroviral therapy Opportunistic infections and malignancies Hormonal deficiencies (thyroid and testosterone) Inflammatory cytokine increase and dysregulation

an HIV infection nutrition has an important role along with antiretroviral and antimicrobial therapies to reduce HIV replication and reduce the risk of opportunistic and other secondary infections that characterize the later stages of the disease. Both the primary, i.e. HIV infection, and the secondary infections stimulate production of pro-inflammatory cytokines which cause fever, breakdown of muscle protein and loss of nutrients from the body. The poor nutritional status in turn will compromise the immune system further (nutritionally acquired immunodeficiency) and, acting synergistically with the HIV infection that directly targets the immune mechanisms, results in rapid progression of the disease and death. Nutritional support can reverse these changes and prolong survival.

9.4 Nutrition and Tuberculosis

TB is one of the most widespread infectious diseases afflicting man. Several factors such as poverty and inequity, poor housing and local environment, poor nutrition and inadequate access to health services all contribute to perpetuate TB in developing countries. The pandemic of HIV/AIDS and the rise of multidrug-resistant TB have further contributed to the spread of this disease. TB is caused by the tubercle bacillus, *M. tuberculosis*, which is an aerobic, non-motile, non-spore forming bacterium that spreads infection through inhalation and ingestion and mainly affects the lung and respiratory tracts, although other organ systems can also be affected. TB remains a major cause of morbidity and mortality worldwide, and particularly so in developing countries. It is generally accepted that the decline in TB in economically developed nations is largely attributable to improved socio-economic factors and better nutrition.

There is a close relationship between a chronic infectious disease such as TB and the nutrition of the host. Poor nutrition status increases risk of infection with TB, although other environmental factors that often underlie poor nutrition, such as poor housing, overcrowding and poverty, also contribute to increasing susceptibility. TB infection in the host, in turn, often results in undernutrition due to loss of appetite and wasting. TB and undernutrition are synergistic processes as poor nutrition not only increases susceptibility to TB infection but also appears to be closely associated with progression from latent to active TB disease, and active TB disease worsens existing nutritional deficits.

The historical record of the association between nutritional status and TB is quite extensive. In 1925 navy cadets in Norway were reported to have a high incidence of TB prior to improvements in their diet by the addition of margarine, cod-liver oil, whole wheat bread, fresh fruit, vegetables and milk. Despite earlier attempts to lower the morbidity associated with TB by improvement of housing and hygiene, it was only the changes in the diet which resulted in reducing the levels of TB. In Harlem in New York supplements of vitamins and minerals reduced the rate of re-infection in families exposed to re-infection with TB. Experience during World War I showed that when diets lacked meat and fish the mortality from TB increased by 30% in Denmark, and in most of Europe. During World War II mortality from TB doubled in Germany. When malnutrition was widespread mortality from TB was very high and this dropped after the war when food supply improved. Similar findings on TB mortality in the Warsaw ghetto during World War II were attributed to the deterioration in the nutritional status.

Undernutrition and tuberculosis

Native resistance, as well as susceptibility to *M. tuberculosis* infection, is determined by a range of host factors including nutritional status. A large retrospective study in Norway between the years 1963 to 1975, covering over 1.7 million individuals, showed an inverse association between body mass index (BMI) (indicating poor nutritional status) and increased risk of developing TB, as well as increased risk of TB-related mortality. Several other cohort studies have shown that poor nutritional status at baseline and failure to demonstrate improvement in anthropometric parameters such as body weight and BMI with therapy are associated with poor prognosis in patients with pulmonary TB. Patients with poor nutritional status have a higher prevalence of more extensive disease and pulmonary TB patients diagnosed with moderate to severe undernutrition (BMI <17.0 kg/m^2) had higher rates of TB-related death than those with only mild to moderate undernutrition (BMI >17.0 kg/m^2). Other studies following up patients on therapeutic regimens have shown that poor nutritional status is also associated with an increased risk of relapse. All of these studies suggest an association between poor nutritional status and disease severity and clinical outcomes, i.e. increased mortality and risk of relapse after treatment.

Anthropometric indicators like BMI are not the only markers used to assess the role of nutritional status in patients with TB. Plasma levels of albumin have been shown to be lowered in TB infection and have been considered as good predictors of clinical outcome, with those being admitted with low plasma albumin levels (<2.7 g/dl) shown to be at increased risk of in-hospital death. Other plasma proteins like pre-albumin, RBP, transferrin and ferritin are also significantly lower in patients with TB compared with healthy controls. The recovery of plasma proteins occurs much more slowly than the clinical recovery noticed in TB patients who are being treated. Amino acid kinetic studies suggest that active TB appears to impose an 'anabolic block' where the host is unable to mount an adequate anabolic response to food intake to re-synthesize proteins and improve the nutritional status rapidly.

Undernutrition in individuals with TB infection shows compromised immune responses manifested as attenuation of DTH, attenuation of responses to DNCB and reduced lymphocyte transformation.

NK-cell activity may be reduced as well as the production of IL-1 and IL-2. Undernutrition in individuals with pulmonary TB is thus characterized by impaired cell-mediated immunity and reduced cytokine production. A significant synergistic interaction between severe undernutrition and TB has also been observed in children. Cell-mediated immunity in children with TB showed the immunosuppressive effect of TB in all children, irrespective of undernutrition. However, well-nourished children with TB had similar cell-mediated immune status irrespective of the severity of the disease, while undernourished children with severe forms of TB showed the lowest cell-mediated immune response. The synergistic interaction of TB infection and undernutrition on immune function is evident here in addition to the contributory role of undernutrition in causing more severe immunosuppression during an infection.

Experimental studies on animal models of the disease suggest that undernutrition impairs host resistance to TB by interfering with the physical containment of mycobacteria within the primary lesion. Undernourished animals show defects in the reaction responsible for local granuloma formation, which is essential to confine and localize the infection and resist the spread of the infection. TNF-α is essential for granuloma formation and it has been demonstrated that TNF-α production is diminished in undernourished animals. Local bacillary replication and extra-pulmonary dissemination are thereby encouraged and result in increased spread of the disease.

Interventions with micronutrients in the treatment of tuberculosis

There is increasing evidence that micronutrients which are well known to influence innate and specific immune responses to infection may be used as therapeutic adjuvants to drugs in the treatment of TB. Historical anecdotes support this, as prior to the era of modern chemotherapy of TB, cod-liver oil, an excellent source of vitamins A and D, was used as therapy for TB.

Vitamin A supplementation

Patients with TB have lowered stores of vitamin A (retinol) which is worsened if there is concomitant co-infection with HIV. The poor vitamin status may be the result of poor appetite and lowered nutrient intakes, although there is evidence to suggest that the chronic inflammatory state associated with the infection may promote excessive urinary loss of retinol.

The existence of a causal relationship between vitamin A deficiency and susceptibility to TB is unclear although there are reports of low retinol levels in patients with TB. Latent TB infection complicated by persistent vitamin A deficiency is associated with a higher likelihood of progression to active TB. Children with active TB infection in the presence of vitamin A deficiency show derangements in cytokine production which may predispose them to being ineffective in controlling the progression of the disease.

Several studies have highlighted the potential role for vitamin A as an adjuvant to conventional drug treatment in influencing the clinical outcome and response to treatment. Controlled trials of vitamin A supplementation along with treatment for TB have been carried out. A study in Indonesian adults newly diagnosed with TB showed that administration of retinol over an 8-week period along with conventional TB treatment resulted in a significantly higher percentage of individuals with sputum smear conversion and a decrease in size of pulmonary lesion observed radiographically, compared with the placebo group. Another study in Tanzanian adults newly diagnosed with TB but complicated by the presence or absence of HIV showed that retinol lowered rates of recurrence and increased body weight with TB treatment, while other parameters including sputum smear conversion and all-cause mortality did not show any difference between the supplemented and placebo group. However, a study in children with TB in South Africa observed no differences in clinical or radiological outcomes with retinol administration. The potential role for vitamin A as an adjuvant to conventional chemotherapy for the treatment of TB needs further careful investigation.

Vitamin D and tuberculosis

Laboratory studies have demonstrated that the active form of vitamin D modulates the immune response by the increased expression of cathelicidin, an endogenous antimicrobial peptide that exhibits activity against mycobacteria. Patients with TB on the other hand have been observed to have lower serum levels of 25-hydroxyvitamin D than healthy controls and the presence of vitamin D deficiency seems to correlate with increased severity of the disease in pulmonary TB.

Cod-liver oil, an important dietary source of vitamin D, has in the past been used to treat TB, and so has the application of ultraviolet light to the skin for the treatment of cutaneous TB since it increases the synthesis of vitamin D. These early observations have provided support for the use of vitamin D as an adjuvant in the treatment of TB. There are many clinical trials ongoing using vitamin D as an adjuvant in the treatment of TB; the one published study showed that high doses of vitamin D provided daily along with conventional treatment of pulmonary TB resulted in a shorter duration for sputum cultures to become negative for the bacillus in the vitamin D-supplemented group as compared with the placebo group. The results of the many ongoing trials will probably influence the future treatment protocols for TB.

Zinc deficiency and tuberculosis

Zinc plays an important role in immune function and the active inflammatory process seen in patients with TB may predispose to zinc deficiency. TB patients have been reported to have lower levels of plasma zinc in Indonesia. Zinc deficiency appears to be common in TB patients and was found to be correlated with the severity of the disease in other studies. However, zinc supplementation trials in the treatment of pulmonary TB reported from India, Indonesia and Tanzania have not always provided consistent clinical benefits.

Other micronutrients and tuberculosis

Chronic infections like TB generate significant oxidative stress in the host and are reflected in the elevated levels of lipid peroxide metabolites. Vitamin A (retinol), vitamin C (ascorbate), vitamin E (α-tocopherol) and selenium are important antioxidant micronutrients and patients with pulmonary TB show decreased blood levels of these antioxidant nutrients compared with controls. While supplementation trials with vitamin E and selenium have been shown to reduce levels of indicators of oxidative stress in TB patients, the possible beneficial effect on clinical outcomes was not reported from this study from Iran. A more recent randomized clinical trial using a micronutrient supplement with vitamins A, B complex, C and E, and selenium, along with drug treatment of pulmonary TB patients (some with co-infection with HIV), reported better clinical outcomes such as signifi-

cantly lower rates of TB recurrence and reduced TB-related mortality. This trial from Tanzania endorsed a role for the use of micronutrients along with TB chemotherapy for better clinical outcomes.

Tuberculosis as a cause of undernutrition

Clinical and nutritional assessment of patients with chronic infections like TB clearly demonstrates the catabolic effect of these infections. Body weight, BMI, subcutaneous fat and muscle mass are all significantly reduced in patients with TB. In addition, they demonstrate functional impairment such as reduction in hand grip strength. Severe and long-standing infection may manifest with severe wasting and asthenia. Some of the poor nutrition is attributable to the poor appetite and reduced intake of food and nutrients. The recurrent febrile episodes increase energy expenditure and energy requirements, and enhance the breakdown of lean tissue and the utilization of stored energy in the fat stores. There is evidence of increased protein breakdown and turnover of proteins, and this catabolic process in combination with the reduced intake results in wasting and poor nutritional status. The 'anabolic block' creates an imbalance between catabolism and anabolism resulting in more lean tissue loss and less re-synthesis of proteins and rebuilding of tissues, prolonging and extending the period of poor nutritional status in those who have been infected and treated.

Further Reading

Beisel, W.R. (2000) AIDS. In: Gershwin, M.E., German, J.B. and Keen, C.L. (eds) *Nutrition and Immunology.* Humana Press, Totowa, New Jersey, pp. 389–401. *Highlights the importance of nutrition in AIDS and the links between nutritionally acquired immunodeficiency and AIDs-related immunocompromise of the host and role of nutritional support in therapy.*

Dreyfuss, M.L. and Fawzie, W.W. (2002) Micronutrients and vertical transmission of HIV-1. *American Journal of Clinical Nutrition* 75, 959–970. *A review that summarizes the epidemiological evidence on micronutrients that influence the vertical transmission of HIV and the potential mechanisms involved.*

Kiure, A. and Fawzi, W. (2004) HIV. In: Gershwin, M.E., Nestel, P. and Keen, C.L. (eds) *Handbook of Nutrition and Immunity.* Humana Press, Totowa, New Jersey, pp. 303–337. *A review that summarizes the various studies that have examined the potential causes of* undernutrition and impaired immune function in HIV-infected individuals.

Singhal, N. and Austin, J. (2002) A clinical review of micronutrients in HIV infection. *Journal of the International Association of Physicians in AIDS Care* 1, 63–75. *An article that reviews the current literature on the role of micronutrients in HIV infection and recommends the use of multivitamins as adjuncts to conventional antiretroviral therapy as a low-cost intervention.*

Case Studies

Case Study 9.1: Multivitamin supplements and their influence on HIV disease progression and mortality.

A randomized controlled trial carried out in Dar es Salaam, Tanzania enrolled pregnant women infected with HIV. The primary aim of the study was to compare the effects of multivitamins (vitamins B, C and E), vitamin A alone or both, with those of a placebo. Antiretroviral therapy was not available to the pregnant women in this study, as was the case with the majority of women in Tanzania at the time the study was conducted.

The four arms of the study thus comprised: (i) a placebo group; (ii) a multivitamin group; (ii) a multivitamin plus vitamin A group; and (iv) a vitamin A only group. Of the 271 women who received only multivitamins, 67 progressed to Stage 4 or died compared with 83 of 267 pregnant women in the placebo control group, i.e. 24.7% compared with 31.1%, providing a significantly reduced relative risk of 0.71 for the multivitamin group.

Some of the significant findings of this trial including markers of disease, clinical outcomes and complications are summarized in Table 9.6.

The multivitamin-supplemented group showed significantly higher CD4+ and CD8+ cell counts and significantly lower viral loads. The numbers reporting several of the important HIV-related complications were also significantly lower in the multivitamin group. The effects on all parameters studied were smaller in the group receiving vitamin A alone and many of the differences were not statistically significant compared with the placebo group. The results of the group who received both multivitamins and vitamin A demonstrated results in between, with reduced benefit compared with the multivitamin group.

This study demonstrated that multivitamins excluding vitamin A improve survival and slow down the progression of the disease in the absence of antiretroviral therapy. Multivitamins may provide additional benefits when given as adjuncts to antiretroviral therapy.

Reference

Fawzi, W.W., Msamanga, G.I., Spiegelman, D., Wei, R., Kapiga, S., Villamor, E., Mwakagile, D., Mugusi, F., Hertzmark, E., Essex, M. and Hunter, D.J. (2004) A randomized trial of multivitamin supplements and HIV disease progression and mortality. *New England Journal of Medicine* 351, 23–32.

Table 9.6. Data on markers of disease, clinical outcomes and complications. (Adapted from Fawzi *et al.*, 2004.)

	Multivitamin group	Multivitamin + vitamin A group	Vitamin A only group
Markers of disease			
Mean difference in CD4+ cell counts/mm^3	48*	41*	−15
Mean difference in log viral load	−0.18*	−0.07	−0.03
Clinical outcome			
RR of progression to Stage 4	0.50*	0.67	0.68
RR of deaths from AIDS-related causes	0.73	0.91	0.93
Complications			
RR of thrush	0.47*	0.58*	0.69
RR of oral ulcers	0.44*	0.54*	0.94
RR of difficult/painful swallowing	0.41*	0.68	1.25
RR of dysentery	0.66*	0.82	0.90

RR, relative risk.
*Statistically significant difference compared with the placebo group.

Case Study 9.2: Vitamin A supplementation of HIV-infected mothers, birth outcomes and mother-to-infant transmission of HIV.

HIV-positive pregnant women were enrolled at 18–28 weeks' gestation into a randomized trial conducted in Blantyre, Malawi. All women received iron and folate from enrolment until they delivered, but half of the HIV-positive pregnant women received in addition vitamin A. The baseline characteristics of the vitamin A and control groups were similar for age, body mass index, $CD4^+$ and $CD8^+$ cell counts and $CD4^+/CD8^+$ ratios, as well as for viral loads. Their plasma vitamin A levels were similar at enrolment.

Table 9.7 summarizes the maternal and infant health outcomes in the vitamin A and control groups. Maternal vitamin A levels (both plasma and breast milk) were significantly higher in the group supplemented with vitamin A, while maternal folate levels were similar in both groups. The mean birth weights were higher and the proportion of low-birth-weight infants was significantly lower in the vitamin A supplementation group. Anaemia was also less of a problem with the infants born to vitamin A-supplemented HIV-positive mothers.

There were no significant differences in the proportion of HIV-infected infants at 6 weeks, 12 and 24 months after birth between the groups. However, the proportion of infants who were not infected at the age of 6 weeks but who were HIV infected at 24 months, i.e. most likely to have been infected via breastfeeding, was significantly higher in the control group.

This randomized trial of HIV-infected mothers shows that antenatal vitamin A supplementation during the second and third trimesters of pregnancy improves birth weight and infant growth and reduces the risk of anaemia in infants. It also corroborates findings from Tanzania and South Africa that vitamin A supplementation has no overall impact on mother-to-child transmission of HIV. This is despite the evidence that low vitamin A status is associated with higher rates of mother-to-child transmission and the increased genital shedding of HIV virus.

Reference

Kumwenda, N., Miotti, P.G., Taha, T.E., Broadhead, R., Biggar, R.J., Jackson, J.B., Melikian, G. and Semba, R.D. (2002) Antenatal vitamin A supplementation increases birth weight and decreases anemia among infants born to human immunodeficiency virus-infected women in Malawi. *Clinical Infectious Diseases* 35, 618–624.

Table 9.7. Data on maternal and infant health outcomes. (Adapted from Kumwenda *et al.*, 2002.)

	Vitamin A group	Control group
Mean birth weight (g)	2895*	2805
Percentage of infants with LBW (<2500 g)	14.0*	21.1
Infant haemoglobin at 6 weeks (g/l)	116*	112
Percentage of infants with anaemia at 6 weeks	23.4*	40.6
Percentage of infants infected with HIV at 6 weeks	26.6	27.8
Percentage of infants infected with HIV at 12 months	27.3	32.0
Percentage of infants who died before 6 weeks	4.2	6.5
Percentage of infants who died by 12 months	20.4	18.8
Percentage of infants HIV-negative at 6 weeks but HIV-positive at 24 months	2.8*	7.7

LBW, low birth weight.
*Statistically significant difference compared with the control group.

Case Study 9.3: Micronutrient supplementation of patients with pulmonary tuberculosis in Indonesia.

Malnutrition is frequently observed in patients with pulmonary tuberculosis (TB). A study carried out in urban Jakarta, Indonesia found poor micronutrient status among patients with TB. Vitamin A and zinc levels indicative of deficiency in both micronutrients were observed more frequently in TB patients compared with matched controls in this study from Jakarta. The same investigators then proceeded to evaluate the effect of vitamin A and zinc supplementation along with standard anti-TB treatment using a double-blind, placebo-controlled supplementation trial.

The intervention group (who received vitamin A and zinc supplements) were comparable to the control group (who received a placebo) in all respects, including body mass index, tuberculin skin test responses, sputum and X-ray findings,

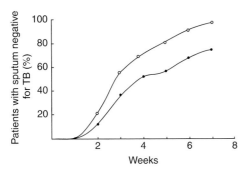

Fig. 9.1. Plot showing the proportion of TB patients in the micronutrient-supplemented group with sputum smears converting to negative (—○—) compared with the placebo group (– –•– –) over the first 8 weeks of anti-TB treatment. (Adapted from Karyadi *et al.*, 2002a.)

Table 9.8. Changes in mean lesion area (cm²) in chest X-ray before and after (2 and 6 months) treatment. (Adapted from Karyadi *et al.*, 2002a.)

	Baseline (pre-treatment)	2 months post-treatment	6 months post-treatment
Placebo controls	221.3	123.9	20.6
Vitamin A and zinc supplement group	233.9	92.9*	21.2

*Statistically significant difference compared with the placebo group.

and plasma albumin and white blood cell counts. After 6 months of anti-TB treatment, subjects in both groups gained weight. The weight gain, erythrocyte sedimentation rate, plasma C-reactive protein levels and micronutrient scores were significantly higher than the baseline pre-treatment levels. Only the micronutrient scores (Karnofsky scores) were significantly different between the intervention and placebo control groups after 6 months of treatment.

However, micronutrient supplementation resulted in an earlier elimination of the tubercle bacilli from sputum (Fig. 9.1). After 2 weeks of treatment the number of patients with sputum smears negative for tubercle bacilli was higher in the micronutrient-supplemented group (23% compared with 13% in the placebo group) and this difference was maintained for up to 7 weeks. This difference was statistically significant.

The mean reduction in the pulmonary lesion area on the chest X-ray was significantly greater in the micronutrient-supplemented group after 2 months (see Table 9.8) and the reduction in the mean lesion

area at 6 months correlated significantly with the plasma retinol levels.

This is the first study in the literature to report a demonstrable benefit to the concurrent supplementation of micronutrients on the treatment outcome of TB patients. The addition of vitamin A and zinc improved the effectiveness of anti-TB drugs during the first 2 months of treatment. It also contrasts with a study in South African children where supplementation with high doses of vitamin A alone along with anti-TB treatment showed no effects on disease outcome.

This study demonstrates the potential for micronutrient supplements in improving therapeutic response to anti-TB treatment of patients with pulmonary TB in developing countries.

Reference

Karyadi, E., West, C.E., Schultink, J.W., Nelwan, R.H., Gross, R., Amin, Z., Dolmans, W.M., Schlebusch, H. and van der Meer, J.W. (2002a) A double blind placebo controlled study of vitamin A and zinc supplementation in persons with tuberculosis in Indonesia: effects on clinical response and nutritional status. *American Journal of Clinical Nutrition* 75, 720–727.

10 Nutrition, Immunity and Infections of Infants and Children

- Childhood undernutrition is a global health problem associated with increased morbidity and mortality that is directly related to compromise in the host's defence mechanisms.
- Undernutrition and micronutrient deficiencies in children increase the incidence of illnesses like diarrhoeal disease, respiratory infections and measles.
- Undernutrition and micronutrient deficiencies in children increase morbidity and mortality associated with infectious diseases.
- Suboptimal breastfeeding increases the risk of infection in children and the morbidity and mortality associated with it.
- Exclusive breastfeeding is important to reduce risk of infectious diseases and their consequences in infants and children.
- Micronutrient deficiencies increase the risk of diarrhoeal disease, pneumonia, measles and malaria.
- Nutrition interventions include the promotion of optimal breastfeeding and appropriate, adequate and safe complementary and supplementary feeding.
- Nutritional interventions to reduce the risk and impact of infectious diseases and their consequences include micronutrient supplementation.
- Other interventions for good child health include de-worming and good hand-hygiene practices.

10.1 Introduction

Nowhere is the impact of poor nutrition, the consequent compromise of immune function and in turn the increase in risk of infection and the morbidity and mortality associated with it, more important than in the health of infants and children. Undernutrition in infants and children under 5 years of age, i.e. pre-school children, is a serious issue of public health significance. Undernutrition in this phase of the life cycle includes LBW and its consequences, which are discussed in Chapter 11 on maternal nutrition and birth outcomes. However, childhood undernutrition largely encompasses the classical forms based on anthropometric indicators, namely underweight (low weight-for-age), stunting (low height-for-age) and wasting (low weight-for-height), along with the range of micronutrient deficiencies related to vitamin and mineral inadequacies.

Infant and child undernutrition is determined by immediate causes, i.e. inadequate nutrient intakes and disease, the latter largely the result of infections in infancy and childhood. The contribution from infections is attributed to underlying causes such as poverty, which are also responsible for inadequacy of nutritional intakes, inadequate care and impoverished household environments with lack of access to appropriate health care. Poverty thus underlies the three proximate determinants of childhood undernutrition – food security, adequate care and health. Micronutrient deficiencies are also linked to poverty in developing countries.

The prevalence of all forms of childhood undernutrition worldwide is quite high and is almost entirely confined to the developing regions of the world. Recent United Nations (UN) estimates indicate that 20% of children in the developing world are underweight numbering a total of 112 million, 32% are stunted numbering 178 million, and 3.5% are wasted accounting for just over 19 million children. Micronutrient deficiencies cover much higher proportions of the population of infants and children in developing countries.

Table 10.1. Risk of child mortality expressed as odds ratio associated with degree of underweight. (Adapted from Black *et al.*, 2008.)

	Weight-for-age Z-score		
	−1 to −2	−2 to −3	>−3
Overall child mortality	1.8	2.5	9.7
Mortality due to diarrhoea	2.1	3.4	9.5
Mortality due to pneumonia	1.2	1.3	6.4
Mortality due to malaria	0.8	1.2	1.6
Mortality due to measles	1.3	2.3	6.4

The synergistic relationship between child undernutrition and infection is well documented. When nutritional deficiency and infectious disease coexist, the consequence is usually greater than that due to the summed effect of the two together. Population-based studies from different countries showed that between 20% and 80% of child mortality had undernutrition as an underlying cause, and in most cases 40 to 60% of mortality was associated with mild to moderate undernutrition. More recent estimates by WHO of child morality attribute about 50% to underlying undernutrition.

It has recently been estimated that 77.5 million children are born each year in 36 countries with the highest burden of undernutrition, of whom about 7.4 million die before reaching 3 years of age. Mortality of children under 5 years old is estimated at 103 deaths per 1000 live births. Table 10.1 summarizes the odds ratios for mortality from infectious disease risk associated with child underweight estimated recently based on data sets from eight low-income countries which include Ghana, Guinea Bissau, Senegal, the Philippines, Nepal, Pakistan, India and Bangladesh. It also presents the cause-specific mortality associated with the infections, i.e. diarrhoea, pneumonia, malaria and measles, and clearly illustrates the increased risks of mortality due to infectious diseases in the presence of child undernutrition.

10.2 Undernutrition, Micronutrient Deficiencies and Infections in Infancy and Childhood

Child undernutrition is a major global public health problem which has been a serious concern for several decades despite the major advances in food production and economic development. It remains a pervasive problem in many low- and middle-income countries and contributes to both the health and economic burden of these nations. Child undernutrition includes underweight, stunting and wasting in addition to micronutrient deficiencies, and is a bigger nutritional problem than food insecurity. In 2005, 20% of pre-school children below 5 years of age had a weight-for-age Z-score of less than −2, accounting for 112 million underweight children in all developing countries. An estimated 32%, i.e. 178 million, were stunted with a height-for-age Z-score of less than −2. For wasting, i.e. weight-for-height Z-score less than −2, the global estimate was 10%, i.e. 55 million children, of whom 19 million had a Z-score of less than −3 indicative of severe wasting. The risk of mortality in undernourished children due largely to infectious diseases increases with the degree of undernutrition. The odds ratios of mortality (both all-cause and due to specific infectious diseases) associated with underweight are presented in Table 10.1. The data show that the risk of mortality rises exponentially when the underweight is severe, i.e. when the Z-score is less than −3.

The associations between undernutrition in the newborn manifesting as LBW due to IUGR and infectious disease morbidity and mortality in the neonatal period are dealt with in Chapter 11, which focuses on maternal nutrition and birth outcomes.

Breastfeeding, complementary feeding, child care practices and risk of infection in children

The recommendation made by UN agencies for optimal growth, good nutrition and freedom from infections in infancy and childhood is to ensure exclusive breastfeeding (i.e. nothing but breast milk) for the first 6 months of life and to continue breastfeeding thereafter through the second year of life. However, the first part of this recommendation is poorly adhered to in much of the developing world, with the percentage of mothers exclusively breastfeeding dropping from the second month after birth to about 30% by 5 month. Table 10.2 presents data comparing the risk of infections like diarrhoea and pneumonia, and mortality attributable to these infections, in infants who were not exclusively breastfed up to 6 months of age. The same analysis showed that continued breastfeeding after 6 months and into the second year of life has benefits related to risk of both diarrhoeal disease incidence and all-cause mortality. Those who were not provided breast milk at all over this period from 6 months to 23 months of age increased their risk of infectious diseases and mortality.

The absence of exclusive breastfeeding is considered as suboptimal breastfeeding and may be either predominant breastfeeding (i.e. only liquids like water in addition to breast milk) or partial breastfeeding (i.e. other liquids or solids in addition to breast milk). When exclusively breastfed infants are compared with predominantly breastfed and partially breastfed infants and with those infants who were not breastfed at all, it is quite evident that the risk of mortality and morbidity increases with suboptimal breastfeeding – with the very highest risk of infections among infants who were not breastfed at all (Table 10.2).

Breastfeeding provides optimal nutrition for an infant up to 6 months of age. After this age, infants require appropriate, adequate and safe complementary foods to continue to grow and develop normally. Failure to provide adequate complementary foods after this age can increase the risk of undernutrition. The risk of stunting appears to be maximal from the age of 6 months to 2 years. This is a period of high nutrient demand for the rapidly growing infant and suboptimal complementary feeding will compromise gain in height and in weight. This is also the period when other foods apart from breast milk are introduced and this increases the risk of infections associated with both inadequate nutrient intakes and unsafe food consumption. This age group is characterized by high rates of infectious diseases like diarrhoea, respiratory illness and measles, which adversely affects growth and the nutritional status of the infant. It has been shown that in relative terms both poor complementary feeds and increase in infectious episodes contribute equally to poor nutrition and growth during this crucial period of infancy.

Complementary feeds must ensure adequate intake of nutrients, both in macro- and micronutrient content. The care practices related to feeding infants in this period need to focus on frequent feeds of highly energy-dense food which is appropriate in quality and digestibility by the young infant and is safe in terms of not having pathogens or toxic agents. Interventions that provide nutrition education to the mother or other caregivers – which emphasizes the importance of frequent, good-quality, energy-dense foods along with some animal-source foods which are rich in micronutrients – seem to have the most beneficial effects on linear growth and weight gain of infants in this critical period of life.

Childhood infections and risk of undernutrition

Episodes of infection in infancy and childhood are important determinants of poor nutritional status and inadequate linear growth in infants. Growth faltering occurs when infants suffer from infections and may result in stunting. Episodes of diarrhoeal illness, respiratory infections and pneumonia, as well as malaria in endemic areas, all contribute to be growth faltering in children. Diarrhoea seems to be particularly important because in addition to the illness, it causes loss of appetite and loss of nutrients due to malabsorption. Long-term follow-up studies in children up to 2 years of age, which have recorded the numerous episodes

Table 10.2. Relative risk[a] of infection and child mortality associated with suboptimal and poor breastfeeding practices. (Adapted from Black *et al.*, 2008.)

	Predominant breastfeeding[b]	Partial breastfeeding[c]	No breastfeeding
Incidence of diarrhoea	1.26	3.04	3.65
Incidence of pneumonia	1.79	2.48	2.07
Child mortality			
All causes	1.48	2.85	14.40
Mortality from diarrhoea	2.28	4.62	10.53
Mortality from pneumonia	1.75	2.49	15.13

[a]The relative risk is based on the comparison between exclusively breastfed from birth until 5 months and any breastfeeding thereafter from 6 to 23 months.
[b]Predominant breastfeeding, only liquids like water in addition to breast milk.
[c]Partial breastfeeding, other liquids or solids in addition to breast milk.

of diarrhoeal illness compiled from several developing countries, seem to suggest that each episode of diarrhoeal illness has a multiplicative effect on stunting. Undernutrition in childhood in turn has multiplicative effects on child mortality.

Micronutrient deficiencies and infections in childhood

Micronutrient deficiencies increase the risk of infections in infancy and childhood. Nutritional interventions that supplemented vitamin A to newborn infants and to children up to the age of 5 years showed a reduction in mortality up to 6 months of age. The reduced mortality from diarrhoeal diseases and measles provides proof that vitamin A deficiency increases the risk of infections in infancy and childhood. It also supports the view that nutritional interventions that supplement vitamin A are of benefit and reduce both morbidity and mortality in children. However, several clinical trails where vitamin A has been supplemented to neonates do not provide convincing evidence of the reduced risk of mortality and morbidity in young infants. Zinc deficiency in children increases the risk of diarrhoea, pneumonia and malaria. Evidence also comes from the benefits seen in zinc supplementation trials where the placebo groups have a higher risk of infections.

The risk reduction observed in supplementation trials has been used to estimate the contribution of micronutrients to child mortality due to infections. Using this method it has been estimated that the relative risk for diarrhoea mortality is 1.47 and that for measles 1.35 as a result of vitamin A deficiency. While the relative risk for infections in the presence of zinc deficiency is estimated at 1.09 for diarrhoea, 1.25 for pneumonia and 1.56 for malaria, the relative risks for under-5 child mortality associated with the same illnesses are 1.27, 1.18 and 1.11, respectively.

Box 10.1. Basics of Nutritional Epidemiology: Basic Terminology, Study Design and Sample Size.

While *epidemiology* is defined as the study of the distribution and determinants of diseases (and health outcomes) in human populations, *nutritional epidemiology*, a sub-speciality of epidemiology, is the study specifically of the dietary/nutritional determinants of disease. The linkages between diet and nutrition and diseases are complex. There are probably multiple determinants including genetic predispositions, the long latent periods of diet-related disease outcomes, and the relatively low frequencies of the disease even among people with high exposure to risk factors, which makes the task of establishing causality more arduous. Many of the associations between diet and disease are small and if the effects are real, they are relatively subtle. It thus makes it difficult if not impossible to determine, from epidemiological studies alone, whether the relatively weak associations between nutritional factors in the diet and disease are real, or whether they reflect some type of subtle bias or measurement error that the researchers were unable to eliminate. While the associations identified by epidemiological studies are useful for generating and testing new hypotheses about the diet–disease relationship, other lines of scientific research such as experimental models and rational mechanistic explanations are needed to provide evidence that a specific dietary/nutritional factor can account for the causation or prevention of the disease outcome. Determining that the observed associations between diet and disease are causal is crucial; otherwise efforts to modify exposure to that factor are unlikely to reduce disease risk.

Epidemiological studies are either descriptive or analytical. *Descriptive epidemiology* is the study of the amount and distribution of diseases and exposures, while *analytical epidemiology* specifically examines the determinants of disease in a population.

Basic terminology

Defining some epidemiological terms is very useful at this stage. They include the following.

- *Exposure* is defined as the contact over time and space between the individual and one or more biological, chemical or physical agent(s). Thus the agent is food, drug, chemical, etc. to which the individual is exposed. In nutritional epidemiology, it includes what an individual eats and the nutrients and non-nutrients in the diet the person is exposed to. It also includes the individual characteristics such as lifestyle, behaviour, etc.
- *Outcome* is the occurrence of the disease, event or health-related state.
- *Risk* is the possibility of suffering harm or loss, and disease or death.
- *Incidence* is the number of new cases of a disease in a specific time period. It is usually expressed as the incidence rate, i.e. the number of new cases

---

over a specified period of time divided by the number of people in the population at risk of developing the disease. The incidence rate enables populations of different sizes to be compared.

- *Prevalence* is the number of existing cases of a disease in a population. Since most diseases do not occur with equal frequency among people of all ages, for a meaningful comparison of disease rates in populations with different age structures it is necessary to take account of the effects of age. This can be done either by comparing age-specific rates or by using a technique called *age standardization*, by which the rates of disease in each age group are weighted by the age distribution of a standard population.

Study design

Epidemiological findings are only as good as the studies that produce them. Hence studies in nutritional epidemiology must be designed and executed with great care to minimize bias. Several different study designs are used in nutritional epidemiology. Each study design serves different purposes and has specific strengths and weaknesses. These include descriptive studies, ecological studies, case–control studies, cohort studies and intervention trials.

Descriptive and ecological studies include studies like comparisons of risks and exposures between population groups; time trends in the same population; and studies in special population groups where the exposure is controlled and on migrants who move from one environment to another, thus changing exposure and the consequent disease outcome.

Study designs in analytical nutritional epidemiology may be broadly categorized as observational or experimental in nature. *Observational studies* are uncontrolled assignments, while *experimental studies* have a controlled assignment. The two types of study design in observational studies are case–control studies and cohort studies. The two types of experimental studies are community trials and clinical intervention trials.

- *Case–control studies* follow up people who have the disease (cases) and otherwise similar populations or people who do not have the disease (controls) and compare the exposures that may have influenced disease risk. This is a quick, inexpensive technique which investigates a wide range of disease risks. Disadvantages include selection and information bias and the need to rely on past exposure.
- *Cohort studies* follow a defined study population over time. They may be *prospective*, i.e. followed

into the future, or *retrospective*, where a cohort characterized in the past is followed to the present. The advantages are that the prospective design minimizes bias, while long-term follow-up and the expense involved may be disadvantages.

- *Intervention trials* are when the researcher recruits individuals and then assigns them randomly to receive or not receive a treatment. These may be individual *clinical trials*; or *community trials* when a whole community/population is assigned to receive the treatment and is then compared with another community that does not receive the same treatment. The advantages of intervention trials are that they can provide direct evidence of cause-and-effect relationships. The disadvantages are that they may take a long time, can be expensive and may raise ethical issues. They can also only assess one or two factors at a time.

Some terminology related to intervention trials may be relevant.

- *Randomized* is when selection of the individual or community to receive or not receive the treatment/intervention is completely random, thus eliminating selection bias.
- *Placebo controlled* is when the randomly selected individual or group who is not to receive the treatment receives instead only the vehicle or some innocuous substance that appears identical to what the individual/group selected for the treatment arm receives.
- *Blinded* is when the selected recipient does not know or is not aware if he/she is receiving the treatment or a placebo. A trial is said to be *double blind* if neither the investigator who dishes out the treatment nor the recipient who receives it knows whether what is administered is a treatment or placebo.

Sample size

For all the study designs outlined above a sample size comprising an adequate number of subjects is crucial to allow effects to be detected. Statistical techniques are used in combination with knowledge of the anticipated strength of the association to derive the adequate sample size for any study. If too many subjects are recruited the study becomes cumbersome and expensive, while too few subjects will make the study under-powered and worthless.

The data analysis and interpretation of epidemiological studies are outlined in Box 11.1.

10.3 Nutritional Interventions and Infections in Childhood

Early initiation of and exclusive breastfeeding

Early initiation of breastfeeding is not a serious problem in developing countries since initiation of breastfeeding is almost universal in the countries studied. However, initiation rates remain low in many high-income countries, particularly among the low-income groups in their populations. Intervention strategies to promote exclusive breastfeeding of infants up to 6 months of age and to sustain continued breastfeeding thereafter up to 12 months of age have been evaluated based on a review that analysed 34 trials of 29,385 mother–infant pairs in 14 countries. This review provided evidence that any form of extra support provided to the mother increased the duration of both partial and exclusive breastfeeding up to 6 months. All forms of additional support affected the duration of exclusive breastfeeding significantly. A review of specific breastfeeding promotion showed that both individual counselling and group counselling of mothers substantially increased (with odds ratios of 1.93 and 5.19, respectively) exclusive breastfeeding at 6 months of age.

A review of intervention trials and observational studies in developed and developing country settings, which examined the potential benefits and drawbacks of exclusive breastfeeding for up to 6 months of age, showed that exclusively breastfed infants had no growth deficits in infant weight gain or in increase in length. The infants experienced less morbidity due to gastrointestinal infection compared with partially breastfed infants.

Interventions that promote child growth and development and prevent undernutrition

Complementary feeding

Complementary feeding is the provision of foods and liquids along with continued breastfeeding of infants, generally after the period of exclusive breastfeeding, when the young infant is introduced to other foods. The nutrient intake of an infant usually deteriorates when complementary foods start to substitute for breast milk. Hence, many of the interventions that are focused on complementary feeding include those that provide additional nutrients, especially micronutrients and energy, and also use nutrition education to ensure appropriate, adequate and safe provision of complementary feeds.

Interventions that improve intake of complementary foods by infants aged 6 to 12 months in developing countries have been shown to have a positive impact on their growth and nutrition. Studies conducted on complementary feeding in developing countries have been reviewed extensively. Although these studies varied in terms of the age of the infant at intervention, the composition of the complementary food and the extent of breastfeeding at the same time, several of them demonstrated an increase in the weight and length of the infant. Nutrition education aimed at improving complementary feeding of infants also showed an increase in height-for-age used as the indicator, compared with control groups who were not targeted. In food-insecure populations in developing country settings however, educational interventions were of benefit only if they were combined with food supplements being provided to the infant.

A review of the impact of complementary feeding interventions on morbidity can be summarized as showing that: (i) educational interventions reduced diarrhoea in Brazil and upper respiratory infections in Vietnam; (ii) milk fortification demonstrated significant effects on both diarrhoea and acute lower respiratory illness in India; and (iii) the use of micronutrient sprinkles showed beneficial effects on diarrhoea and fever in Pakistan.

Supplementary feeding

Supplementary feeding implies the provision of extra food to infants and children over and above the normal ration of their daily home diets. This intervention merits evaluation since several community-based programmes in many parts of the world have a component of supplementary feeding aimed at improving child health and nutrition. A review focusing on evaluation of the effectiveness of supplementary feeding of pre-school children at the community level was unable to draw any useful conclusions on the effectiveness and benefits of supplementary feeding. Universal and untargeted supplementary feeding programmes may not be cost-effective and beneficial.

Behaviour and practices of caregivers

The practices of caregivers (i.e. people who take care of others including infants and children, most often they are family members) are crucial in ensuring the nutrition and health of children. Caregivers provide food, health care, psychosocial stimulation and the emotional support necessary for the healthy growth and development of children. These care-giving practices and the ways in which they are performed are critical for survival, optimum growth and proper development of children and in the prevention of undernutrition. A WHO review concluded that interventions that incorporate care components are effective and identified several important conditions to maximize their impact. They concluded that benefits accrue if interventions are targeted at the early phase of the life cycle – both prenatally and in infancy. Targeting children in poor households, employing several types of interventions with more than one delivery channel and with a high level of parental involvement were preconditions for success. A study in Ghana showed a close association of better scores for care practices with lower levels of stunting and underweight in children, emphasizing the importance of care practices on the nutritional status of infants and children.

Micronutrient supplementation on child growth and risk of infection

Micronutrient supplementation – either singly or as micronutrient mixes – has been used as an intervention strategy to improve child nutrition as well as to reduce the infectious disease burden which in turn has an impact on child undernutrition. Micronutrients have also been added to interventions with complementary foods or during supplementary feeding interventions in the community.

Iron supplementation resulted in weight gain in anaemic children but had variable impact on improving height, while the risk of diarrhoeal disease apparently seemed to increase. These interventions with iron supplements to children demonstrate the adverse effects of additional iron on infectious diseases risk with no major gains with regard to growth.

Zinc supplementation or fortification of foods, on the other hand, reduces morbidity and mortality due to diarrhoeal disease and respiratory illness. A meta-analysis of 25 studies provided good evidence of an overall small but significant impact on height of children with zinc supplementation. This effect was only seen in children who had evidence of stunting.

Vitamin A supplementation of young infants is expected to reduce morbidity and mortality but the overall findings are largely variable, with several randomized controlled trials failing to show any benefit on risk of infections and growth. However, several randomized trials with vitamin A supplements to children between the ages of 6 months and 5 years showed that child mortality was reduced, as was mortality associated with diarrhoeal disease and measles. Supplementation of vitamin A to newborn infants reduced mortality in the first 6 months of life.

Multiple micronutrient supplements also provide variable impact, with improvements noted in stunted children in Vietnam and Mexico but no impact on growth in Peru and Guatemala.

Considering the major infectious diseases that contribute both to mortality and morbidity in children separately may provide helpful insights. A critical review of randomized trials of nutritional interventions on ALRTI morbidity and mortality in children indicates that: (i) zinc supplementation in zinc-deficient children prevents 25% of ALRTI episodes; (ii) promotion of breastfeeding reduces ALRTI morbidity; (iii) iron supplementation alone does not reduce ALRTI incidence; and (iv) vitamin A supplementation does not reduce ALRTI incidence or mortality.

DIARRHOEAL DISEASE. Micronutrient intervention trials have also been aimed at the reduction of the incidence of diarrhoeal disease in children and the morbidity and mortality related to it. The results can be generally summarized as indicating that: (i) zinc supplementation significantly lowers the incidence of diarrhoeal disease and reduces its risk, also reducing the incidence of persistent diarrhoea; (ii) zinc is a useful adjuvant in the management of diarrhoeal illness in children along with oral replacement therapy, helping to reduce the duration of diarrhoea and promoting early recovery; (iii) vitamin A reduces diarrhoeal disease incidence and severity in pre-school children, reduces morbidity and mortality, and protects against diarrhoeal disease risk; (iv) iron shows a modest probably, non-significant effect on diarrhoeal disease risk, although in endemic areas it increases risk of clinical malaria; and (v) breast-feeding promotion and proper complementary/supplementary feeding are paramount in reducing risk of diarrhoeal diseases in children.

MEASLES. Measles is another important infectious disease that contributes to raising the infectious disease morbidity and mortality in children. Summarizing intervention studies suggests that: (i) vitamin A (in high doses) improves recovery, decreases the duration of the illness, reduces the risk of secondary complications post-measles and decreases mortality; and (ii) the few studies conducted to address the question of clinical benefits with zinc supplementation have shown no difference in the clinical outcome of measles. It is of course important to remember that immunization against measles is a major preventive measure.

MALARIA. Apart from the crucial role that iron supplementation has on the incidence and risk of malaria and malaria parasitaemia, a proper evaluation of the role of other micronutrients on malarial infections in children is not possible at the current time. However, the few studies in the literature suggest the following: (i) a meta-analysis of iron intervention studies concluded that iron supplementation did not significantly increase the incidence of infections; (ii) vitamin A supplementation to malaria-exposed children reduced the risk of malarial episodes in Papua New Guinea, but not in Ghana; and (iii) similarly, intervention studies with zinc in children found a reduction in the risk of malaria episodes in Papua New Guinea that was not confirmed in a similar study in Burkina Faso.

Other interventions to prevention and treat infections in children

Treatment of infections and parasitic infestations also has a positive impact on child growth and nutrition. De-worming and use of anti-helminthics is particularly effective in children. A systematic review of 25 studies has documented the impact of single and multiple doses of anti-helminthics on the growth of children. A single dose of anti-helminthic was associated with increases in body weight and height of children; a benefit that was not improved upon by several doses a year.

Other interventions that are beneficial include those that promote hand-washing, water quality treatment, sanitation and health education. All of these interventions reduce the risk of diarrhoeal disease and thus have an impact on promoting child nutrition and health. These are clearly strategies that emphasize the role of poor environments and poor hygiene as important underlying causes of child undernutrition and its vicious and cyclic interaction with infectious disease.

Adapted from and based on the international recommendations recently published by the Maternal and Child Undernutrition Study Group, Table 10.3 summarizes the interventions for better infant and child nutrition, optimal growth and good health.

Table 10.3. Interventions for optimal infant and child nutrition, growth and health in developing countries. (Adapted from Bhutta et al., 2008.)

Educational and promotional strategies for breastfeeding	Exclusive breast-feeding recommended for first 6 months
Educational strategies for better and safe complementary feeding	Breastfeeding to be continued up to 2 years when complementary foods are introduced and added to diet of infants and children
Ensure adequate micronutrient intakes during complementary feeding – strategies include supplementation, dietary diversification and fortification	Evidence of positive impact of improved zinc, vitamin A, iron and iodine micronutrient status. Includes decreased mortality, reduction in incidence of diarrhoea and respiratory infections, and reduced diarrhoeal morbidity. Reduced mortality and disease burden in infants and children. Multiple micronutrient supplements and fortified foods beneficial
Prevent infections: hygienic interventions – hand-washing, clean water and sanitation; de-worming in childhood	Hygienic interventions like hand-washing reduce gastrointestinal infections. De-worming improves micronutrient status and promotes growth
Encourage use of probiotics	Probiotics reduce risk of diarrhoea

Further Reading

Bhutta, Z.A., Ahmed, T., Black, R.E., Cousens, S., Dewey, K., Giugliani, E., Haider, B.A., Kirkwood, B., Morris, S.S., Sachdev, H.P.S. and Shekar, M., for the Maternal and Child Undernutrition Study Group (2008) Maternal and child undernutrition: what works? Interventions for maternal and child undernutrition and survival. *Lancet* 371, 417–440. *A recent comprehensive review of interventions that affect maternal and child undernutrition and nutrition-related outcomes.*

Black, R.E., Allen, L.H., Bhutta, Z.A., Caulfield, L.E., de Onis, M., Ezzati, M., Mathers, C. and Rivera, J., for the Maternal and Child Undernutrition Study Group (2008) Maternal and child undernutrition: global and regional exposures and health consequences. *Lancet* 371, 243–269. *A recent comprehensive review that estimates the effects of risks related to measures of undernutrition and poor breastfeeding practices on mortality and disease.*

Langseth, L. (1996) *Nutritional Epidemiology: Possibilities and Limitations.* International Life Sciences Institute Europe, Brussels. *A valuable monograph and source book in nutritional epidemiology written for students with a general background in life sciences.*

Case Studies

Case Study 10.1: Summary of epidemiological studies on exclusive breastfeeding and clinical outcomes.

Table 10.4 summarizes data from some of the important studies carried out in developing country settings that have investigated and documented the benefits of exclusive breastfeeding on infectious disease morbidity related to diarrhoea and acute respiratory infections (ARIs) and on child mortality.

Irrespective of the location of the study in the developing world or the general economic development status of the country and the socio-economic

Table 10.4. Summary data on the benefits of exclusive breastfeeding on infectious disease morbidity. (Adapted from Bhutta *et al.*, 2003.)

Location and studies	Intervention	Clinical outcome
WHO Study Team; pooled analysis of studies from Brazil, Gambia, Ghana, Pakistan, Philippines and Senegal	EBF versus MF or FF	OR for mortality 5.8 in non-breastfed infants <2 months of age
India, urban hospital setting; prospective cohort study	EBF versus MF	Similar birth weights but better weight gain in 2 months in EBF group. EBF had only 40 sickness episodes versus 69 in MF. Diarrhoea 1 per 100 child-months in EBF versus 20 per 100 child-months in MF group
India, hospital setting; randomized clinical study	Morbidity and mortality based on record of first 7 days in rural hospital setting	EBF lowest mortality (29%) compared with no breastfeeding (64%)
Brazil, urban hospital setting; case–control study	Cases of infant deaths identified and compared with 2 matched controls for each	MF infants had RR for death from diarrhoea of 4.2 compared with EBF infants. Those receiving no breast milk at all had RR of 14.2. RR for death from respiratory infections 1.6 for MF and 3.6 for not breastfed at all compared with EBF
Philippines, urban hospital setting; prospective clinical study	9886 newborn infants followed up	Infants with diarrhoea: 90% FF, 6% PBF, 4% EBF. Infant deaths: 96% FF compared with 3% EBF

WHO, World Health Organization; EBF, exclusive breastfeeding/exclusively breastfed; MF, mixed feeding/mixed fed; FF, formula feeding/formula fed; OR, odds ratio; RR, relative risk; PBF, partial breastfeeding/partially breastfed.

and geographical setting (urban or rural) of the community investigated, the limited summary in Table 10.4 confirms the enormous health benefit to infants who are exclusively breastfed. They have significantly less morbidity due to diarrhoeal disease and in one study from Brazil for ARI compared with partially breastfed (or mixed-fed) infants or infants who were not breastfed at all and had formula feeds only. In two studies at least (Brazil and the Philippines) and based on the odds ratio (5.8) observed in the World Health Organization collaborative study, the worst clinical outcomes with infectious disease morbidity and child mortality are in the non-breastfed or formula-fed group.

Reference

Bhutta, Z.A., Ahmed, T., Black, R.E., Cousens, S., Dewey, K., Giugliani, E., Haider, B.A., Kirkwood, B., Morris, S.S., Sachdev, H.P.S. and Shekar, M., for the Maternal and Child Undernutrition Study Group (2008) Maternal and child undernutrition: what works? Interventions for maternal and child undernutrition and survival. *Lancet* 371, 417–440.

11 Maternal Nutrition, Infections and Birth Outcomes

- Maternal undernutrition and micronutrient deficiencies are associated with increased morbidity and mortality that are directly related to compromise in the host's defence mechanisms.
- Nutritional deficiencies in the mother can lead to intrauterine growth retardation, resulting in low birth weight and other poor birth outcomes.
- Intrauterine growth retardation and small for gestational age are associated with reduced immune function and increased neonatal and post-neonatal morbidity and mortality.
- Intrauterine growth retardation and low birth weight have other consequences, including increased risk of adult-onset diseases.
- Nutritional interventions can improve birth weight and reduce incidence of low birth weight.
- Nutritional interventions in pregnancy can improve maternal health and reduce maternal morbidity and mortality.

11.1 Introduction

In most developing countries maternal undernutrition is pervasive and is an important contributor to maternal morbidity and mortality and poor birth outcomes. The prevalence of maternal undernutrition and micronutrient deficiencies is high in many regions of the world. Maternal undernutrition characterized by short stature and/or low body weight and low BMI is a major cause of adverse pregnancy outcomes since the nutritional status of a woman before and during pregnancy is an important determinant of healthy birth outcomes. Short stature in women of reproductive age is a risk factor for assisted delivery or delivery by Caesarean section, a situation compounded by poor access to medical care and increasing the risk to mother and infant. Access to proper obstetric care also implies increased risk of maternal morbidity and even mortality due to the operative intervention and hospitalization.

Lower-than-appropriate maternal body weight, indicated by low pre-pregnancy BMI and inadequate weight gain during pregnancy, and maternal micronutrient deficiencies, are associated with IUGR and LBW which increases risk in the newborn. Maternal micronutrient deficiencies will influence the micronutrient stores in the newborn. While maternal undernutrition has no impact on breast milk output, maternal micronutrient deficiencies will be reflected in the composition of the milk and hence will be an important determinant of the micronutrient status of the breastfed infant.

The high prevalence of undernutrition and micronutrient deficiency diseases in pregnant women has led to interventions to supplement nutrients as well as micronutrients or to reduce loss due to infections (malaria, worms, etc.) with therapeutic regimes like de-worming or chemoprophylaxis as for instance against malaria. These interventions in women of reproductive age are expected to improve maternal nutrition in pregnancy and reduce maternal mortality, and in turn have beneficial impact on birth outcomes and child nutrition.

11.2 Intrauterine Growth Restriction and Low Birth Weight

Maternal undernutrition and its consequent impact on fetal and infant nutrition is a major public health problem in developing countries. Birth weight is one of the best indicators of nutritional status of the newborn infant. A newborn infant weighing less than 2500 g is considered to be an

Box 11.1. Basics of Nutritional Epidemiology: Data Analysis, Expression of Associations and Interpretation.

On completion of an epidemiological study or clinical trial, the data collected and cleaned will then be subject to analysis and interpretation using rigorous statistical techniques.

Data analysis and expression of associations

The objectives of the data analysis are to determine whether associations exist between exposures and outcomes and also to assess the strength of these associations. The direction and the strength of this association will provide information on the causal linkages, if any, between the exposure and the outcome. These associations are often expressed as relative risk or odds ratios.

- *Relative risk*: Relative risk (RR) is the ratio of the outcome rate among individuals who are exposed to a factor/causal agent divided by the outcome rate among other individuals who are not exposed to the factor/agent. If the RR is >1.0 then those individuals who are exposed to the factor or agent are at increased risk of the outcome, while RR of <1.0 implies that those exposed are less at risk of the outcome and may suggest that there is a protective effect of the factor. While the direction of the relative risk indicates deleterious or protective effects, the strength of the association is also a useful indicator. For instance, an RR of 10.0 may indicate a strong association compared with an RR of 1.5. Also, an RR of 2.0 implies a 100% increase or a doubling of risk, while an RR of 0.37 implies only a third of the risk. The strength of the association is useful in helping to prioritize public health measures. RR is also referred to as the *risk ratio*.
- *Odds ratio*: In case–control studies an odds ratio (OR) may sometimes be used instead of RR and signifies the odds of exposure for cases to the equivalent odds for controls. The OR is particularly useful when investigating relatively rare conditions or diseases. Like with RR, an OR of >1.0 implies increased risk and an OR of <1.0 signifies reduced risk.

Two more parameters used to analyse the results of an epidemiological study or clinical trial are attributable risk and population attributable risk.

- *Attributable risk* is the extent to which the occurrence of a disease or outcome can be attributed to that particular factor/agent. Attributable risk is different from RR or OR.
- *Population attributable risk* (PAR) indicates the proportion of all cases in a defined population

which may be attributed to the specific factor/agent. PAR reflects both the RR and the frequency of the factor in the population. This is a useful measure because it helps one decide whether efforts in modifying the factor are likely to have substantial impact on public health.

The data analysis must also consider three factors as follows.

- *Chance*: One must consider the possibility that an observed association between an exposure and an outcome may be due purely to chance. Statistical tests of significance can assess this possibility. A finding is considered significant if there is only a 5% likelihood that it is due to chance.
- *Bias*: Bias is a systematic error that may result in over- or underestimation of the strength of an association between an exposure and an outcome.
- *Confounding*: Confounding results from factors that are unequally distributed in a population and give rise to spurious associations. Statistical techniques can be used to adjust for confounding.

Interpretation

Interpretation of the results is the final step to be carried out once the effects of chance, bias and confounding have been taken care of. Two techniques are used for interpreting the results of several studies that assess a set of related research hypotheses.

- *Meta-analysis*: The interpretation of epidemiological findings becomes difficult if studies do not always conform and the results conflict with one another. In this situation inconsistency is resolved through meta-analysis. This is a quantitative technique in which the statistical results of several studies are pooled to yield overall conclusions. A pooled analysis of the results providing an overall estimate of the effect is the meta-analysis, and a meta-analysis should be based on a systematic review of all the available literature.
- *Systematic review*: Results from different study designs do not offer information of equal weight; the strongest evidence of association comes from experimental trials while it is weakest with ecological and cross-sectional studies. The findings of any study must be considered in the context of those from other literature reports on the topic. A systematic approach is required to take into consideration the various studies and their results. This process of carrying out a thorough and complete analysis of all the data is referred to as a systematic review.

LBW infant. There are two types of LBW infants: (i) those born *premature*, i.e. before the completion of 37 weeks of gestational age; and (ii) those having IUGR who are born *small for gestational age* (SGA). SGA is also defined based on a cut-off of birth weight below the 10th percentile of weight-for-gestational-age. SGA infants are born at full term but are underweight.

Causes of intrauterine growth restriction and low birth weight

According to the WHO, 30 million infants are born each year with LBW, which accounts for nearly 24% of all births and almost 95% of them in developing countries. There are many causes of IUGR – some fetal, some maternal and others due to problems with the placenta (Table 11.1). Fetal causes of LBW include birth defects, which often cause premature births, and fetal infections like cytomegalovirus and rubella. The maternal causes of IUGR include: chronic health problems like hypertension and diabetes mellitus; smoking, particularly during pregnancy, which can double the risk of IUGR; excess alcohol consumption in pregnancy, which limits fetal growth and may cause birth defects; maternal infections, both those affecting the reproductive system like urinary tract infections and generalized infections like malaria, TB and HIV/AIDS; and nutritional deficiencies.

Nutritional deficiencies in pregnancy that increase risk of IUGR-related LBW are associated with poor socio-economic circumstances and poverty and are an important cause of the high incidence of LBW in developing countries. In developed countries IUGR-related LBW is attributed mostly to adolescent pregnancy where there is competition for nutrients between the young mother who is still growing and the fetus, resulting in her inability to mobilize energy stores to enhance fetal growth which are reserved for her own continued growth. Adolescent pregnancy is also an important cause of LBW in developing countries.

The nutritional causes of LBW are short stature, low pre-pregnancy body weight and BMI, inadequate weight gain during pregnancy, and micronutrient deficiencies like anaemia. Maternal anaemia and low haemoglobin levels are associated with increased risk of LBW. In developing countries maternal iron deficiency is also positively associated with LBW, with numerous studies indicating an association between maternal indicators of iron

Table 11.1. Causes of IUGR.

Maternal causes	Chronic health problems, e.g. hypertension and diabetes mellitus
	Smoking during pregnancy
	Excess alcohol consumption in pregnancy
	Maternal nutritional deficiencies
	Short stature
	Low body weight and low BMI
	Inadequate weight gain in pregnancy
	Micronutrient deficiencies, e.g. iron and possibly zinc
	Maternal infections
	Affecting the reproductive system, e.g. urinary tract infections
	Generalized infections, e.g. malaria, TB and HIV/AIDS
Fetal causes	Birth defects and genetic disorders
	Fetal infections, e.g. cytomegalovirus and rubella
Placental causes	Inadequate placental growth
	Uterine malformations
	Decreased utero-placental blood flow
	Multiple gestations

status and birth weight of the offspring. Some studies suggest that maternal zinc deficiency may possibly contribute to increasing risk of LBW.

The immune system of infants develops mostly during intrauterine life but continues to grow and mature during infancy, i.e. the first few months after birth. Infants born prematurely and those with LBW as a result of IUGR are unlikely to have a fully developed immune system that is functional at birth. Nutrient deficiencies in the mother can induce changes in the immune system of her offspring. IUGR-related LBW is associated with compromised cell-mediated immunity and lymphocyte function. IUGR infants demonstrate a reduced cell-mediated immunity and reduced numbers of T lymphocytes. These infants may continue to show reduced cell-mediated immunity for several months or even years thereafter. On the other hand, a premature LBW infant develops the ability to mount an immune response by the age of 3 months.

SGA infants have a higher morbidity and frequent illnesses due to the immune system abnormalities. A comparison of the frequency of infective episodes in IUGR-LBW infants with those in full-term, normal-weight infants shows that the first

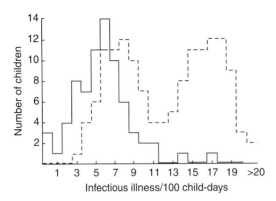

Fig. 11.1. Morbidity due to infectious illness episodes in infants with normal birth weight (—) compared with infants with LBW (– – –). (Adapted with permission from Chandra, 1988.)

peak almost coincides with that of the normal-weight children; this represents the morbidity due to infective episodes in these infants (see Fig. 11.1). The second peak represents the frequency of illness in LBW children who experience a higher morbidity due to more frequent illnesses. It is this group of LBW infants who have a much higher frequency of immune system abnormalities than normal infants.

Breastfeeding can supply a large number of protective factors. Maternal IgA in breast milk has a broad spectrum of antimicrobial activity, providing protection against a range of bacteria, viruses and even fungi. Breastfeeding is hence crucial in the nutrition of a newborn infant, especially an LBW infant.

Consequences of intrauterine growth restriction and low birth weight

The high proportion of births in developing countries which fall into the category of IUGR-LBW, while not in itself a direct cause of neonatal death, contributes indirectly to neonatal mortality caused by birth asphyxia and infections. Sepsis, pneumonia and diarrhoea are three infections that account for 60% of neonatal deaths. Estimates based from data collected from five studies in developing countries showed that LBW infants weighing between 1500 and 2000 g were eight times more likely, while those with birth weights between 2000 and 2500 g were nearly three times more likely, to die in the neonatal period compared with infants from the same communities who had normal birth weight, i.e. >2500 g. Examination of the cause of

neonatal death in these same studies showed that the relative risk of death due to infectious diseases was 4.2 in the 1500–2000 g group and 2.0 in those neonates who had a birth weight of 2000–2500 g. Table 11.2 shows the association between birth weight and neonatal and post-neonatal mortality in infants, expressed as relative risk.

The links between LBW and childhood morbidity and mortality have long been recognized. LBW is the major underlying risk factor for increased mortality during infancy as well as increased morbidity and the consequent increased risk of subsequent childhood undernutrition. Weight at birth is a good predictor of size in later adult life; IUGR infants demonstrate poor catch-up growth and thus the incidence of LBW is reflected in an increased prevalence of underweight in children. IUGR infants are also at greater risk of stunting during childhood and adolescence, and, like other children stunted due to poor nutrition, end up as short statured adults. Short stature pre-pregnancy is in turn a risk factor for IUGR and LBW, thus leading to the 'intergenerational' perpetuation of LBW and its consequences (see Fig. 11.2).

Poor maternal nutrition and the consequent fetal growth restriction result in poor birth outcomes. Not only is LBW an important factor that imposes an increased risk of morbidity, mortality and undernutrition in infancy and childhood, it is also now recognized to be a crucial determinant of an increased risk of adult-onset diseases. Extensive research has now established that adult mortality and morbidity are programmed by fetal nutrition and birth weight. LBW is related to adverse outcomes in adulthood including obesity, hypertension, diabetes mellitus and coronary artery disease. The evidence also seems to support the view that rapid catch-up growth of SGA infants may increase their risk of adult-onset diseases, evidence of which is indicated by higher blood pressures and higher

Table 11.2. Estimated relative risk of neonatal and post-neonatal mortality associated with birth weight. (Adapted from Ashworth, 1998.)

Birth weight (g)	Neonatal mortality	Post-neonatal mortality
>3500	0.3	0.5
3000–3499	0.4	0.5
2500–2999	1.0	1.0
2000–2499	4.0	2.0
1500–1999	18.0	5.0

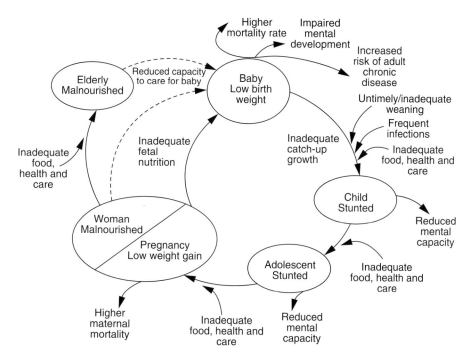

Fig. 11.2. Nutrition through the life cycle showing the effects of LBW, including increased risk of adult-onset diseases and the intergenerational effects of undernutrition. (Adapted from Report of the ACC/SCN Commission on the Nutrition Challenges of the 21st Century, 2000.)

blood glucose levels already evident in childhood. It is also well documented that undernourished children, particularly those who are stunted, show signs of increased risk of obesity and metabolic abnormalities in childhood.

Nutritional interventions to reduce low birth weight related to intrauterine growth restriction

Nutritional interventions have an important role to play in improving birth outcomes, and these interventions will have to target women both before and during pregnancy. Some interventions have been aimed at reducing maternal undernutrition at conception (manifested as small maternal size, i.e. short stature, underweight and low BMI), low gestational weight gain as well as micronutrient deficiencies, which are the principal attributable risk factors for IUGR and LBW. The evidence from well-designed intervention studies which address these issues in maternal nutrition and pregnancy outcomes will have to be examined and evaluated carefully to select those interventions that are suitable for up-scaling in large

communities and national populations. Table 11.3 summarizes the important nutritional intervention trials that have shown a benefit in birth weight or a reduction in incidence of LBW or both.

Interventions with energy and protein supplementation

Maternal food supplements that provided balanced protein and energy were the only community nutritional interventions that seem to have improved pregnancy outcome measured as improved birth weight. Antenatal intervention trials with balanced protein–energy supplements significantly improved fetal growth, reduced LBW and reduced the risk of fetal and neonatal deaths. Many of these nutritional intervention trials were largely conducted in developing countries and in some cases in poor inner-city communities in industrialized countries where the risk of LBW was high. Compared with nutritional interventions providing balanced protein–energy supplementation, protein supplements alone when provided during pregnancy were shown to be of negligible benefit.

Table 11.3. Interventions for improving birth weight and reducing LBW. (Adapted from Shetty, 2009.)

Interventions with additional protein–energy or food supplementation	Randomized controlled trials in Gambia, Thailand, Taiwan, Colombia and India (plus iron–folate) Quasi-experimental trials in Indonesia, Guatemala (two trials), Gambia and Colombia
Interventions with micronutrients	
Antenatal iron supplementation	Randomized controlled trials in India and Gambia
Antenatal folate supplementation	Randomized clinical trial in South Africa
Antenatal zinc supplementation	Randomized clinical trial in India
Antenatal iodine supplementation	Prospective cohort study in Zaire
Antenatal vitamin A supplementation	Randomized clinical trial in Malawi (plus iron–folate)
Antenatal multiple micronutrient supplementation	Randomized clinical trials in Nepal, Tanzania and South Africa

NUTRITIONAL INTERVENTIONS FOR ADOLESCENT MOTHERS. Pregnant adolescents are at increased risk of inadequate gestational weight gain and micronutrient malnutrition due to inadequate intakes in their diets to support healthy fetal growth and promote good birth outcomes. Reviews of community interventions in developed societies show a predominance of medical models providing prenatal care with little emphasis on nutrition education to alter prenatal dietary behaviours of adolescents. Positive effects on birth outcomes were evident when the approaches were driven by multidisciplinary teams supporting the nutritional and psychosocial needs of pregnant teenagers while individualized education and counselling encouraged optimal dietary intakes and appropriate gestational weight gain. However, as explained earlier, increase in gestational weight gain in adolescent pregnancy is no indication that optimal fetal growth has occurred since an adolescent mother's metabolism is geared to promote her own growth and the mobilization of nutrients to the developing fetus is not prioritized.

Interventions with micronutrient supplementation

Since micronutrient deficiencies are common in developing countries and some like anaemia seem to be associated with LBW, the impact of prenatal micronutrient supplementation – singly, in combination or as multiple micronutrient supplements – given to women in the reproductive age group in developing countries needs to be assessed carefully.

IRON SUPPLEMENTATION. In developing countries, maternal iron deficiency is positively associated with LBW and hence interventions to tackle iron deficiency in pregnancy are important. Meta-analysis of iron supplementation trials in pregnancy showed no detectable effect on birth outcome despite a significant reduction in maternal anaemia. Community-based iron supplementation trials in developing countries have also failed to demonstrate any improvement in birth weight apart from a study in India which showed a reduction in LBW rates with iron–folate supplementation from before 20 weeks of gestation, and another from rural Nepal where iron–folate supplementation slightly reduced the prevalence of LBW. Oral iron supplementation may improve maternal anaemia but has no clear demonstrable impact on birth weight – a conclusion that is drawn largely as a result of the paucity of robust trials of iron supplementation in community settings in developing countries.

FOLATE SUPPLEMENTATION. A study in South Africa in a tertiary hospital setting is the only one to show a significant decrease in the incidence of LBW births. Along with iron supplements, folic acid has a demonstrable impact on improving maternal haemoglobin levels. The evidence is very strong that periconceptual folate supplementation reduces neural tube defects and other birth defects, whereas its impact on other beneficial birth outcomes resulting from supplementation during pregnancy is doubtful. However, the combined administration of iron and folate in pregnancy seems to reduce the incidence of LBW.

ZINC SUPPLEMENTATION. A review of zinc supplementation trials showed that birth weight increased in four out of ten trials, but the composite results of the analysis of all ten trials on maternal zinc supplementation revealed no differences in birth outcome. Evidence from other community-based studies suggests that zinc supplementation does not have any impact on birth weight. Interestingly, two of the studies did show a reduction in incidence of infectious disease morbidity among LBW infants and mortality among SGA infants born to zinc-supplemented mothers. This obviously has enormous implications for reducing infant mortality and childhood malnutrition, particularly given that LBW infants are at increased risk of both these consequences.

OTHER MICRONUTRIENTS. Reports are available only for two other micronutrients – iodine and vitamin A. Neither iodine nor vitamin A supplementation trials have demonstrated any benefit on birth outcomes; although the studies show that iodine supplementation even in mid-pregnancy reduces deaths in infancy and early childhood, while vitamin A supplementation of pregnant mothers reduces maternal mortality.

MULTIPLE MICRONUTRIENT SUPPLEMENTATIONS. The benefits of multiple micronutrient supplements during pregnancy may be potentially high given the increased demand on nutrients for fetal growth. However, community-based intervention trials have not provided clear evidence from studies in developing countries because either the data are limited or the community intervention programmes under evaluation are so varied. In addition, many of the trials are complicated by the provision of additional energy or protein or food supplements alongside the micronutrient supplements.

A recent review has shown that multiple micronutrient supplementation during pregnancy resulted in a decrease in both LBW and SGA infants. There is also some evidence that suggests that multiple micronutrient supplements are not superior to iron–folate supplements alone. A meta-analysis comparing multiple micronutrients with folic acid and iron combination reported a small increase in birth weight with the iron–folate supplementation reducing the risk of LBW. However, another recent report highlights the fact that the effects of antenatal multiple micronutrient supplementations during pregnancy on the fetus persist into childhood, with increases in both body weight and body size in those infants born to mothers who were supplemented.

Other maternal interventions to reduce intrauterine growth restriction and low birth weight

Other interventions during pregnancy that may have a beneficial effect on birth outcomes include those that reduce the risk of maternal infections, particularly ones that may increase the risk of nutritional deficiencies. These include interventions to reduce infections like malaria and worm infestations, which cause maternal anaemia.

Prevention of maternal infections

Maternal infections have an adverse impact on birth outcomes. These infections include malaria, which greatly increases the risk of maternal anaemia and increases the risk of preterm birth, LBW and neonatal mortality. The estimated population attributable risk of LBW among primigravidae with malaria is 10 to 40%. Hookworm infections and the associated maternal anaemia is another problem, and so too are maternal STDs like HIV, syphilis and gonorrhoea.

Malaria chemoprophylaxis of mothers has been the main option in malaria-endemic areas, although its efficacy is uncertain compared with intermittent presumptive treatment. A review of 15 trials has shown that infants born to mothers on malaria chemoprophylaxis were heavier, especially so if they were born to primigravidae (first pregnancy). In rural Uganda, primigravidae on chloroquine (used here as a chemoprophylaxis for malaria) had a significantly lower LBW rate (2% in the treatment group versus 9% in the control or placebo group). Other studies in Africa also support the findings of a benefit related to improved birth weights associated with malaria chemoprophylaxis during pregnancy. The increase in birth weight observed in almost all studies provides strong evidence for the beneficial effect of malaria chemoprophylaxis on birth weight in malaria-endemic areas. Compared with chemoprophylaxis, use of insecticide-treated bed nets as a preventive measure has been shown to have little impact on birth weights although they were effective in reducing maternal mortality and morbidity from malaria.

De-worming is an accepted strategy to tackle helminthic infections like hookworm, which affect maternal health and haemoglobin status. The summary evidence based on several small trials does favour de-worming as being effective in reducing maternal anaemia, improving maternal haemoglobin status and having some benefit in improving birth weights. Maternal treatment of urinary tract infections and STDs with antibiotics also has been shown to have benefits with regard to improving birth outcomes.

Other interventions to promote maternal health

Data on the effect of cessation of smoking during pregnancy on birth outcomes are largely from industrialized countries and they seem to present mixed results on birth outcomes such as preterm birth or LBW rates. The important related issue from a developing country perspective is to study the impact of maternal environmental exposure to smoke and the beneficial effects of the reduction to solid-fuel smoke exposure. This topic has not been examined systematically in developing countries and hence no firm conclusions can be drawn, although one would expect it to benefit the mother and reduce the risk of maternal morbidity and illness.

11.3   Nutrition, Maternal Mortality and Morbidity

Estimates by WHO along with other international bodies indicate that worldwide 536,000 maternal deaths occurred in 2005, 99% of which were in developing countries. Half of these deaths occurred in sub-Saharan Africa, with South Asia not far behind. One of the Millennium Development Goals is to reduce maternal mortality ratio (MMR) by three-quarters by the year 2015. MMR is highest in developing countries at 450 maternal deaths per 100,000 live births, compared with 9 deaths per 100,000 live births in developed countries.

Maternal deaths may be the result of *direct obstetric deaths*, i.e. resulting from obstetric complications of pregnancy, or from *indirect obstetric deaths*, i.e. those resulting from previous pre-existing disease or diseases that developed during pregnancy. The term *pregnancy-related death* includes all maternal deaths as it encompasses any death that occurs during pregnancy, child birth or postpartum. The four major causes of maternal deaths are: (i) severe bleeding, mostly postpartum; (ii) infections, also mostly after delivery; (iii) hypertensive disorders of pregnancy, including eclampsia; and (iv) obstructed labour. Unsafe abortions also contribute to infections and death. Pre-existing maternal health conditions, including anaemia, malaria and HIV/AIDS, have further impact on the principal causes of maternal mortality.

Maternal infections are responsible for 15% of maternal deaths. Maternal nutritional status and immune function will influence the risk of puerperal infections, one of which is maternal tetanus.

However, it is important to recognize that risk of maternal infection is largely influenced by the quality of health care, such as following the basic rules of asepsis during labour. Inadequate sterilization and disinfection and limited access to medical supplies and drugs aggravate the problem. Lowering the rates and severity of maternal infection is crucial. Obstructed labour, another important cause of maternal mortality, is related to a woman's age and parity; young and adolescent mothers and birth of the first child are important risk factors. Nutritional factors include maternal height and cephalo-pelvic disproportion, the latter often evident in short stature or nutritionally stunted mothers. Toxaemia of pregnancy, or pregnancy-induced hypertension and eclampsia, is another important cause of maternal mortality where again micronutrients like calcium, zinc and magnesium may be implicated.

Micronutrient deficiencies and maternal mortality and morbidity
Maternal anaemia, mortality and morbidity

It is estimated that about half of the pregnant women in the world are anaemic; hence even in the developed world anaemia in pregnancy is a problem of public health significance. Estimates of MMR attributable to anaemia may be high in many developing countries. The relative risk of maternal death in anaemic women compared with that in non-anaemic mothers in developing country situations may be as high as 5.9 in rural areas and 2.0 in urban areas. Along with obstetric haemorrhage, anaemia may be responsible for between 17 and 46% of maternal deaths, although this may depend highly on the underlying cause of anaemia such as iron deficiency, HIV, etc. It is even more difficult to quantify the part played by anaemia in maternal morbidity.

Iron deficiency anaemia causes abnormalities in immune function and increases the risk of premature labour and LBW. The increased demand for iron in pregnancy increases the risk of anaemia in this physiological state. Adequate iron stores can cope with this increased demand, but supplementation of iron helps meet the extra need. Vitamin A deficiency in pregnancy can also contribute to anaemia since this nutrient plays an important role in haematopoiesis and is required for mobilization and utilization of iron by the body. Folate and B_{12}

Table 11.4. Interventions for optimal maternal health and birth outcomes in developing countries. (Adapted from Bhutta *et al.*, 2008.)

Intervention	Outcome(s)
Maternal supplementation with balanced energy–protein supplements in pregnancy	Reduction in IUGR births
	Reduced risk of stillbirths
Food fortification including iodization of salt	Improved micronutrient status in women of childbearing age
	Reduced goitre prevalence
Iron–folate and multivitamin supplements in pregnancy	Improved micronutrient status
	Reduced maternal anaemia
Maternal calcium supplementation	Reduced risk of pre-eclampsia
	Maternal mortality or serious morbidity reduced
Delayed cord clamping	Improved iron status of neonate
Malaria chemoprophylaxis	Increases birth weight
	Reduces LBW
	Reduces maternal anaemia
Insecticide-treated bed nets	Reduces risk of delivering LBW infant
De-worming in pregnancy	Improved micronutrient status
	Less decline in haemoglobin during pregnancy

deficiencies can also contribute to the problem of anaemia in pregnancy. Infections like malaria and HIV, and helminthic infestations of the gastrointestinal tract, can cause or aggravate the problem of anaemia in pregnancy.

Iron deficiency anaemia is associated with compromise of immune function manifested as reduced cell-mediated immunity, reduced bacterial killing ability and lowered proportions of T and B lymphocytes. These immunological abnormalities increase the risk of maternal infections, in addition to the other problems associated with anaemia such as the higher risk of antepartum haemorrhage as reported from Kenya.

Nutritional interventions to reduce risk of maternal mortality

Consumption of foods fortified with iron, or supplementation with iron and folate or iron alone, is assumed to reduce the risk of maternal anaemia and hence reduce the risk of maternal mortality by 23%. Two studies which assessed the impact of iron fortification in women of childbearing age and one in pregnant women demonstrated a significant increase in maternal haemoglobin levels. Iron–folate supplementation during pregnancy resulted in a rise in haemoglobin and a 73% reduction in anaemia at the end of pregnancy. Trials with vitamin A and β-carotene in Bangladesh and Nepal showed inconsistent results related to maternal mortality. The same was apparently the case with zinc supplementation of mothers.

Chemoprophylaxis for malaria prevention in pregnancy showed a reduction of 12% in maternal anaemia, while use of insecticide-treated nets to reduce risk of malaria did not seem to benefit maternal anaemia although risk of malaria was reduced considerably. A single-dose treatment of helminthic infections during pregnancy, which are responsible for anaemia, is more effective in reducing maternal anaemia than providing iron plus folate supplements alone throughout pregnancy.

Micronutrients like calcium, zinc and magnesium may play a role in pregnancy-induced hypertension and eclampsia in pregnancy. A review of 12 intervention trials with over 15,000 pregnant women showed that calcium supplementation during pregnancy reduced the risk of pre-eclampsia significantly (relative risk = 0.48). The effects of calcium supplementation were best seen in pregnant women who were either at high risk of hypertensive disorders of pregnancy (relative risk = 0.22) or had low serum calcium levels to begin with (relative risk = 0.36). Calcium supplementation also significantly reduced the risk of maternal mortality and serious morbidity. Zinc and magnesium supplementation have shown inconsistent results with regard to reducing the risk of pregnancy-induced hypertension.

Intervention strategies that aim to improve maternal nutrition and health are the most significant interventions since they also confer better pregnancy outcomes. An adequate and diversified diet promotes weight gain in pregnancy, and hence food supplements or balanced energy–protein supplementation may be used to target vulnerable groups such as undernourished low-BMI pregnant women and adolescent mothers. Multivitamin supplements have shown to be effective in improving not only maternal health and birth outcomes, but also subsequent infant growth and health.

Table 11.4 summarizes the most important interventions for maternal health and good pregnancy outcomes that are supported by evidence from intervention studies and trials. The table is based on the international recommendations published recently by the Maternal and Child Undernutrition Study Group.

Further Reading

Bhutta, Z.A., Ahmed, T., Black, R.E., Cousens, S., Dewey, K., Giugliani, E., Haider, B.A., Kirkwood, B., Morris, S.S., Sachdev, H.P.S. and Shekar, M., for the Maternal and Child Undernutrition Study Group (2008) Maternal and child undernutrition: what works? Interventions for maternal and child undernutrition and survival. *Lancet* 371, 417–440. *A recent comprehensive review of interventions that affect maternal and child undernutrition and nutrition-related outcomes.*

Black, R.E., Allen, L.H., Bhutta, Z.A., Caulfield, L.E., de Onis, M., Ezzati, M., Mathers, C. and Rivera, J., for the Maternal and Child Undernutrition Study Group (2008) Maternal and child undernutrition: global and regional exposures and health consequences. *Lancet* 371, 243–269. *A recent comprehensive review that estimates the effects of risks related to measures of undernutrition and on Maternal mortality and disease.*

Langseth, L. (1996) *Nutritional Epidemiology: Possibilities and Limitations.* International Life Sciences Institute Europe, Brussels. *A valuable monograph and source book in nutritional epidemiology written for students with a general background in life sciences.*

Case Studies

Case Study 11.1: Community-based studies of intrauterine growth retardation and mortality and morbidity.

This case study examines the association between infant and child mortality and birth weight. These community-based epidemiological studies have been made in developing country settings and have followed up a cohort of full-term infants some of whom have low birth weight (LBW) due to intrauterine growth retardation (IUGR). As shown in Table 11.5, the outcomes are either all-cause mortality or morbidity associated with

Table 11.5. Data on the association between infant and child mortality and birth weight. (Adapted from Ashworth, 1998.)

Study location (year)	Age (months)	Birth weight range (g)	Clinical outcome	Relative risk
Brazil (1996)	0–6	3000–3499	All-cause mortality	1.0
		1500–2499		6.6
India (1979)	0–11	>2500	All-cause mortality	1.0
		2000–2499		2.6
India (1978)	0–11	>2500	All-cause mortality	1.0
		<2500		1.7
Guatemala (1978)	0–11	>2500	All cause mortality	1.0
		<2500		1.7
Brazil (1996)	0–6	3000–3499	Diarrhoea	1.0
		1500–2499		1.3
Ethiopia (1994)	3–40	>2500	All infectious morbidity	1.0
		<2500		1.5
India (1993)	0–3	>2500		1.0
		1500–2499	Diarrhoea	2.4
			Respiratory infection	3.6
Guatemala (1991)	0–3	>2500	Sepsis and respiratory	1.0
		<2500	infection	3.0

diarrhoeal disease or lower respiratory tract infections, and are expressed as relative risk compared with that in infants of normal birth weight (relative risk = 1.0).

Careful scrutiny of the data in Table 11.5 shows that the relative risk of all-cause mortality is high among the IUGR infants. The risk of infectious disease morbidity and illnesses such as diarrhoeas and respiratory infections is higher in the LBW infants.

Reference

Ashworth, A. (1998) Effects of intrauterine growth retardation on mortality and morbidity in infants and young children. *European Journal of Clinical Nutrition* 52, S34–S42.

Case Study 11.2: Maternal iron and folate supplementation interventions.

In developing countries there is a strong association between maternal iron deficiency and low birth weight (LBW). Systematic reviews and meta-analysis suggest that the evidence is insufficient to infer that iron supplementation in pregnancy increases birth weight. A careful examination of the data in Table 11.6 obtained

from randomized controlled trials using iron (with or without folate) supplementation from developing countries illustrates this inconsistency in the data.

The evidence from developing countries does not support the benefits of iron (and folate) supplementation in improving birth weights and reducing the incidence of LBW infants. However, it is important to recognize that iron supplementation during pregnancy will improve iron and haematological status, thereby contributing to maternal health and reducing the risk of maternal morbidity and mortality. Anaemia and iron deficiency in women of reproductive age is a serious public health problem in developing countries. Hence iron (and folate) supplementation has been included as one of the important recommended interventions to be undertaken as a public policy because it improves maternal micronutrient status and reduces maternal anaemia (see Table 11.4) and will also contribute to improving infant micronutrient status and reduce risk of anaemia in the infant.

Despite the lack of evidence from developing countries, a recent well-conducted randomized trial in the USA has shown a remarkable increase in birth weights in iron-supplemented mothers with no evident differences in haemoglobin or ferritin status compared with the placebo group.

Table 11.6. Data on iron supplementation in pregnancy and birth weight. (Adapted from Shetty, 2009.)

Study location (year)	Intervention	Outcome	Other effects
Niger, peri-urban (1997)	Iron supplement versus placebo control	Iron-supplemented group associated with increase in birth length but not birth weight	Significant effect in reducing maternal anaemia; drastic reduction in neonatal deaths
Gambia, rural (1994)	Iron supplement versus placebo control; folic acid given weekly for both groups	Iron supplement had no significant effect on birth weights or LBW rates	Significant increase in haemoglobin and plasma iron levels
Sri Lanka, rural (1994)	Fortified food supplement with iron + folate every day	No effect on birth weight	Iron + folate supplements improved maternal haemoglobin status
India, rural (1991)	Supplement of iron + folate daily for 100 days	Significantly heavier babies in iron + folate group; 46% decrease in LBW	Iron + folate supplementation group had increased haemoglobin and serum ferritin levels
South Africa, hospital based (1970)	Iron alone or iron + folic acid daily	Iron + folic acid supplementation group had lower number of infants weighing <2.3 kg	

LBW, low birth weight.

Reference

Shetty, P. (2009) Community-based approaches to address childhood undernutrition and obesity in developing countries. In: Kalhan, S.C., Prentice, A.M. and Yajnik, C.S. (eds) *Emerging Societies – Coexistence of Childhood Malnutrition and Obesity*. Nestlé Nutrition Institute, Vevey, Switzerland and Karger, Basel, pp. 227–258.

12 Nutrition, Immunity and Infections in the Elderly

- Elderly individuals are at increased risk of infection and disease.
- Undernutrition and micronutrient deficiencies are a serious problem among the elderly.
- There are several causes for undernutrition in the elderly.
- The ageing process affects both the nutritional status and the immune function and response of elderly persons.
- The interactions between nutrition and immune function in the elderly and aged are complex.
- Understanding the changes in immune function due to the ageing process requires elderly individuals who are very healthy and free of any underlying nutritional deficiencies.
- Cell-mediated immunity is compromised with ageing while humoral immunity is less affected.
- Several nutrients influence immune function in the elderly, which may or may not be related to the age-related changes in immune function.
- Nutritional interventions with multiple micronutrients or single nutrients can alter and influence immune function in the elderly.
- Nutritional interventions with multiple micronutrients do not seem to show definite health benefits related to infectious disease episodes in the elderly.

12.1 Introduction

The proportion of elderly individuals is increasing rapidly in both developed and developing countries. Future projections indicate that the numbers of people of both sexes aged over 65 years will continue to increase worldwide. One major consequence of this change in the demographic profile of populations worldwide is the significant increase in age-related illness and disease and consequently in health-related expenditure.

The ageing process is influenced by several factors – both genetic and environmental – which include nutritional factors and exposure to antigens throughout life. Nutrition is considered to be an important influence on age-related diseases. Although there is a tendency to focus on non-communicable chronic degenerative diseases in elderly and aged people, it is important to remember that infection remains a major cause of morbidity and mortality in this vulnerable group. Poor nutrition and increased risk of undernutrition in the elderly and aged increases their susceptibility to

a wide range of infections and is a major contributor to the morbidity and mortality in this population group.

It has been known for some time that a substantial proportion of older adults who are either homebound or institutionalized in developed countries have some nutritional deficit (see Box 12.1). Some studies have reported that over two-thirds of hospitalized and institutionalized elderly have some form of malnutrition, usually evidence of undernutrition or micronutrient deficiencies. This underlying poor nutritional status compounds the immunological changes with age to increase this population's susceptibility to infections and consequent poor health.

Age-associated physiological and psychological changes in the individual compounded by social and economic factors may thus adversely affect the immunological and nutritional status of the elderly person, which is then reflected in his/her susceptibility to illness, poor health and reduced quality of life. The incidence of infections as well as that of other

Undernutrition or malnutrition is common in the ageing population; about 2–4% of the independent, self-sufficient elderly population in developed societies has severe undernutrition. The situation is worse in the institutionalized elderly, such as among nursing home patients, and when the aged are hospitalized, with malnutrition rates exceeding 50%. Poor nutritional status in the elderly and aged is usually associated with acute progressive diseases in both independent and hospitalized populations. Undernutrition in elderly hospitalized individuals indicates poor prognosis; the risk of death is four to six times greater in the elderly than in the undernourished hospitalized young.

Several groups of elderly and aged people are increasingly vulnerable and are at particular risk of undernutrition. These include persons living alone, those who are handicapped or disabled, and those who are poor or socially and geographically isolated. Elderly people who are hospitalized, or who have chronic disease, and very aged individuals are also vulnerable. Those elderly people who are selective about diet, or who have a poor appetite, or have gastrointestinal disorders, are also at increased risk of undernutrition. Finally, elderly and aged people are often on drugs and medication causing drug–nutrient interactions and modifications in taste and appetite that, in turn, can increase nutritional vulnerability.

Ageing is accompanied by physiological changes dominated by sensory impairment that affects the sense of taste and smell, which in turn affects appetite and food intake. Visual and hearing impairment and the likelihood of osteoarthritis, which restricts mobility and activity, add to this by affecting the ability to shop, cook and provide nourishing meals for oneself. Loneliness and social isolation and the risk of

mental depression and dementia compound this situation, which may be worsened if financial and economic constraints coexist. Poor oral health and dental problems cause difficulty in chewing and swallowing, increasing the likelihood of the habitual consumption of poor-quality and nutritionally inadequate diets. The presence of other chronic diseases and their medication can make this situation worse by affecting appetite, digestion and absorption of nutrients.

The decrease in energy requirements with ageing and the reduced physical activity levels reduce food intake, which may meet macronutrient (energy and protein) adequacy but not that of essential micronutrients. The age-related decline in muscle mass and lean tissue decreases functional ability and increases dependence on others to perform activities of daily living. The cumulative effect of all these changes predisposes to a progressive undernutrition in elderly and aged individuals.

Undernutrition in the elderly increases the risk of complications such as increased risk of infection, poor or slow wound healing, decreased muscle strength, poor cognition, increased dependency and increased mortality.

The general measures recommended for the elderly population in the UK include general nutritional advice and the use of nutritional supplements, which is more effective than nutritional advice alone; dealing with inability to shop or prepare meals by referring to social services or providing meals on wheels; improving the food intakes of the elderly by altering the meal environment (by increasing the number of people eating together) and improving the palatability of meals; and the treatment of existing conditions like poor oral health and dental problems to help improve nutritional intakes.

chronic diseases increases in old age. The ageing process is accompanied by a complex interaction of the age-related alterations of the immune system with the changes in dietary intake and nutritional status that are also influenced by increasing age. Thus an examination of immunity and infection in the elderly will have to examine separately the effect of ageing on immune function and nutrition, and then evaluate their interactions in the individual. The role played by correction of nutritional deficiencies on restoring immune function and thus aiding the prolongation of optimal health in the elderly will need to be considered too.

12.2   Changes in Immune Function with Ageing

A marked decline in immune function with increasing age has been considered to be a normal feature of the process of ageing. However, more recent evidence suggests that some immune responses do not decline with age and may in fact even increase in old age. It is hence now believed that the decline in immune function with age is not inevitable. Rather, it is currently considered that the influence of ageing on immune function is one of dysregulation rather than a general decline.

In addition, the story is complicated by the fact that many of the studies conducted have been unable to clearly separate the effects of changes in the nutritional status of elderly persons from those effects due purely to increasing age. Careful selection of very healthy elderly does not provide evidence of age-related decline except in those who are older than 90 years (the aged). Thus only examination of such healthy elderly individuals will enable us to understand the effects of the ageing process on immune function and thus help separate the effects of other environmental influences including nutritional on the immune responses of these apparently healthy elderly subjects. These immune function changes seen in very healthy elderly individuals with no other underlying causes are referred to as *primary ageing immune deficiency* (see Table 12.1).

Changes in clonal proliferation and T-cell production

Involution of the thymus starts relatively early, i.e. at puberty, and thymic function is lost by the age of 60 years. The ability of stem cells to undergo clonal proliferation decreases although stem-cell generation does not decline with age. The ability of these cells to mature into lymphoid tissue is also reduced, largely as a result of reduced function of the thymus with age. Elderly and aged people have fewer mature T lymphocytes and increased numbers of immature T cells. The inability to produce adequate numbers of mature T cells compromises considerably the ability of these individuals to respond effectively to infections.

Changes in cell-mediated immune function

Circulating lymphocytes are decreased in aged persons but the decline is small. Although T-cell numbers are not affected, there is a decrease in the numbers of fully mature T cells and an increase in the numbers of immature T cells. It is believed that this is likely to be the effect of the end of T-cell maturation which occurs in middle age rather than being linked to old age. There is also an aged-related lowering of the proliferative ability of T cells. The inability to rapidly generate mature T cells by the elderly often accounts for the lymphopaenia seen when they have a severe infection.

There is a decrease in naïve T-cell numbers, an increase in memory T cells and a decrease in cytotoxic

Table 12.1. Summary of main changes in immune function with ageing (primary ageing immune deficiency).

Changes in cell-mediated immunity and T lymphocytes	Loss or marked reduction in thymic function
	Fewer mature T lymphocytes and increase in immature T cells
	Decrease in naïve T cells, increase in memory T cells, decrease in cytotoxic T cells
	Decreased lymphocyte proliferation in response to stimulation (by mitogens/antigens) – functional ability of T cells reduced
	Decreased effectiveness of CD4+ Th cells and CD8+ T suppressor cells
	Cell-mediated immunity declines and decrease in DCH responses seen
Changes in B lymphocytes	Less compromised than cell-mediated immunity
	B-lymphocyte responses unaltered
	Plasma levels of IgA and IgG increase; decreased IgM production
	Antibody response to vaccines reduced
	Relative increase in production of autoantibodies
	Decreased response to specific antigenic challenge
Changes in macrophages and NK cells	Function well preserved
	Phagocytosis and lysosomal activity maintained
	Macrocytes produce more prostaglandins and free radicals
Changes in cytokines	Probably comparable IL-2 secretion as young adults
	Th2 cytokine secretion increases
	Production of interleukins (IL-3, IL-4) increases
	During infections IL-1, IL-6 and TNF-α secretion increases

T cells. Even this change is attributed to maturation of the immune system rather than attributable to ageing. This shift in naïve to memory T-cell ratios with ageing leads to a lower lymphocyte proliferation response in the elderly. However, very healthy elderly have comparable proliferative responses to those of young adults, and hence this may not be a significant change due to ageing that may then result in compromised immune function. Even the secretion of IL-2 appears to be comparable to that of young adults. Similarly, the earlier observation that INF-γ secretion is reduced with age has also been shown not to occur in the very healthy elderly, suggesting that this is also not related to ageing. Since these are Th1 functions it raises the question whether Th1 function declines with age. It does not, and hence seems to support the general belief that Th1 function is replaced by Th2 function with age, as immune function matures in all individuals. Many studies have provided evidence that Th2 cytokine secretion increases with age; a feature that seems to start in middle age and which may be related to the antigenic pressures that have occurred throughout life.

Along with the reduction in lymphocyte proliferation with ageing, the functional ability of peripheral circulating T cells also decreases with age. Some of the reduced T-lymphocyte proliferation is attributable to the decreased ability of the circulating T cells to react to a mitogenic or an antigenic stimulus. Reduced functional ability of the peripheral T cells also compromises cytotoxicity and response to DCH tests, or graft rejection. It appears that this compromise in the function of circulating T lymphocytes may be a consequence of hormonal changes that occur with ageing.

Some immune system functions are enhanced with ageing. For instance, cytokine production increases with ageing – particularly production of IL-3 and IL-4, and during infections IL-1, IL-6 and TNF. These cytokines have widespread metabolic effects. The increase in cytokine production during an infective episode is aimed at stimulating lymphocyte activity, but has adverse effects on elderly and aged individuals. The deleterious effects include muscle protein breakdown and depletion of body reserves of nutrients. They thus contribute to the dramatic wasting that occurs in the elderly during an infectious illness.

In summary, cell-mediated immune responses decline with age but may be retained in very healthy elderly individuals. It occurs sooner in older individuals and is probably related to the antigenic pressures encountered by those individuals throughout life.

Humoral immune responses

Humoral immune responses are less compromised than cell-mediated immune responses in elderly and aged people. The proliferative response of B lymphocytes to mitogenic stimuli is largely unaltered. Plasma levels of IgA and IgG are increased, while levels of IgM may be mildly reduced. The antibody responses that are affected are the responses that require T-cell mediation (Th cells) for the antibody production – these responses show a decline.

Primary antibody responses to vaccines are decreased with ageing and this decrease is attributed to age-related decreases in Th-cell function. It is also attributed to the increased production of anti-idiotype antibodies, which results in the synthesis of antibodies with lower antigen affinities. There is some deregulation of B-cell function and the humoral response, with a decrease in cells responsible for antibodies to foreign antigens and a relative increase in cells that produce autoantibodies. Thus ageing is associated with a characteristic increase in autoantibody levels.

In summary, the humoral responses are much less affected by ageing and although similar levels of antibodies are produced, they probably exhibit less antigen specificity.

Macrophage function

The functions of macrophages and of monocytes are often well preserved and probably enhanced with ageing. The phagocytic capacity of leucocytes is intact, and lysosomal activity – the metabolic activity that occurs following phagocytosis – is also maintained. Macrophages of aged individuals produce more prostaglandins and free radicals. Since prostaglandin E$_2$ (PGE$_2$) suppresses T-cell functions and as the lymphocytes of aged individuals are sensitive to the actions of PGE$_2$, this may result in a suppression of T-cell function in the elderly. Here again is an example of age-related dysfunction of the immune system.

12.3 Changes in Nutritional Status with Ageing

In general, elderly and aged individuals, including those who do not appear to be undernourished, have inadequate intakes of macronutrients such as energy and protein as well as of micronutrients. Both intakes and plasma levels of a wide range of vitamins and minerals are lower than recommended in the elderly. Very often, nutritional deficiencies in this group of people are multi-nutrient deficiencies with single micronutrient deficiencies being rare.

The intakes of micronutrients which have an antioxidant role, such as vitamin E, vitamin C and zinc, were reported to be below two-thirds of the recommended levels in half of the healthy non-institutionalized elderly population surveyed in the USA. This same group of healthy elderly had only marginal deficiencies in the intake of protein and energy compared with their recommended daily allowances. The intakes and levels of vitamin C were found to be below recommended levels in UK elderly aged over 75 years in both sexes, which was associated with reduced intakes of fruits and vegetables. However, among those aged over 65 years, women had better vitamin C status than men. While no age-related changes in β-carotene levels were observed, dietary intakes and levels of vitamin B_6 (pyridoxine) were well below recommended values. Since pyridoxal phosphate, the active form of vitamin B_6, is a cofactor in muscle metabolism, the changes in muscle mass with ageing may contribute additionally to the age-associated reduction in this vitamin. Marginal zinc deficiencies are also seen in the elderly and may be related to a reduced consumption of the more expensive animal- and marine-source foods as a result of their social and economic circumstances. Levels of selenium may also be lowered in the elderly.

The poor nutritional intake in the elderly which increases their risk of undernutrition is the result of many related causes (Table 12.2). With reduced levels of physical activity and a lowering of energy requirements, unchanged quality and nutritional content of the diet may result in a proportionate reduction in micronutrient intakes when energy intakes are reduced. In the elderly and aged, particularly those who are institutionalized or hospitalized, a combination of factors such as chronic disease, depression, dementia and sensory impairment such as reduced taste, smell, vision and hearing contribute directly to reduced appetite and to consuming a nutritionally poor diet. In addition unappetizing foods (quite often presented without proper care and attention), and poor dentition, frequently combined with the side-effects of medication, will conspire to influence what and how much the elderly eat, predisposing them to the risk of undernutrition which can sometimes be quite severe. Studies show that the prevalence of under-nutrition among long-term nursing home residents ranges from 10 to 40%, while micronutrient malnutrition such as vitamin deficiencies occur in up to 50% of elderly residents.

Table 12.2. Causes of poor nutrition with ageing.

Reduced intake and intake of nutritionally imbalanced diets	Sensory impairment leading to altered or decreased sense of taste and smell, contributing to reduced appetite
	Poor oral health and dental problems, leading to difficulty in chewing and inflammation, resulting in poor quality of diet
	Decreased vision and hearing, reducing the ability to purchase and prepare food
	Immobility and disability, reducing access to purchasing and cooking food
	Psychosocial factors that promote isolation and living alone, which decrease appetite and the urge and motivation to eat
	Environmental influences such as financial and economic factors, leading to limited access to food, inadequate cooking and consumption of poor-quality diets
	Medication that predisposes to loss of appetite
Reduced physical activity	Reduced energy requirements, contributing to a diet inadequate in other nutrients
	Decreased physical activity levels, causing progressive depletion of lean body mass and also contributing to reduced appetite, decreased energy needs and a diet poor in other nutrients
	Muscle loss (sarcopaenia), resulting in decreased functional ability and the need for assistance with activities of daily living
Altered absorption and metabolism of nutrients	Age-related changes in gastrointestinal digestive function and absorption and alterations in the metabolism of nutrients

12.4 Effects of Nutrient Supplementation on Immune Function in the Elderly

With age-related changes in both immune function and nutritional status, elderly and aged people are likely to exhibit a more profound interaction between these two factors. With ageing, the immune system becomes more sensitive to changes in nutritional status than it is in young adults, and the combination of ageing and nutritional deficiency tends to exert a cumulative influence on the immune system. Undernutrition enhances the age-related compromise seen in the immune function of the elderly. It is now well recognized that undernutrition in elderly and aged individuals exerts a marked influence on the immune response: there is a reduction in all parameters of cell-mediated immunity, well beyond that attributable to the ageing process alone. The degree of cell-mediated immune deficit parallels the severity of the undernutrition.

A comparison of the immune function of the very healthy elderly with those apparently healthy but with underlying low nutritional status showed that lymphocyte proliferation was lower in the latter group. While many immune functions like percentage of $CD3^+$ cells, mitogenic response, IL-2 production and antibody response to vaccine were not affected, others like percentage of $CD4^+$ cells and DTH responses were impaired in those with low nutritional status. Low plasma albumin levels used as a marker of poor nutritional status were important determinants of the compromise in immune function noticed in this group of elderly. Folate status also seems important since treatment with folic acid induced increases in immune responses in the elderly. Nutritional supplements improved the immune function changes seen in this group of apparently healthy elderly, and it also appears that the immune system of the aged is more sensitive to nutritional status than that of young adults.

Supplementation of *n*-3 polyunsaturated fatty acids

Supplementation of *n*-3 PUFAs decreased the production of all inflammatory cytokines in healthy elderly; the decrease was more marked in the elderly than in young adults who were also similarly supplemented with PUFAs. Proliferation response of mononuclear cells in response to mitogenic stimulation was slower among the elderly compared with young adults. PUFA supplementation reduced this period of the proliferative response in the elderly. PGE_2, which suppresses T-cell function, was decreased following *n*-3 PUFA supplementation of the elderly. These effects may be related to the magnitude of the PUFA supplementation-induced changes in circulating plasma fatty acids (EPA and DHA), which were more marked in the elderly.

Micronutrient supplementation

Several micronutrients play an important role in immune function and many specific micronutrient deficiencies also modify the immune functions of elderly and aged people. Although single nutrient deficiencies are infrequent some single nutrient deficiencies may be important. The similarities in the compromises in immune function with ageing and from micronutrient deficiencies raise the issue of whether the immunological changes associated with ageing may be remedied by multiple vitamin and mineral supplements.

Supplementation of elderly Canadian subjects (aged 65 years and over) with a micronutrient mix over a 1-year period resulted in reducing several micronutrient deficiencies (vitamins A, B_6 and C, iron and zinc) noticed at the onset of the supplementation. Immunological parameters such as numbers of T cells and NK cells increased following the supplementation, as did lymphocyte proliferation, production of IL-2, NK activity and antibody response to influenza vaccination. Another similar supplementation study showed at the end of 1 year that DTH responses were significantly increased in the elderly. Both these studies suggest that micronutrient deficiencies may account for much of the immunomodulation seen in healthy elderly individuals. However, the role of individual vitamins or minerals in influencing the immune responses of the elderly requires supplementation studies with individual micronutrients; the evaluation of such studies follows.

β-Carotene

Two placebo-controlled randomized trials of β-carotene supplementation over a short (3 weeks) and long (10–12 years) duration failed to show either an enhancing or a suppressive effect of the supplement on T-cell-mediated immune functions of healthy elderly subjects. However, the subjects on the long duration supplementation showed a significantly greater NK-cell activity. It has been suggested that the latter may contribute to an immunosurveillance role in the elderly, thus providing a possible link to the protective role of β-carotene in the prevention of some cancers.

Vitamin E

Vitamin E deficiency is associated with inadequate immune response and its supplementation has been used to improve immune function in the elderly. Several supplementation studies have shown that vitamin E or α-tocopherol supplementation of the elderly increases DTH responses and IL-2 production, and in some doses can increase antibody responses to hepatitis and tetanus toxoid vaccines. The exact mechanism by which vitamin E exerts its immunomodulatory effects is not known, although it is speculated that it possibly reduces prostaglandin synthesis and also alters free radical formation. Vitamin E deficiency impairs cell-mediated immunity and other non-specific immune functions as well as compromising the body's antioxidant functions; all these effects are reversed on supplementation.

Vitamin B$_6$ (pyridoxine)

Vitamin B$_6$ is important since its deficiency is common among the elderly and leads to impaired cell-mediated immunity. Studies on B$_6$ supplementation of the elderly resulted in proliferation of both T and B lymphocytes, with those elderly who had the lowest B$_6$ status showing the greatest lymphoproliferative response. A study that initially induced B$_6$ depletion prior to repletion by supplementation showed that B$_6$ deficiency significantly impaired T- and B-lymphocyte proliferation and IL-2 production, which were restored on repletion and supplementation. It is likely that B$_6$ supplementation functions by facilitating nucleic acid synthesis.

Vitamin C

Vitamin C administration has been shown to improve DTH responses to various antigens and significantly increased IgG, IgM and complement C3 levels. It is likely that the immunostimulatory effects of vitamin C are mediated through its antioxidant function.

Zinc

Zinc deficiency is common in the elderly group and results in a cell-mediated immunodeficiency that manifests as poor DTH responses. This is largely attributable to a decrease in the synthesis of the thymic hormone – thymulin – and therefore a reduction in thymulin activity, which is markedly decreased in elderly and aged individuals. Zinc supplementation in the elderly results in significant increase in DTH response to several recall antigens and also increases IgG antibody response to tetanus vaccine. Those receiving zinc had significantly greater numbers of cytotoxic T cells. However, in contrast to these supplementation studies which showed positive effects in antibody production, there are others where no significant difference in antibody production to influenza vaccine was observed. Mildly zinc-deficient subjects demonstrated significantly lower IL-2 production, and zinc supplementation in these elderly subjects increased both thymulin activity and production of IL-2.

Selenium

Selenium is an important trace element and is essential for maintenance of the immune response. A carefully conducted selenium supplementation trial in institutionalized elderly showed significantly greater lymphoproliferative response which was limited to B cells. Since the effect was greatest in those with lowest selenium level to start with and there were no effects on T-cell proliferation, it was assumed that selenium was not effective in changing the age-associated defects in T-cell function. Selenium probably acts to influence immune function largely due to its important role as an antioxidant, being an integral part of the glutathione peroxidase system.

Nutritional rehabilitation of undernourished elderly people restores both nutritional and immune status. It improves cell-mediated immunity, humoral antibody responses, macrophage function and cytokine secretions. Studies that have investigated the immune responses of healthy elderly individuals to supplementation with a single nutrient are also very promising. They demonstrate that supplementation permits enhancement of the immune responses, and thus raises the important question of whether or not elderly and aged individuals need a supplemental intake of micronutrients.

Supplementation trials with all known micronutrients (vitamins, minerals and trace elements) at levels up to three times the recommended allowances for periods of over 1 year have produced positive results. These studies resulted not only in a reduction in micronutrient deficiency but also improved immune responses. They confirm not only that micronutrient deficiencies are deleterious to immune function in the elderly, but also that the recommended micronutrient intakes are probably low for the elderly, particularly for those micronutrients that function as antioxidants. In addition, these studies also showed some reduction in the morbidity and frequency of infective episodes in the elderly; this is examined in more detail in the following section.

12.5 Nutritional Interventions and Risk of Infections in the Elderly

The evidence that micronutrients play an important role in maintaining immune function in the elderly is fairly strong as evidenced by supplementation studies that are able to reverse some of the impaired immune responses. Whether this in turn influences risk of infection and alters the parameters of morbidity such as the incidence, duration and severity of the infection needs to be evaluated.

The 1-year multivitamin and mineral supplementation of non-institutionalized elderly in Canada resulted in significantly fewer days (23 versus 48 days in the control group) of infection. A repeat of this supplementation protocol in two trials in smaller groups of individuals also confirmed the health benefit by halving the number of days of illness. A short (4 month) randomized controlled trial in non-institutionalized elderly from France with twice the daily recommended levels of vitamin and mineral supplements failed to confirm any benefit, with no differences in the incidence of infection between the intervention and placebo groups. Another supplementation trial in France among institutionalized elderly subjects who received trace elements and/or vitamins at twice the recommended intake for 2 years showed a reduction in respiratory tract infections but no effect on either urogenital infections or survival. A much larger recent intervention in the Netherlands with multivitamins over a 15-month period showed no benefit with regard to infections in the elderly. However, when those receiving high doses of vitamin E were compared with those not receiving the vitamin E supplement, the former showed significant increases in illness severity such as duration of illness, number of symptoms, presence of fever and restriction of activity.

In summary, the interventions with micronutrient supplements in the elderly were equivocal with regard to clinical disease and infection. The data are clearly inconclusive and seem to depend on the number of individual subjects in the trials and their micronutrient status at baseline before the intervention. Nevertheless, it would appear that there is a place for multivitamins and mineral supplementation as a beneficial strategy to improve nutritional status, since the prevalence of nutrient deficiencies is high among this vulnerable group. However, despite the effects of these interventions on the immune response among elderly and aged people, evidence of clinical benefit is limited. There is a need for more trials to confirm a clear health benefit from nutritional intervention in elderly and aged individuals.

12.6 Immune Function in Severe Malnutrition in the Elderly

Risk of severe malnutrition is high among the elderly, and particularly among those hospitalized or institutionalized (see Box 12.1). Severe PEM affects all immune responses in the elderly, manifesting as decreased cell-mediated immunity, humoral immunity and innate immunity. Malnutrition accentuates age-related decline in lymphocyte counts, lymphocyte proliferation and cytokine release. The effects of malnutrition and ageing thus appear to be cumulative on the immune system. Aged individuals with malnutrition show lowered cell-mediated immunity, a reduction in $CD2^+$, $CD3^+$ and $CD4^+$ cells, and a decrease in IL-2 and IL-6 production. The decrease in humoral immune response is manifested by a lower antibody response to vaccines, while compromise of other non-specific immune responses is seen in the reduction in leucocyte and macrophage functions.

The changes in macrophage function in severely undernourished elderly subjects may have considerable clinical significance. In the healthy elderly, macrophage functions are retained while T-cell function starts to decline – a disequilibrium which favours the release of cytokines by macrophages to stimulate T-cell responses during an infection in the elderly. The increased release of macrophage-derived cytokines may however be harmful to the host as they induce mobilization of the body's nutritional stores to meet the increasing demands of the activated cells. Since ageing disturbs the normal balance of muscle tissue breakdown (catabolism) followed by re-synthesis (anabolism), tissues are not fully restored in older adults unlike in the young. Hence any infective process in the elderly results in muscle loss which is not fully restored during recovery. If an undernourished elderly person gets an infection, although the cytokine response is lower and this may cause less tissue breakdown, the lowered immune response prolongs the illness and hence the hypercatabolic state and ultimately does more harm. Thus severe undernutrition in the elderly not only lowers specific and non-specific immune responses but also prolongs the hypercatabolic state, and, compounded by the age-associated changes in protein metabolism, increases risk of morbidity and mortality. Nutritional supplementation and interventions are important clinical interventions that are required in these situations.

Further Reading

Burns, E.A. and Goodwin, J.S. (1994) Aging: nutrition and immunity. In: Forse, R.A., Bell, S.J., Blackburn, G.L. and Kabbash, L.G. (eds) *Diet, Nutrition and Immunity.* CRC Press, Boca Raton, Florida, pp. 59–72. *An excellent, though dated review of age-related changes in immune functions and nutritional changes with ageing.*

Lesourd, B., Reynaud-Simon, A. and Mazari, L. (2002) Nutrition and ageing of the immune system. In: Calder, P.C., Field, C.J. and Gill, H.S. (eds) *Nutrition and Immune Function.* CAB International and The Nutrition Society, Wallingford, UK, pp. 357–374. *A good review that distinguishes primary from secondary ageing immune deficiency and provides a good account of the changes in immune function in the healthy elderly.*

Meydani, S.N. and Santos, M.S. (2000) Aging: nutrition and immunity. In: Gershwin, M.E., German, J.B. and Keen, C.L. (eds) *Nutrition and Immunology: Principles and Practice.* Humana Press, Totowa, New Jersey, pp. 403–421. *Provides an excellent account of the effects of a range of nutrients on immune function in the elderly.*

Case Studies

Case Study 12.1: Vitamin E supplementation and immune function in healthy elderly.

Few intervention studies have been successful in influencing age-associated decline in immune function. The double-blind, placebo-controlled, randomized clinical trial with vitamin E featured in this case study is one that shows significant changes in cell-mediated immune response in healthy elderly.

Free living elderly were randomly assigned either to a placebo or one of three groups receiving 60, 200 or 800 mg of vitamin E per day for 235 days. Delayed cutaneous hypersensitivity (DCH) responses and antibody production to hepatitis B, tetanus, diphtheria and pneumococcal vaccines were investigated both before and after the

Table 12.3. Data on vitamin E supplementation, DCH responses and antibody production. (Adapted from Meydani *et al.*, 1997.)

	Placebo	Vitamin E (60 mg)	Vitamin E (200 mg)	Vitamin E (800 mg)
DCH response (induration, mm)				
Before	22	24	17	17
After	24	29*	27*	26*
Antibody titre to hepatitis B vaccine (U/ml)				
Before	4.0	4.0	4.0	4.0
After	7.3	10.4*	23.9*	9.2*
IgG antibody levels to pneumococcal vaccine (PN19F) (μg/ml)				
Before	1.3	0.9	1.1	1.6
After	2.6	2.6	3.4	3.3

*Statistically significant difference compared with baseline.

supplementation period. After the intervention, data were obtained at different times for each of the variables; only the data for PN19F pneumococcal and hepatitis B vaccine are reported here (see Table 12.3).

Clinically relevant indices of cell-mediated immunity examined in the study showed improvement with vitamin E supplementation. Elderly subjects on 60, 200 and 800 mg of vitamin E daily had a 41%, 65% and 49% increase in DCH response, respectively, compared the placebo group which showed only a 17% increase. The increase in antibody titre to hepatitis B vaccine was threefold (60 mg), sixfold (200 mg) and 2.5-fold (800 mg) higher in the vitamin E groups compared with placebo controls, who showed less than a twofold increase. The group receiving 200 mg of vitamin E daily showed the best response to all indicators including antibody titres to tetanus vaccine. There was a good relationship between tertile of serum vitamin E (α-tocopherol) and both antibody titre to hepatitis B vaccine and the percentage of seropositive subjects (see Fig. 12.1). This study showed that

increased levels of vitamin E enhance *in vivo* indices of T-cell-mediated immune function in healthy elderly.

Reference

Meydani, S.N., Meydani, M., Blumberg, J.B., Leka, L.S., Siber, G., Loszewski, R., Thompson, C., Pedrosa, M.C., Diamond, R.D. and Stollar, B.D. (1997) Vitamin E supplementation and *in vivo* immune response in healthy elderly subjects: a randomized controlled trial. *Journal of the American Medical Association* 277, 1380–1386.

Case Study 12.2: Daily multivitamin and mineral supplementation and risk of infections in the elderly.

While the earlier case study (12.1) demonstrated significant changes in immune responses following daily supplementation of key nutrients, how this translates into altering risk of infection in the elderly becomes an important issue. The evidence hitherto demonstrating the efficacy of multivitamin–mineral supplements in the elderly is limited and inconclusive.

This case study looks at the incidence and severity of acute respiratory infection (ARI) using data from a randomized, double-blind, placebo-controlled trial in non-institutionalized elderly subjects in the Netherlands. This clinical trial compared four groups with daily supplementation of: (i) multivitamin–minerals at physiological doses; (ii) vitamin E (200 mg); (iii) both multivitamin–minerals and vitamin E; against (iv) a placebo group.

Table 12.4 summarizes the data on incidence and severity of acute respiratory tract infections in the elderly population studied.

The incidence rate ratio was lower for the multivitamin–mineral supplementation group than for other groups but the difference was not statistically significant. The severity of ARIs was not influenced by multivitamin–mineral supplements. Comparison of the multivitamin–mineral group with the vitamin E alone group showed significantly better results for illness duration, number of symptoms, presence of fever and restriction of activity. The vitamin E group fared the poorest; a comparison of the data for those with and without vitamin E suggests the vitamin E administration had an adverse effect on illness

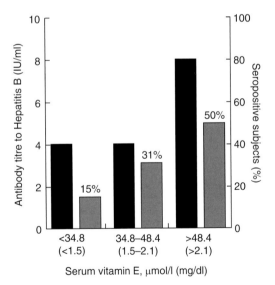

Fig. 12.1. The relationship between tertile of serum vitamin E and antibody titres to hepatitis B (■) and the percentage of subjects who were seropositive (▨). Used with permission from the *Journal of the American Medical Association* 277(17), 1380–1386. Copyright © 1997 American Medical Association. All rights reserved.

Table 12.4. Data on incidence and severity of acute respiratory tract infections. (Adapted from Graat *et al.*, 2002.)

	MV-M	Vitamin E	MV-M+ Vitamin E	Placebo
Mean incidence of infections per year	1.48	1.73	1.63	1.53
Incidence of infection rate ratio	0.96	1.13	1.06	1.0
Severity of infections				
Total illness duration (days)	14	19	19	14
Number of symptoms	5	5	6	4
Fever (%)	25.0	37.5	36.0	25.5
Restriction of activity (%)	34.8*	49.5	54.9	48.5
Episode-related medication (%)	30.2	26.8	35.1	33.3

MV-M, multivitamin–mineral supplements.
*Statistically significant difference compared with the placebo group.

severity. This is in striking contrast to the beneficial *in vivo* findings in the previous case study (12.1) for the same dosage administered every day. It needs to be kept in mind that the clinical benefits may relate to infections other than ARIs in the elderly.

Reference

Graat, J.M., Schouten, E.G. and Kok, F.J. (2002) Effect of daily vitamin E and multivitamin–mineral supplementation on acute respiratory tract infections in elderly persons. A randomized controlled trial. *Journal of the American Medical Association* 288, 715–721.

13 Nutrition, Immunity and Chronic Diseases

- Nutrients in the diet interact with the immune system in several chronic diseases in man.
- The diet is an important determinant of some types of cancer and nutrients play a role both by influencing the normal cell cycle and also through the presence of carcinogenic agents in the diet.
- Chronic inflammation can induce cell damage and increase risk of cancer.
- Micronutrients that affect the immune system can also play a role in chronic inflammatory responses and in cancer.
- Autoimmune disease like type 1 diabetes and rheumatoid arthritis may be influenced by diet and nutritional factors.
- Nutrients and diet may have an important role in the prevention or treatment of autoimmune diseases like rheumatoid arthritis.
- Infections may predispose risk to diet-related diseases like cardiovascular disease.
- Mild immune impairment may be a feature of obesity in man.

13.1 Introduction

This chapter reviews the relationship between nutrition, immunity and non-communicable or chronic diseases like cancer and autoimmune diseases. The term 'chronic diseases' is preferred to 'non-communicable diseases' since some types of so-called non-communicable diseases including cancer may have an infectious origin or aetiology. The chapter discusses the separate roles of nutrition and immune systems in cancer and their interactions. Autoimmune diseases result from loss of tolerance to self-antigens, leading to an immunological response that damages host tissues. The probable role nutrition plays in a few autoimmune disorders is presented. There is increasing evidence that infections may contribute to the causation of chronic diseases like cardiovascular disease which are believed to be largely due to alterations in the diet and lifestyles of individuals. The last section briefly addresses this issue.

13.2 Nutrition, Immunity and Cancer

Nutrition and cancer

Food plays an important role both in carcinogenic initiation, i.e. the formation of a neoplastic or cancerous cell, and in the promotion and progression of cancer once it is initiated. The putative role that

food plays in the development of cancer requires that we have a basic understanding of the cell replication and proliferation process (Box 13.1).

Role of nutrients in the normal cell cycle

Several nutrients play an important role in the various stages of a normal cell cycle. Macro- and micronutrients are needed for the biosynthesis of the various cell components as they proliferate and divide. They contribute energy for the process and enable the synthesis of new proteins and other cellular components as the cell advances through the cycle of replication. Specific nutrients may also function to modulate and regulate this process. These include folic acid, which is required for DNA replication, while vitamin A or retinoids can act to arrest the cycle in G_1 phase. Folate is also a necessary cofactor for DNA synthesis and folate deficiency can reduce cell proliferation by decreasing DNA synthesis.

Initiation of cancer or carcinogenesis

The process of division of cells through the cell cycle is beset with the potential for error in the replication of the DNA. These mutations can result in either non-functioning genes or changes in the

Box 13.1. The Normal Cell Cycle.

The normal cell cycle is the sequence of changes which a cell goes through to divide into two daughter cells. Normal cells require external signals which stimulate them to initiate the process of cell division. These signals are from growth factors, but often it is the microenvironment around the cell and the balance of the signals that promote or inhibit cell division and cell growth that ultimately determines what happens. Growth inhibitory signals are as important as growth stimulating signals. In adults, most cells in the body are not actively dividing and are in a quiescent or inactive phase or resting state, referred to as G_0. The move from this inactive/quiescent stage to one of active cell division is determined by the stimuli from growth factors, the sufficiency of space and nutrients for the cell division to occur.

Once induction to the normal cell cycle occurs, the cell moves from G_0 to the next phase designated G_1. In the G_1 phase where the chromosomes are prepared for replication, the cell synthesizes protein and RNA and increases in size. At the end of this first phase the cells must pass through a G_1 checkpoint which arrests the cell cycle if DNA damage is detected, thus ensuring that such cells with damaged DNA are not replicated. These arrested cells can either repair their DNA or undergo programmed cell death, i.e. apoptosis.

On passing through the G_1 checkpoint the cell enters the next phase referred to as the S phase for synthesis of DNA. During this phase the DNA inside the cell is replicated. The S phase ends when the DNA content of the cell is doubled and the chromosomes are replicated; the cell now enters the G_2 phase, a preparatory phase for cell division. In the G_2 phase the cell further increases in size and synthesizes new proteins. The G_2 checkpoint functions to arrest the cell cycle if the DNA is damaged or unreplicated at this stage. Again cells at this stage can also undergo DNA repair or apoptosis.

If the cell passes the G_2 checkpoint it can divide into two daughter cells during the phase of mitosis, hence called the M phase. There is also an M checkpoint which ensures that each new daughter cell has received the correct DNA. The normal cell cycle is controlled by proteins called cyclins and their specific enzymes called cyclin-dependent kinases (CDKs). Cyclins joins their CDKs to form cyclin–CDK complexes to activate transcription factors which lead to the transcription of genes during the normal cell cycle.

---

amino acid sequences of proteins synthesized from the altered genes. The latter can lead to altered cell function. DNA is continuously exposed to damage from a variety of agents, which include agents in food (see Table 13.1); these are called carcinogens when they are responsible for causing cancer.

Nutrients and DNA repair

The normal cell cycle also informs of the potential for DNA repair during the normal cell cycle should defects be identified by the checkpoints. Just as agents in food can induce cancer, nutrients can also influence and aid the DNA repair process. The nutrients involved in DNA repair include vitamin A or retinoids, vitamin D, folate and selenium.

Immune system and cancer

The linkages between the immune system and cancer operate via several likely pathways and nutrition may be an important modulator of this relationship.

Table 13.1. Carcinogens in food.

Source	Examples
Naturally occurring	Mycotoxins
	Alkaloids (pyrrolizidine alkaloids)
	Allyl isothiocyanates
	Safrole, estragole
Contaminants	DDT (dichlorodiphenyl-trichloroethane)
	Trichloroethylene
Additives	Aramite, thiourea/thioacetamide
	Non-nutritive sweeteners like Dulcin
	Food colours like butter yellow
Formed in food	
During processing	Nitrosamines
	Aryldiazonium compounds
During preparation	Benzopyrene
	Heterocyclic amines
	Acrylamides
Formed *in vivo*	Nitrosamides/nitrosamines

Box 13.2. Carcinogenesis and Characteristics of Cancer Cells.

Cancer results from altered expression of the genes which affects the normal cell cycle. The altered gene expression is the result of damage to DNA that changes the characteristics or pheno-type of the cell, converting it from a normal to cancerous cell. The hallmark of cancer cells is their unlimited replication resulting in enhanced cell proliferation. Unlike normal cells which can divide only a finite number of times (usually 60–70 times) before they are no longer able to divide – a proc-ess referred to as *senescence*, the cancer cell acquires the ability to replicate endlessly. This pre-ordained limit to cell divisions is controlled by structures in the chromosomes called telomeres, which shorten each time the cell divides; cancer cells, on the other hand, maintain the length of their telomeres despite frequent cell divisions. In addition cancer cells are neither dependent on external growth factors to stimulate the cell cycle nor sensitive to growth inhibitory signals. Thus, unlike normal cells, cancer cells demonstrate the following six characteristics which are considered the hallmarks of cancer:

1. growth signal autonomy (self-sufficiency in growth signals);
2. insensitivity to growth inhibitory signals;
3. unlimited replication potential;
4. evasion of apoptosis;
5. sustained angiogenesis;
6. invasion and metastasis.

The development of cancer or carcinogenesis requires a series of cellular changes, as no single gene is likely to be responsible for cancer. It appears to be a multi-step process of accumulation of errors in genes that control cellular processes. One mutation may result in the acquisition of one new trait by a cell which imparts advantage over other cells and is passed on to its progeny. However, cancer develops only when several genes are altered which then confer growth and sur-vival advantages over normal cells.

The first stage of carcinogenesis is the *initiation* process when the exposure of the cell to an agent, i.e. carcinogen, initiates DNA damage and induces a genetic mutation. The DNA damage is usually by the formation of DNA adducts (a piece of DNA covalently bound to a cancer-causing chemical) which, if left uncorrected, are transferred to the daughter cells during cell division. Initiation alone does not lead to cancer. An initiated cell forms a clone of initiated cells and this clonal expansion then increases the risk of developing cancer.

The stage of *promotion* involves exposure of the initiated cell or its clones to promoting agents which then alter the rate of proliferation or cause addi-tional DNA damage and further mutations. Finally these cells grow and expand to form a visible growth or tumour. These cells with accumulated DNA damage and mutations acquired during this multistage process, and now forming a tumour mass or abnormal growth, bear all the above hall-marks of cancer.

Chronic inflammation and cancer risk

While an acute inflammatory response to a patho-gen, chemical or trauma may be beneficial to the body, chronic inflammation increases the risk of damage to DNA and hence promotes cancer. The inflammatory cells infiltrating chronically inflamed tissues produce a range of bioactive chemicals which include cytokines, ROS and reactive nitro-gen species (RNS), cyclooxygenase (COX) and lipoxygenase products.

ROS is a normal product of cellular metabolism and its production in excess is harmful. Excess ROS is released during environmental stress such as ultraviolet or heat exposure of the organism. Excess ROS leads to oxidative stress and can dam-age cell structure and the DNA of cells, thus predis-posing to cancer. Several nutrients function in the body as antioxidants and defend the cells from damage by these highly reactive oxidative mole-cules. RNS, on the other hand, are antimicrobial molecules derived from nitric oxide and the enzymes required for this action are expressed by macro-phages. Together with ROS they can induce cell and DNA damage and are often referred to as RONS (reactive oxygen and nitrogen species).

COX are enzymes that convert fatty acids to a group of biological mediators called prostanoids, which include prostaglandins. The inhibition of COX by pharmacological agents can relieve pain and inflammation. Lipoxygenases are a family of iron-containing enzymes also involved in fatty acid metabolism and in the metabolism of prostaglandins and leucotrienes. This environment of chronic inflammation full of harmful chemicals will influ-ence cell metabolism and cell division, resulting in an increase in cell proliferation and cell differentiation. It also results in the formation of new blood vessels (angiogenesis) and inhibition of the programmed death of cells, a normal process referred to as 'apoptosis'.

Two examples of cancer resulting from chronic inflammation are ulcerative colitis and Barrett's oesophagus. It is estimated that 5% of patients with ulcerative colitis, a form of irritable bowel disease, will develop cancer of the colon. Barrett's oesophagus is the result of reflux of acid from the stomach into the oesophagus that causes changes to the mucosal lining and can ultimately lead to cancer. It is estimated that 1% of individuals with this condition develop oesophageal cancer, which is very much higher than the risk of oesophageal cancer in the general population.

Cancer induced by chronic inflammation is sensitive to nutritional influences since nutrients can function as antioxidant defences, influence the immune system and act to suppress the inflammatory process. It may also help explain geographical differences in the patterns of cancer incidence. Cancers like liver and cervical cancer caused by infective agents are more common among populations in developing and low-income countries with poor nutritional status. Macronutrient and numerous micronutrient deficiencies in these populations may affect the immune system and promote chronic inflammation which predisposes to cancer development. In contrast, in economically developed and industrialized societies, hormone-related cancers such as breast and prostate cancer are more common.

Immunological surveillance

It has been hypothesized for a long time that immunosurveillance exists against the development of cancer. Since cell division is a constant and continuous process that occurs in the body, it can often result in mutant clones of cells which may be potentially neoplastic. The immune response has to have the capacity to deal with this. The hypothesis was further developed to suggest that the immune system mounts a surveillance operation against tumour-associated antigens. The 'immunosurveillance' hypothesis thus envisages that the immune system constantly surveys for newly formed cancer cells and then eliminates them, thus preventing the onset and progression of cancer.

The ability of the immune system to recognize cancer cells from normal cells is dependent upon the expression of different proteins on the surface of the cancer cells compared with normal cells of the same type. These proteins are referred to as 'tumour antigens'. The tumour antigens generate an immune response much like that to a foreign protein of a pathogen. Hence tumour antigens have to be proteins expressed only by cancer cells, or proteins that have mutated during the development of the cancer, or be expressed due to differentiation of cancer cells, or be expressed in abnormal quantities by cancer cells. It is now known that highly immunogenic tumours may be effectively dealt with by the immunosurveillance mechanism, although in general most tumours are only weakly antigenic. Thus tumours can escape the host's immune response and not be detected by the immunosurveillance system because they are not immunogenic. The relevance of this process of immunological surveillance may thus be to protect against virus-induced tumours which are immunogenic. However, the absence of an increase in tumours among those who are immunosuppressed or have immunodeficiencies seems to diminish the importance of this process in man.

Immune response in a person with cancer

The immune system may be compromised or even suppressed in a person with cancer. This may be a generalized phenomenon resulting from crowding out of the immune cells by the cancerous cells or the result of suppression of the immune system resulting from treatment for the cancer such as chemotherapy and radiotherapy. On the other hand the immunosuppression may be specific to the tumour or cancer cells, which produce a number of chemicals like prostaglandins that may exert an immunosuppressive effect. In addition, the immune response may be impaired by the poor nutritional status of a host with cancer which may in turn increase morbidity and mortality.

Nutrition, immunity and cancer

There is no doubt that generalized undernutrition as well specific nutrient deficiencies compromise the immune response of the body. There is also evidence that the immune system plays a role in altering the risk of some types of cancer. The question that needs to be considered is what are the interactions between nutrition, immunity and the risk of cancer?

Both the type and the amount of fat in the diet influence immune function and interacting together they may promote or inhibit tumour growth. While the role played by dietary fats on immune function is well studied, clarifying the exact role of how the composition of fat in the diet connects immune function to cancer risk seems be a difficult question to resolve. This situation is further complicated by the recognition that fat intake per se is not to be considered a risk factor for cancers of the breast and colorectum as was previously believed. The level of evidence has now been downgraded as being limited and only suggestive of the linkage with fat intakes.

Micronutrients like vitamin A and carotenoids, vitamins E, D, C and minerals like selenium play an important role in immune function. Here again the demonstration of the interactions with immune response and cancer risk is an impossible task. However, since many of these micronutrients function as potent antioxidants they not only prevent or reduce oxidative damage but also provide the important antioxidant defence, thus reducing the potential for cell and DNA damage and thus cancer.

Restriction of energy or calorie intake lowers the incidence and delays the onset of spontaneous and induced tumours in animals. Calorie restriction and/or increase in physical activity can reduce body weight and body fatness, and all three of these factors – i.e. body weight (increased), body fatness (increased) and level of physical activity (decreased) – are now clearly implicated as providing convincing evidence for increasing risk of several cancers in man. These include cancer of the oesophagus, pancreas, breast (postmenopausal), endometrium and kidney.

13.3   Nutrition and Autoimmune Diseases

When the immune system targets a pathogen, it is usually very specific and does not cause damage to normal host tissue. However, some collateral or bystander damage is unavoidable and often occurs but is self-limited. In autoimmune diseases the immune system is activated by self-components and damage occurs specifically to the host tissues. This attack of the host's own tissues occurs in an auto-amplifying and self-sustaining manner lead-

ing to self-tissue destruction. Thus autoimmune diseases result from loss of tolerance to self-antigens and this loss of tolerance results in an immunological response that causes damage to host tissues.

Autoimmune diseases may be tissue (or organ) specific, e.g. type 1 or insulin-dependent diabetes mellitus, myasthenia gravis, and Graves disease or thyrotoxicosis. They may also be systemic and directed against molecules widely distributed in the body. The tissue damage in this case may be the result of widespread tissue damage compounded by the deposition of immune complexes at sites such as the skin, joints and kidneys. The latter includes conditions like rheumatoid arthritis and scleroderma. Only a few autoimmune diseases where the role of nutrition has been reasonably well elucidated are discussed here, with one example each of tissue-specific and systemic autoimmune disease being presented.

Type 1 diabetes mellitus

Diabetes mellitus is a metabolic condition characterized by abnormal blood glucose levels due to alterations in insulin production, insulin action or a combination of both. Diabetes is of two types: (i) type 1 or insulin-dependent diabetes, which accounts for about 10% of all diabetes, characterized by the destruction of insulin-producing β cells of the pancreas; and (ii) type 2, accounting for 90% of all diabetes, which is late in onset, associated with obesity and characterized by insulin resistance. Most cases of type 1 diabetes mellitus are immune mediated and the result of selective autoimmune destruction usually occurring early in life, with the onset of disease occurring between 5 and 15 years of age.

The aetiology or causation of type 1 or insulin-dependent diabetes is probably related to both genetic and environmental risk factors being associated with its development. Viral infections and toxins as well as dietary factors have been implicated as putative environmental risk factors. The recognition of the role of diet in the onset and progression of type 1 diabetes, an autoimmune disease, reveals the interaction between immune systems and the diet, and raises the prospect of preventing this disease and contributing to its better treatment.

Type 1 diabetes mellitus is the result of autoimmune destruction of β cells, and there is abundant evidence of inflammation and autoimmune attack of these specific cells in the pancreas. Chemicals including cytokines produced by the islet cells infiltrating inflammatory cells are considered the mediators of this damage to the β cells.

Diet and type 1 diabetes

The evidence seems to support an important role for the diet in infancy and early childhood in causation of the autoimmune damage that results in type 1 diabetes. Short duration of breastfeeding (less than 3 months) is an important risk factor. So too are the early introduction of cow's milk and exposure to cow's milk before 4 months of age, which have both been identified as significant risk factors. Breastfeeding seems to protect against diabetes although the exact mechanisms are not clear. Breast milk provides both cellular and immune factors as well as growth factors which may all play a role in protecting the infant. Infants who are breastfed for short durations and weaned early are possibly deprived of key developmental signals and immune-related bioactive factors and may be burdened with precocious exposure to antigens, all of which may contribute to the development of diabetes.

A hypothesis referred to as the 'milk hypothesis' has arisen from these observations and postulates that early exposure to proteins present in cow's milk may trigger the autoimmune diabetes. This hypothesis is not without controversy, as there are as many studies showing this relationship as there are those failing to show it. Studies using animal models of autoimmune diabetes confirm that diet composition is an important determinant of the development of diabetes, but show that cereal-based diets generally promote the disease while semi-purified diets based on cow's milk proteins prevent or delay onset of diabetes. The interesting similarities between insulin-dependent diabetes and coeliac disease, both of which have a high incidence in Northern Europe, makes the observations between cereal-based diets and diabetes in experimental models interesting. However, conclusive evidence from human subjects is lacking. Hence the data from human studies can best be summarized as follows. The possible association between short duration of breastfeeding and/or the early introduction of cow's milk with type 1 diabetes is controversial and most human studies have focused on the early exposure to cow's milk pro-

teins. Most importantly, the mechanisms of how diet modulates the development of type 1 diabetes are not well understood.

Other aspects of diet and its linkages to type 1 diabetes relate to the consumption by pregnant mothers of processed meat such as smoked, cured mutton, which is known to contain nitroso compounds. These observations are also controversial, although a large study in Swedish children showed a higher consumption of foods containing nitrosoamines by those newly diagnosed with type 1 diabetes.

Rheumatoid arthritis

Rheumatoid arthritis is a generalized or systemic autoimmune disease characterized by symmetric and multiple joint involvement with pain, swelling and functional impairment of the joints. It affects about 1% of the adult population in the West and is more common among women. Rheumatoid arthritis usually shows signs of systemic inflammation evidenced by an elevation in plasma levels of cytokines and acute-phase proteins. Both the synovial fluid (fluid in the joints) and the synovial cells from patients with rheumatoid arthritis contain high levels of pro-inflammatory cytokines like TNF-α and interleukins.

Eicosanoids like prostaglandins, thromboxanes and leucotrienes are important mediators of inflammation as they modulate the intensity and duration of the inflammation. They are derived from PUFAs, with arachidonic acid being the main precursor of eicosanoid synthesis. The important role that fats and fatty acids as nutrients play in the immune and inflammatory response is outlined in Chapter 3. Oily fish and fish oils contain very-long-chain PUFAs, important among which are EPA and DHA. Consumption of these fish oils results in their incorporation into the phospholipids of immune cells, and the consequent alterations in the fatty acid composition of the membranes influence immune cell function and the inflammatory process itself. Several studies have shown that these fatty acids (EPA and DHA) when consumed in high quantities decrease antigen presentation, T-cell proliferation and the consequent production of cytokines. Their increased consumption also results in decreased production of eicosanoids like prostaglandins and thromboxanes by inflammatory cells and alters the potency of several other mediators like leucotrienes. They also seem to cause the synthesis of novel anti-inflammatory mediators and inhibit the production of inflammatory cytokines. These studies have provided a sound basis for trials with these specific PUFAs in patients with rheumatoid arthritis.

Almost all the clinical trials that have used these *n*-3 PUFAs or fish oils in rheumatoid arthritis patients has shown some benefit and clinical improvement, which includes reduced duration of morning stiffness, reduced joint pain, reduced number of tender or swollen joints, reduced time to fatigue, increased grip strength and most importantly reduction in the use of non-steroidal anti-inflammatory drugs. Well-conducted meta-analysis of all the available studies confirmed the robustness of the efficacy of dietary fish oil consumption in rheumatoid arthritis, which is it now regarded as part of the standard therapy for this systemic autoimmune disease.

13.4 Nutrition, Immunity and Other Chronic Diseases

Although the role of diet, nutrition and physical activity in the aetiology of chronic diseases like cardiovascular disease (CVD) – including stroke and coronary heart disease – is well documented, increasingly evidence is emerging that infections and the response of the immune system may play a part. These early observations also raise the prospect of an interaction between nutrition and the immune function as a likely contributor in their development. Infections associated with arterial and cardiovascular diseases include specific infections like *Chlamydia pneumoniae* and *Helicobacter pylori* infections of the stomach, and non-specific infections like periodontal infections and respiratory tract infections. Early reports seem to show an association between some of these infections and chronic diseases. However, recent meta-analysis have shown that associations of serum markers of *C. pneumoniae* and *H. pylori* with arterial disease, their risk factors or potential intermediary mechanisms for disease are weaker than was first suggested by the early reports. Infection with hepatitis A virus has also been linked with the prevalence of CVD. But CVD risk markers in a large population-based sample of patients who are at high risk of developing CVD did not show that hepatitis A seroprevalence influences CVD progression in patients at risk.

It has been suggested that infections may be responsible for an accelerated development of atherosclerosis, which results from a focal accumulation of lipids. Diet and plasma lipid levels are important determinants of atherosclerosis and the consequent CVD. Recent data suggest that periodontal disease may increase the risk of CVD. It is now apparent that lipid metabolism may be altered by local and acute systemic infections which result in unregulated levels of cytokines. Bacterial infections mediated via the actions of TNF-α and interleukins (IL-1β) lead to increases in free fatty acids, low-density lipoproteins and triacylglycerols. Thus infections or other agents that increase these cytokines have the potential to cause hyperlipidaemia. High serum levels of total cholesterol, low-density lipoprotein cholesterol and triacylglycerols have been observed in patients with periodontal disease and although it is not clear whether this is a cause-and-effect relationship, the associations draw our attention to the fact that the changes in lipid profiles seen are suggestive of increasing risk of CVD in periodontal disease.

Several reports have suggested that human obesity causes immune dysfunction. This is largely the result of reports suggestive of a higher incidence of infectious disease episodes and increased infection-related mortality among the obese. Comparative studies of indicators of immune function between obese and non-obese have failed to demonstrate differences of any significance in immune response. However, there are reports which indicate that obesity specifically affects some immune functions such as the release of macrophage migration inhibitory factor and in the responsiveness of lymphocytes to stimulation, both of which appear to be impaired. In summary, the evidence seems to point towards a variable but modest impairment of the immune system in human obesity.

Further Reading

Scott, F.W. (1994) Food, diabetes and immunology. In: Forse, R.A., Bell, S.J., Blackburn, G.L. and Kabbash, L.G. (eds) *Diet, Nutrition and Immunity*. CRC Press, Boca Raton, Florida, pp. 73–95. *A good review on the role of diet in the development of type 1 diabetes mellitus.*

Tice, D.G. and Meguid, M.M. (1994) Cancer: nutrition and immunity. In: Forse, R.A., Bell, S.J., Blackburn, G.L. and Kabbash, L.G. (eds) *Diet, Nutrition and Immunity*. CRC Press, Boca Raton, Florida, pp. 97–113. *A critical review attempting to examine the links between immune status, nutrients and cancer.*

Case Studies

Case Study 13.1: *n*-3 Polyunsaturated fat supplements and rheumatoid arthritis.

A randomized trial was carried out in rheumatoid arthritis patients with active disease in Brazil to compare the effects of supplementation with fish oils rich in *n*-3 PUFAs with a placebo, i.e. soy oil. The oil supplements were provided as capsules along with their usual medication of anti-rheumatic and non-steroidal anti-inflammatory drugs. Assessment based on standardized clinical indicators was undertaken at baseline and at 12 and 24 weeks of the supplementation trial. The groups were comparable at the start of the trial in terms of the sex distribution, age, disease duration and medication prescribed.

The data related to the clinical indicators used to assess progress in patients with rheumatoid arthritis during and at the end of 24 weeks of supplementation are summarized in Table 13.2.

The beneficial effects of fish oil in addition to standard treatment were observed more consistently after 24 weeks rather than 12 weeks of supplementation. Significant improvements by the fish oil group were also reported in the daily activities undertaken such as bending down to pick up clothing from the floor and getting in and out of a car. This study demonstrated and also confirmed other reports of the beneficial effects of marine or fish oils supplementation in rheumatoid arthritis patients.

It needs to be mentioned that the report provided in this case study pertains only to part of the clinical trial. The study also examined the impact of adding olive oil, which is rich in MUFAs, i.e. oleic acid, to fish oils. The study demonstrated added benefits over fish oil when olive oil was provided in addition to fish oil in a third group of patients who were also studied at the same time.

Reference

Berbert, A.A., Kondo, C.R.M., Almendra, C.L., Matsuo, T. and Dichi, I. (2005) Supplementation of fish oil and olive oil in patients with rheumatoid arthritis. *Nutrition* 21, 131–136.

Table 13.2. Data on clinical indicators in rheumatoid arthritis patients before, during and after supplementation. (Adapted from Berbert *et al.*, 2005.)

Clinical indicator		Baseline	12 weeks	24 weeks
Morning stiffness (min)	Soy oil	38	46	51
	Fish oil	44	21	5*
Joint pain intensity	Soy oil	1.77	1.77	1.83
	Fish oil	2.31	1.46	1.23*
Onset of fatigue (min)	Soy oil	19.5	19.3	21.4
	Fish oil	20.9	17.1	16.3*
Grip strength (right hand)	Soy oil	62	60	68
	Fish oil	54	91	105*
Patient global assessment	Soy oil	1.25	1.42	1.31
	Fish oil	1.54	1.62	1.23

*Statistically significant difference compared with the placebo (i.e. soy oil) group.

14 Probiotics, Prebiotics and Immunity

- The normal bacterial microflora of the gut fulfils several important metabolic, trophic and defence functions in the body.
- Interactions of the microbial flora of the gut with the gut-associated lymphoid tissue are an important component of the immune system of the body.
- Exogenous bacterial supplements can function like commensal bacteria by both enhancing the barrier function of the intestinal mucosa and influencing the normal functioning of the immune system.
- Probiotics provide beneficial effects in reducing the incidence and duration of acute diarrhoeal episodes in infants and children.
- Probiotics are useful in reducing antibiotic-associated diarrhoea in the elderly.
- Probiotics have a non-specific immune-modulating role and confer health benefits.
- Prebiotics and synbiotics are other approaches to provide beneficial health effects by exploiting the normal role of the intestinal microflora in modulating immune function and reducing risk of infection.

14.1 Introduction

The human gastrointestinal tract is home for between 300 and 500 species of bacteria, most of them inhabiting the large intestine. The upper intestinal tract (i.e. the stomach and small intestine) contain only a few species and some in transit, and does not provide an ideal environment for bacterial proliferation. This is largely due to the composition of its contents, made up of acid in the stomach and bile and alkaline pancreatic secretions in the upper small intestine. The large intestine, on the other hand, has a dynamic and high-density microbial ecosystem estimated at 10^{10} or 10^{12} cells per gram of luminal content. The majority of these microbes are anaerobes, i.e. they survive in an environment without oxygen. The commensal bacteria in the gut which constitute the gut flora are vital for the health of the host, unlike some pathogenic organisms which can cause significant harm to the host. The gut flora is generally of benefit to the host and synthesizes vitamins like folic acid, vitamin K and biotin; it also ferments undigested complex carbohydrates that reach the colon. These commensals also inhibit the growth of pathogenic bacteria.

Many factors affect the bacterial composition of the gut flora in man. These include age and immu-nological status, as well as local factors such as pH, gut transit time, interactions between microbes in the flora, and the availability of fermentable nutrients in the gut. Non-digestible dietary residues, mostly complex carbohydrates that pass the upper intestinal tract and enter the large intestine, along with components of digestive secretions and sloughed epithelial cells constitute the substrates for this microbial flora. The main non-digestible residues that are fermentable by these microbes include dietary fibres, resistant starches, oligosac-charides and other unabsorbed sugars. Proteins and fats contribute less to the substrate pool of these microbes in the large bowel.

The gut of the fetus is sterile and is inoculated primarily by organisms originating from the moth-er's vagina and faeces and the surrounding environ-ment during and after birth. Thus colonization of the newborn gut occurs from birth to within a few days after birth. Infants delivered by Caesarean sec-tion have far fewer lactobacilli than those delivered vaginally and acquire the process of colonization from the immediate environment, including other persons and infants in the birth environment. Bacterial populations of the gut develop during the first few days of life and they create a highly

©Prakash Shetty 2010. *Nutrition, Immunity and Infection* (P. Shetty)

reduced environment that favours the growth of strictly anaerobic species.

The microbial flora of exclusively breastfed infants is different from that of formula-fed infants, with breastfed infants having a substantially lower risk of gastrointestinal infections. Most studies show that the major difference in the microbial flora of breastfed infants compared with formula-fed infants is due to the dominance of bifidobacteria, lower counts of bacteroides and almost complete absence of clostridia. Thus exclusively breastfed infants seem to have a faecal flora dominated by bifidobacteria while the flora is more complex in formula-fed infants. The huge presence of bifidobacteria in breastfed infants is probably responsible for the better health of these infants, although it must be remembered that breast milk provides a variety of factors including antibodies that protect the newborn. With the introduction of weaning and solid foods the microbial flora of the infant becomes more complex. By the age of 2 years or so the gut microflora of a child stabilizes and is now closer to that of an adult.

Gut microbes fulfil many physiological functions which can be categorized as: (i) metabolic; (ii) trophic; and (iii) protective. The *metabolic* activities include the salvage of energy and absorbable nutrients and the fermentation of non-digestible dietary residues and substrates including endogenous secretions that enter the large bowel. The non-digestible substrates are mostly complex carbohydrates and include large polysaccharides like resistant starches, cellulose, hemicellulose, pectins and gums and oligosaccharides that are not digested. The end products of their fermentation are short-chain fatty acids (SCFAs; i.e. acetate, propionate and butyrate) which are used by the host cells, thus providing an important source of energy and nutrients. These SCFAs increase absorption of water and nutrients like calcium, magnesium and iron, and influence the growth of epithelial cells. They even modulate the sensitivity of insulin and lower glycaemic response. The colonic microflora also plays a part in the synthesis of vitamins like folic acid and vitamin K, and may also influence the absorption and storage of lipids.

The large intestinal bacteria also exhibit important *trophic* effects on intestinal epithelial cells and on the gut's immune structure and function. The SCFAs that are the result of fermentation by the colonic flora exert trophic effects on intestinal epithelial cells by promoting epithelial cell proliferation and differentiation. There is even evidence suggesting that these SCFAs may promote reversion of cancer cells to normal cells. The gut mucosa is an important interactive phase between the external environment and the immune systems of the gut, since the GALT contains the largest pool of immunocompetent cells. This interaction and dialogue between the microbial flora and the GALT is crucial and is evidenced by low densities of gut lymphoid tissue and low circulating immunoglobulin levels in germ-free animals. Microbial colonization affects GALT and manifests as expansion of lymphocyte numbers and increase in concentration of serum immunoglobulins. These early interactions between GALT and the microbial flora appear to be crucial for the development of complex mucosal and systemic immunoregulatory mechanisms. More importantly, these interactions continue into adulthood and are constantly altered and reshaped. There is evidence to suggest that the nature of the cytokine responses is different, enabling discrimination between potential pathogens from commensal bacteria resident in the colon.

The normal microbial flora also fulfils a *protective* function and provides a line of resistance to the host tissue from the invasion of pathogenic bacteria, as evidenced by germ-free animals which are highly susceptible to infection. The normal flora provides resistance to colonization not only by pathogens but also by opportunistic bacteria, thus conferring stability under normal conditions. These stable conditions can be easily perturbed; for instance, following the use of antibiotics which disrupt the existing ecological balance. Normal flora may affect the entry of pathogenic bacteria owing to their attachment to epithelial cells, thus providing competition for attachment by enteroinvasive pathogens. They may compete for nutrients and also secrete antimicrobial substances called bacteriocins, thus preventing the colonization by pathogens.

14.2 Probiotics

Probiotics are defined as 'live microorganisms which when administered in adequate amounts confer a health benefit on the host'. These are live microbial food supplements that beneficially affect the host by improving the intestinal microbial balance. In man this includes fermented milk products and the now popular commercial preparations that contain lyophilized bacteria. The common micro-organisms in probiotic foods are lactic acid producers like lactobacilli and bifidobacteria as well as some species of gram-positive cocci (see Table 14.1). An effective and useful probiotic exhibits certain properties and characteristics and provides several health-related beneficial effects to the host, many of which are summarized in Table 14.2.

Table 14.1. Examples of probiotics, prebiotics and synbiotics. (Adapted from Collins and Gibson, 1999.)

Probiotics	Lactobacilli
	Bifidobacteria
	Gram-positive cocci
Prebiotics	Fructo-oligosaccharides
	Inulin
	Galacto-oligosaccharides
	Lactulose
	Lactitol
Synbiotics	Bifidobacteria + fructo-oligosaccharides
	Bifidobacteria + galacto-oligosaccharides
	Lactobacilli + lactitol

Table 14.2. Probiotics: properties and beneficial effects.

Properties/characteristics of effective probiotics	Non-pathogenic and non-toxic
	Contains large numbers of viable cells
	Capable of surviving and metabolizing in the human gut
	Remains viable during storage and use
	Good sensory properties
	Isolated from the same species as in the human host
	Exerts a beneficial effect on the human host
Putative health benefits of probiotic intake	Improves digestion
	Stimulates gastrointestinal immunity
	Increases natural resistance to infectious diseases of the gut
	Alleviates symptoms of lactose malabsorption and intolerance
	Suppresses cancer
	Reduces serum cholesterol concentration

Probiotics and the immune system

Since probiotics are supplements of living microorganisms they influence the composition of the microbial flora of the gut by colonization and restoration of the balance, particularly in situations where the normal indigenous flora has been perturbed following the administration of antibiotics or following colonization by invasive pathogens. Thus probiotics play an important role in restoring and augmenting the beneficial physiological effects of the normal indigenous flora of the gut; and one such important function is that of the immune system. Gut-dwelling microbes are important players in the immune systems of the body, especially that associated with the gut. The beneficial role of probiotics is merely a physiological exploitation of the normal gut microbial interactions with the immune system.

The interactions of the gastrointestinal tract with its gut-dwelling microbes which constitute the normal microbial flora or exogenously administered probiotics have a significant impact on health. Children raised in environments rich in early bacterial exposure such as lactobacilli-containing foods seem to be prone to develop fewer immune dysfunctional diseases. This would suggest that early stimulation by appropriate bacterial signals may influence the development of the immune system and reduce the chances of developing immun-opathologies like atopic reactions and mucosal allergies. Studies have shown that supplementing the diets of newborn infants with probiotics made up of *Lactobacillus rhamnosus* can reduce the incidence of atopic eczema in infancy and early childhood. Evidently the administration of exogenous bacteria, which augments the normal microbial flora of neonates, provides the bacterial signals essential to combat allergic sensitization. The same lactobacillus appears to alleviate immune-mediated atopy in infants, and reduces the incidence and severity of infant diarrhoea.

The probiotic bacteria attach themselves to the gastrointestinal epithelial cells that are immuno-competent as they colonize the mucosa; a response which is enhanced when these cells are activated by cytokines during an inflammatory reaction. These gut epithelial cells not only communicate in turn with intra-epithelial lymphocytes, but also secrete anti-inflammatory mediators. Thus it would appear that gut-dwelling microbes and intestinal epithelial cells play an active role in the maintenance of gut homeostasis and thus in regulating intestinal

Box 14.1. Probiotics – The 'Good' Bacteria.

Vast numbers of many different types of bacteria inhabit the intestinal tract, most of them living in the large intestine. It is estimated that the number of bacteria in the human large intestine is about 10^{12} per gram of large intestinal contents, thus contributing to over 222 trillion microorganisms. The widely diverse bacterial flora of the human intestinal tract is classified into groups such as eubacteria, clostridia, bacteriodes, bifidobacteria and lactobacilli. Of these bacteria the later two categories, i.e. bifidobacteria and lactobacilli (as well as specific species of some Gram-positive cocci like *Lactococcus lactis*, *Streptococcus salivarius* and *Enterococcus faecium*), constitute the probiotic organisms or the 'good' bacteria. Bifidobacteria make up about 5% of large intestinal bacteria, while lactobacilli – although constituting less than 1% of intestinal bacteria – are more important in terms of their probiotic effects to the host.

In the human intestines, bacteria are considered good if their metabolism is geared to the breakdown of carbohydrates – referred to as being *saccharolytic*. These bacteria break down carbohydrates that enter the large bowel anaerobically (in the absence of oxygen) and produce short-chain fatty acids (SCFAs) as end products. This process is known as *fermentation* and leads to the production of hydrogen and carbon dioxide. The bacteria derive their energy from this process and grow and multiply to form the biomass in the human intestine. The process of fermentation is considered to be good for the host and none of the end products of fermentation are harmful to the host. In addition these good bacteria produce essential vitamins and contribute to the development of the immune system of the gut. Other bacteria in the intestines such as clostridia may be considered as being bad since they break down proteins in the absence of available carbohydrates that leads to end products like sulfides, amines and ammonia as well as SCFAs. These additional end products of protein metabolism are harmful to the gut epithelium. This process has been historically referred to as *putrefaction*. It has

been known for a very long time that putrefaction occurs in alkaline conditions, while lactic acid bacilli produce acidic conditions in the gut. This has contributed to the theory that the ageing process and the associated ill health is the result of putrefaction in the large intestine. The healthy gastrointestinal flora is considered to be predominantly saccharolytic with significant numbers of bifidobacteria and lactobacilli. In newborns and breastfed infants bifidobacteria dominate the intestinal flora.

The main role of the good bacteria, i.e. bifidobacteria and lactobacilli, is in providing the right environment in the gut, favouring fermentation with a proper intestinal microbial balance. They also provide a first line of defence in the gut against invading pathogens like *Salmonella* and *Campylobacter*. The reported health advantages associated with bifidobacteria in the gut of infants and adults include inhibition of pathogen growth, immunomodulation, the restoration of gut flora after antibiotic therapy, production of digestive enzymes, positive effects on antibiotic-associated diarrhoeas, and the repression of rotaviruses.

Probiotics are consumed as live microbial food supplements that beneficially affect the host by improving the intestinal microbial balance. The number of commercial probiotics available has increased dramatically in the last decade. They are marketed as yoghurts, yoghurt drinks, and even as supplements in the form of capsules or tablets. They have been evaluated for their benefits in a variety of gastrointestinal disorders like irritable bowel syndrome, ulcerative colitis, Crohn's disease, acute diarrhoeas, lactose intolerance and constipation. They have also been used for digestive comfort, prevention of infectious diseases and for improving athletic performance. Since probiotics are safe and have no side-effects with good consumer acceptance, they are being marketed widely as natural products for better health. The principal health claims of these commercial probiotic products are that they keep the gut healthy and support the body's natural defences.

---

inflammation. Gut-dwelling microbes also have contact and interaction with leucocytes directly within the lymphoid patches in the gut and thus enable direct immunoactivation. This latter interaction can lead to systemic immune activation as the lymphoid follicles drain into the mesenteric lymph nodes. It would thus appear that although

the primary site of immunological signalling is at the intestinal mucosal interface, the immunomodulatory effects of bacteria or probiotics can be manifest systemically. It is now evident that probiotics can influence lymphocyte proliferation, cytokine secretion, phagocytic activity of leucocytes, cellular killing by macrophages and NK cells, as well as antibody production. In view of their local and systemic actions, probiotics are capable of modulating the immune system by both immunostimulation and immunoregulation, thus having the potential to confer health benefits to the host.

Probiotics and gastrointestinal infections in infants and children

Diarrhoeal diseases are common in infants and children, being one of the major causes of child mortality in developing countries. Probiotics have been evaluated in clinical trials for both the prevention and the treatment of diarrhoeal diseases in infants and children. One of the earliest preventive interventions was a randomized controlled trial of infants who were either given an infant formula with bifidobacteria or a placebo formula. Over a 3-month period only 10% of the infants on the probiotic-supplemented infant formula had experienced one episode of acute diarrhoea compared with 60% of infants on the unsupplemented placebo formula. A longer period of follow-up of 17 months in infants showed that only 7% of the probiotic-supplemented (*Bifidobacterium bifidum* and *Streptococcus thermophilus*) group developed acute diarrhoea compared with 31% of the controls. It was also observed over the same 17-month period that only 10% of the probiotic-fed infants compared with 39% of the control infants shed rotavirus (a pathogen known to be responsible for acute diarrhoea in children) at some time in their stools.

Probiotics have been more extensively evaluated in the treatment of acute diarrhoeas in infants and children. In a study conducted in well-nourished children with acute diarrhoea (82% due to rotavirus), when oral rehydration was followed with probiotic (*Lactobacillus casei*), those groups receiving the probiotic in addition to rehydration fluids orally recovered from the illness much quicker. The duration of the diarrhoeal illness was reduced to 1.4 days compared with 2.4 days in the control group. There was no evidence of damage to the gut mucosa or its permeability following administration of the probiotic. Furthermore, the same investigators observed that administration of the probiotic (*L. casei*) along with live oral rotavirus vaccine caused an elevated response in rotavirus-specific IgM-secreting cells and an improved anti-rotavirus IgA seroconversion. It is also evident now that the benefit incurred with probiotics is not confined just to diarrhoeas of viral aetiology, but also affects bacterially induced gastroenteritis such as those due to *Escherichia coli*, *Salmonella* and *Shigella*. Probiotics like bifidobacteria also reduce the growth of *Candida albicans*, a commensal fungus or yeast normally present in the gut flora but sometimes growing abnormally and manifesting as an infection referred to as 'thrush' in infants.

A review of nine randomized controlled trials assessing the effects of *Lactobacillus* spp. on acute diarrhoea in infants and children concluded that probiotic administration shortens the diarrhoeal illness by an average of 1 day; not an insignificant reduction given an average episode lasts only 3–4 days. Probiotic administration also reduced the severity of the diarrhoea and there was strong evidence of a dose–response relationship. A more recent review of 23 randomized controlled trials with probiotics, mostly in children, has confirmed that probiotics are beneficial in the management of acute infectious diarrhoeas and that they affect the duration and severity of the diarrhoea. The review showed that the relative risk of diarrhoea lasting more than 3 days was reduced significantly, as well as demonstrating a significant reduction in the mean duration of the diarrhoea and in stool frequency.

Probiotics are effective in severe life-threatening conditions like necrotizing enterocolitis which occurs in premature infants. Necrotizing enterocolitis manifests as acute diarrhoea and is associated with death of sections of the large intestine in a premature infant. A review of nine studies in infants with this condition concluded that probiotics were beneficial and that mortality was reduced by 57% in infants with enterocolitis given probiotics compared with those who did not receive the same.

In addition to their main effects on improved immune function and of immunomodulation, it is hypothesized that probiotics reduce diarrhoea and gastroenteritis by other mechanisms too. These include a reduced gut pH through stimulation of lactic acid-producing microbes, direct antagonistic effects on pathogens, competing for binding and receptor sites that pathogens may occupy, and competition for available nutrients and other growth factors.

Probiotics may have an important role in the prevention of diarrhoeal disease and in reducing the incidence or shortening the duration of acute diarrhoeal episodes in developing countries. However, difficulties with regard to shelf-life and lack of refrigeration need to be addressed. Non-viable microorganisms may offer a stable alternative and there is evidence that heat-inactivated lactobacilli are effective in shortening the duration of rotavirus diarrhoeas. Live and viable bacteria are certainly more effective than killed bacteria, largely by their ability to translocate from the gut into the mesenteric lymph nodes and other extra-intestinal sites. Hence the latter are preferable as probiotics. In many developing countries the use of lactic acid-fermented weaning foods is part of the food culture, and this could hence be exploited to provide the right and safe probiotic foods in developing countries.

Probiotics and antibiotic-associated diarrhoea in the elderly

The elderly are more vulnerable to the side-effects of antibiotics such as antibiotic-associated diarrhoea (AAD). This may be the result of the balance of the intestinal flora undergoing changes with ageing, with the number of bifidobacteria declining and fermentation being replaced by protein breakdown and an increase in the so-called 'bad' bacteria. Elderly individuals when given antibiotics are at risk of AAD; it is estimated that a third of the elderly admitted to hospitals and administered antibiotics develop AAD, which can often be fatal. Several reviews have collated the results of trials with probiotics in the prevention of AAD not just in the elderly but also in children, and have confirmed the beneficial effects. Administration of probiotics along with and starting with the first dose of the antibiotic reduces the risk of AAD significantly compared with those administered antibiotics alone.

The commonest cause of AAD appears to be an association with a toxin produced by *Clostridium difficile* which manifests as a severe diarrhoea. Cases of *C. difficile* infections have been increasing in the UK and have been responsible for an increase in mortality. A randomized trial showed that the administration of a probiotic drink containing lactobacilli reduced the number of elderly who developed AAD to 12%, compared with the 34% seen in the control group. In addition, none of those who received the probiotic drink developed *C. difficile* infection.

Other non-specific immune benefits of probiotics

In addition to the convincing evidence that probiotics have an important role in both the prevention and treatment of diarrhoeal illness in the elderly and infants and children, it is apparent that probiotics may have other health benefits related to immunity and infection. Consumption of probiotic-supplemented yoghurt by elderly individuals over a period of a year has been shown to lower circulating levels of IgE and reduce nasal allergies. The administration of probiotics to elderly individuals also appears to enhance their immune response to the administered flu vaccine. Long-distance athletes who are more prone to frequent upper respiratory tract infections showed a reduction in the incidence and severity of respiratory infections when given probiotics daily.

The immunomodulatory role of probiotics is supported by other studies related to food allergies and atopic eczema in infants and children. The 'hygiene hypothesis' (see Chapter 15) attributes the increase in these conditions in the Western world to the lack of microbial stimulation favouring the development of IgE-mediated allergies especially at a time when intestinal colonization takes place in infancy. It also appears that the balance of beneficial and potentially harmful bacteria is altered in the large intestine of allergic infants, with less colonization by bifidobacteria and lower prevalence of lactobacilli in this group. Clinical trials with probiotic supplementation resulted in significant improvement in atopic dermatitis in infants, with significant decreases in inflammatory markers like TNF-α and α_1-antitrypsin levels that were elevated at baseline. Even when the mothers of exclusively breastfed infants received probiotics the incidence of chronic relapsing atopic eczema in the infants was significantly lowered.

There is good evidence that probiotics provide health benefits by the modulation of non-specific immune responses. Several trials with a variety of probiotics over varying periods of time have shown that their regular consumption increases phagocytosis by polymorphonuclear leucocytes and monocytes, increases bactericidal activities and increases NK-cell activity. They also seem to influence delayed hypersensitivity responses, cytokine production and immunoglobulin levels. The anti-inflammatory effects of probiotics seem to be the result of normalization of intestinal permeability, modification of the degradation and targeting of food antigens and by their direct anti-inflammatory activities, rather than by modulation of intestinal flora towards a more beneficial bacterial composition. It would appear that probiotics help the normal immune function of an individual and reduce the risk of several common infections as well as reducing inflammation. Since they are administered orally, probiotics also affect gastrointestinal function directly by improving gut transit and relieving digestive discomfort.

Probiotics and vaginal microflora

Lactobacillus spp. is the predominant bacterium in the vaginal microbial flora in women in the reproductive age group, while in peri- and postmenopausal women lactobacilli are frequently absent. The vaginal microflora, much like the gut, is a dynamic and viable ecosystem, and a lactobacilli-dominated vaginal flora is considered normal. A reduction in lactobacilli and its replacement by other organisms result in a condition called bacterial vaginosis. A number of probiotics administered as vaginal suppositories are able to effectively normalize the vaginal microflora and treat urogenital infections. Oral administration of probiotics also produces similar results. In a randomized controlled trial, oral consumption of a lactobacillus-based probiotic over 60 days brought about a significant increase in vaginal lactobacilli and a decrease in yeasts and coliform bacilli.

There is evidence to suggest that vaginal lactobacilli provide some protection against HIV infection. A positive association has been seen between abnormal vaginal flora and seropositivity to HIV-1 in several cross-sectional studies in Uganda, Kenya, Malawi, Thailand and the USA. The risk of seroconversion increased with the severity of the disturbance in the vaginal flora in these studies. In addition, data from Kenya suggested the risk of gonorrhoea and *Trichomonas* infection was also higher among women with abnormal vaginal flora. These data seem to suggest a role for probiotics as potential interventions to reduce a woman's risk of acquiring STDs including HIV infection.

14.3 Prebiotics

Prebiotics are substances that selectively modify the microbial flora of the gut and are defined as 'a non-digestible food ingredient that beneficially affects the host by selectively stimulating the growth and/or activity of one or a limited number of bacterial species already resident in the colon' (Table 14.1). Like probiotics, by selectively favouring the growth and activity of 'good' bacteria already resident in the human colon, prebiotics confer health benefits to the host. For a food ingredient to be considered a prebiotic it must not be digested, i.e. hydrolysed, or absorbed in the upper part of the gastrointestinal tract, and must hence pass into the large intestine largely unaffected, ending up as a selective substrate for one or a limited number of potentially beneficial microbes normally resident there. These food ingredients must stimulate the bacteria to grow and/or become metabolically active and hence must be able to alter the microbial flora to a healthier composition. They have also hence been defined as 'a non-viable food component that confers health benefit on the host associated with the modulation of the microbiota'. Although any food ingredient entering the large intestine is a potential prebiotic, it is the selectivity of the fermentation in the mixed culture environment of the large intestine that is most critical. Current focus is largely on the selective growth and/or activity of lactic acid-producing microorganisms, although it is not unlikely that future interests may cover those that selectively act on pathogenic organisms and attenuate their invasiveness and virulence.

Prebiotics are sugar-like carbohydrates which are mostly oligosaccharides (see Table 14.1) and are present in the diet in foods like cereals, soybeans, beans, onions and artichokes. They are present naturally in breast milk and are also used in food manufacturing and processing. Lactulose has been known to increase number of lactobacilli in the intestine of infants and has been used in infant formulas, although its ability to specifically enhance only these microorganisms is not proven. Consumption of fructo-oligosaccharides is known to stimulate bifidobacteria in adults. The administration of 15 g of fructo-oligosaccharide daily in healthy adults increased the proportion of bifidobacteria from 17% to 82% within 15 days. Addition of prebiotics to mixed cultures of bifidobacteria and pathogenic bacteria like *E. coli* results in increase of the former while the pathogenic organisms are reduced. Clinical trials with prebiotics suggest that their regular consumption may influence the incidence of traveller's diarrhoea and that they may have a beneficial effect on calcium absorption from the gut, favouring increases in bone mineral density. They are also known to affect the absorption and bioavailability of other minerals like zinc and iron favourably. In experimental animals, prebiotics like oligofructose exhibit immunomodulatory activities such as changes in lymphocyte subsets, increased phagocytic activity and enhanced IgA secretion. Prebiotics are potentially beneficial to the host from both a specific immune system perspective as well as on health more broadly.

14.4 Synbiotics

Products that contain a combination of both a probiotic and a prebiotic are referred to as synbiotics. The live microorganisms are used in conjunction with their specific substrates for growth; this combination is likely to improve the survival and multiplication of the probiotic organism, thus conferring benefit to the host. The usual combinations may be fructo-oligosacharides with bifidobacteria or lactitol with lactobacilli (see Table 14.1).

A randomized controlled trial using a synbiotic mixture of oligosaccharide (inulin–oligofructose) with bifidobacteria in patients with acute ulcerative colitis showed dramatic effects in reducing inflammation of the gut and mucosal regeneration of the gut epithelium. Markers of inflammation such as TNF-α and IL-1 were also significantly reduced following administration of the synbiotic for 1 month.

The ability to influence the microbial flora of the human intestine by the consumption of probiotics and prebiotics or both (synbiotics), and thereby modulate the immune system of the host to confer health benefits, is an exciting area where much research in nutrition and immune function is likely to take place in the years to come. There are clearly benefits to health with both the prevention of illnesses and the effective treatment of these conditions. Although the focus has been in the prevention and treatment of diarrhoeas and gastrointestinal disorders in infants, children, adults and the elderly, there are potential benefits of strengthening the immune system and improving digestive function by consuming these nutritional products.

Further Reading

Collins, M.D. and Gibson, G.R. (1999) Probiotics, prebiotics and synbiotics: approaches for modulating the microbial ecology of the gut. *American Journal of Clinical Nutrition* 69, 1052S–1057S. *This review provides an overview of how probiotics, prebiotics and synbiotics contribute to the nutritional modulation of the gut microecology.*

Cummings, J.H. (2009) Probiotics: better health from 'good' bacteria. *Nutrition Bulletin* 34, 198–202. *An excellent overview of the subject based on the Annual BNF Lecture delivered by the author.*

Gill, H.S. and Cross, M.L. (2002) Probiotics and immune function. In: Calder, P.C., Field, C.J. and Gill, H.S. (eds) *Nutrition and Immune Function.* CAB International and The Nutrition Society, Wallingford, UK, pp. 251–272. *A good comprehensive review of the topic from an immune mechanism perspective.*

Case Studies

Case Study 14.1: Probiotics in the prevention of antibiotic-associated diarrhoea.

A randomized, double-blind, placebo-controlled study was carried out in adult and elderly patients hospitalized in London, UK. The intervention group received a probiotic drink twice daily during a course of antibiotics and for 1 week after the antibiotic course was over. The control group received a sterile milk shake instead.

The incidence of antibiotic-associated diarrhoea (AAD) was significantly lower in the probiotic group and provided an odds ratio of 0.25 for use of the probiotic and an absolute risk reduction of 21.6%. Some of the data are summarized in Table 14.3.

None of the patients in the probiotic group had diarrhoea caused by *Clostridium difficile* while 17% of the controls developed *C. difficile* diarrhoea.

This study concluded that the consumption of a probiotic drink along with antibiotic treatment can reduce diarrhoea related to antibiotics and *C. difficile*. It can hence contribute to reduce morbidity, mortality and health costs associated with hospitalization of patients older than 50 years of age.

Table 14.3. Data on probiotics and AAD incidence. (Adapted from Hickson *et al.*, 2007.)

	Probiotic	Control
Percentage of hospitalized patients with diarrhoea	12*	34
Percentage of hospitalized patients with no diarrhoea	88	66
Percentage of patients positive for *C. difficile* toxin	0*	17
Percentage of patients negative for *C. difficile* toxin	100	83

*Statistically significant difference compared with the control group.

Reference

Hickson, M., D'Souza, A.L., Muthu, N., Rogers, T.R., Want, S., Rajkumar, C. and Bulpitt, C.J. (2007) Use of probiotic Lactobacillus preparation to prevent diarrhoea associated with antibiotics: a randomised double blind placebo controlled trial. *British Medical Journal* 335, 80–84.

Case Study 14.2: Effects of probiotic administration on persistent diarrhoea in children.

A study was conducted in children in India admitted to hospital with persistent diarrhoea (defined as an episode of diarrhoea which starts with an infection and lasts for at least 14 days), a recognized common cause of undernutrition in children.

This randomized, double-blind, hospital-based study provided randomly either oral rehydration salts (ORS) alone (considered as a control group) or ORS mixed with a powder containing 60 million cells of *Lactobacillus rhamnosus* for the intervention group. Table 14.4 summarizes the findings.

The findings in the case and control groups show that the mean frequency of diarrhoea dropped significantly by day 5 in the group receiving the probiotic, and the differences with the control group persisted until day 9 of hospitalization and treatment. In the control group the frequency of diarrhoea was similar to that of the probiotic group only on day 10. The mean duration of the diarrhoea (5.3 versus 9.2 days) was significantly lower in the probiotic group, but no differences were observed in the mean duration of vomiting (2.0 versus 1.9 days). The duration of hospitalization was also significantly lower in the probiotic group (7.3 versus 15.5 days).

This study not only demonstrates the efficacy of probiotics provided along with ORT in the management of diarrhoeal illness in children in developing countries, but also implies substantial reduction in health care costs in low-income countries.

Reference

Basu, S., Chatterjee, M., Ganguly, S. and Chandra, P.K. (2007) Effect of *Lactobacillus rhamnosus* GG in persistent diarrhea in Indian children. A randomized controlled trial. *Journal of Clinical Gastroenterology* 41, 756–760.

Table 14.4. Data on probiotics and persistent diarrhoea. (Adapted from Basu *et al.*, 2007.)

	Cases (ORS + probiotic)	Controls (ORS only)
Mean frequency of diarrhoea (day 1)	10.4	10.8
Mean frequency of diarrhoea (day 3)	10.4	10.5
Mean frequency of diarrhoea (day 5)	5.2*	10.2
Mean frequency of diarrhoea (day 7)	0.9*	7.5
Mean frequency of diarrhoea (day 9)	1.0*	4.3
Mean duration of diarrhoea (days)	5.3*	9.2
Mean duration of vomiting (days)	2.0	1.9
Mean duration of hospital stay (days)	7.3*	15.5

*Statistically significant difference compared with the control group.

15 Food Allergy

- Adverse reactions to foods are increasingly common and related to changing food consumption practices.
- Adverse reactions to food are immune-mediated (food allergy) or non-immune-mediated (food intolerance).
- Food allergy is largely mediated through IgE-mediated immune reactions.
- Food allergies can manifest as mild symptoms like itching and swelling to fatal anaphylactic reactions.
- Several factors like processing of foods and early introduction of foods can influence the occurrence of food allergies.
- The management of food allergies needs to focus on both prevention and treatment of the allergy.

15.1 Introduction

Food allergies are becoming increasingly common. The adverse response to food varies from mild manifestations at one end of the spectrum to a non-fatal or fatal anaphylactic response at the other end. This often raises the question as to why some foods elicit adverse reactions in human subjects. Adverse reactions to food are not all due to food allergies. Food allergy in turn has to be distinguished from food intolerance. *Food allergy* has an immunological basis as it is an immune-mediated reaction, while *food intolerance* does not have an immunological cause and is an adverse reaction to either the chemical or toxin in the food or the result of an enzyme deficiency in the host (see Box 15.1).

The prevalence of food allergy varies widely in different countries, largely the result of perceptions rather than incidence of the problem. It is estimated that about 20–30% of people in the UK think they have a food allergy while the true prevalence may be 1–3% or less. Geographical differences in food allergy may be attributable to genetic predispositions and to environmental factors such as the high consumption of certain foods or the introduction of novel foods. More recently the increasing prevalence of allergies including food allergy has been attributed to the increasing use of cleaning and hygienic products – often referred to as the 'hygiene hypothesis'.

In countries where the consumption of commonly allergenic foods like milk or peanuts is high, the incidence of allergy to these foods is also likely to be high. Cow's milk allergy is high in countries in North America (USA and Canada) and Northern Europe (Sweden, Denmark, Netherlands, UK) where the consumption of cow's milk is high. High consumption is also responsible for increase in peanut allergy and is probably the case in the USA, where the prevalence of peanut allergy is high compared with countries in Asia and Africa. However, consumption of peanuts is also high in China although the prevalence of allergy is much lower than in the USA. This difference is attributed to the cooking method used such as boiling and frying of peanuts which is common in China and has been shown to decrease the allergenicity of peanut protein.

Exposure to novel foods and the increasing use of chemicals, additives and dyes in processed food may be other factors that have contributed to the increase in food allergies in industrialized societies. Another important factor is the cross-reactivity between other allergens in the air (aeroallergens) and allergens in food. Sensitization to allergens in the air such as to birch pollen seems to confer allergy to the ingestion of fruits and vegetables that share molecules with similar structures to these pollens, thus conferring food allergy by cross-reaction. This chapter confines its discussion to food allergy which is immune mediated.

Box 15.1. Food Intolerance.

Food intolerance is a general term describing an abnormal physiological response to an ingested food or food additive. It is non-psychological and is a reproducible but unpleasant reaction to specific foods. This reaction is not immunological in nature and hence needs to be distinguished from the reactions to food considered as due to food allergy. The European Academy of Allergy and Clinical Immunology defines food intolerance as 'non-immune mediated adverse reaction to food'.

Food intolerance may be either caused by factors present in food or determined by the characteristics of the host. The food-related factors that cause food intolerance include the presence of toxic contaminants in the food or result from the pharmacological properties of the food. Characteristics of the host that result in food intolerance include metabolic disorders and enzyme deficiencies, a good example of which is lactase deficiency.

On this basis food intolerance is classified as follows.

- *Pharmacological food intolerance* may be caused by biogenic amines and other chemical compounds found in food and beverages. These include histamine in fish; tyramine in aged cheeses; phenylethylamine, tyramine or sulfites in wine; serotonin in bananas; caffeine in coffee; theobromine in chocolates; and theophylline in tea. Toxic contaminants and toxins in tinned food is another cause of food intolerance. Some food additives and histamine-releasing factors present in food may also cause pharmacological food intolerance. Some types of fish like tuna and mackerel acquire enriched histamine content as a result of bacterial action when improperly refrigerated. Toxins may be secreted by infectious agents like *Salmonella*, *Shigella* and *Campylobacter*. Sulfites in red wine may cause conditions like migraine.
- *Enzymatic food intolerance* is due to characteristics of the host such as lactase deficiency leading to lactose intolerance. Other forms of enzymatic food intolerance include rare conditions like galactosaemia, alcohol intolerance and glucose-6-phosphate dehydrogenase deficiency presenting as favism.
- *Undefined food intolerance* is an adverse reaction to certain food additives, the mechanisms of which

are largely unknown. The prevalence of this category of food intolerance is largely unknown but is assumed to be less than 1% in the general population. The range of additives used in processed food include colorants like azo and non-azo dyes, preservatives and antioxidants like sodium benzoate and bisulfites, emulsifiers and stabilizers like EDTA (ethylenediamine-*N*,*N*,*N′*,*N′*-tetraacetic acid) and gum acacia, fillers and flavours or sweeteners.

Lactose intolerance

Lactose intolerance is an adverse reaction to ingested milk. It is a commonly diagnosed food intolerance among adults and adolescents. The sugar in milk, i.e. lactose, requires the enzyme lactase in the gastrointestinal tract to break it down into its constituent sugars, glucose and galactose, for absorption. When the levels of lactase are low, large quantities of undigested dietary lactose remain in the gut, inducing osmotic diarrhoea, and when passed into the large intestine become subjected to bacterial action in the colon. This can lead to bloating and flatulence as well as abdominal pain and diarrhoea. A reduced level of lactase does not always imply that lactose is not digested at all and consequently only about a third of the people with lactase deficiency manifest with lactose intolerance. Hence lactose intolerance appears to be dose dependent and some individuals are more sensitive than others to lactose in the diet. It is estimated that 75% of adults worldwide show some decrease in lactase activity. About 5% of North Europeans show some lactase deficiency while it is much more common among Southern Europeans. Among other populations and racial groups such as Asians, Africans and Native Americans, lactase deficiency may exceed 90%.

Lactose intolerance due to lactase deficiency is genetically inherited and affects both males and females equally, although it varies with racial or population group. The prevalence of lactose intolerance varies from 1–2% among the Dutch and Swedes, to over 5% among native British, 12% among European Americans, over 40% among Southern Italians, 75% among African Americans, nearly 90% among Africans, over 95% among Chinese and South-east Asians and almost 100% among Native Americans.

15.2 Mechanism of Immune-mediated Food Allergy

The mechanism of an immune-mediated reaction to food is in many ways similar to the immunological response to a foreign protein or infectious agent. The contact with the component or chemical in food triggers an allergic response by the body. The immune-mediated adverse reaction to food or its component can be one of four types of allergic reaction. The commonest type is an allergic response that is mediated through the immunoglobulin IgE and hence is referred to as IgE-mediated or Type I allergic response. The other allergic responses are less common and are those that trigger other types of allergic responses (Types II, III and IV); together they are referred to as non-IgE-mediated allergic responses. The non-IgE immune-mediated responses are responsible for other immune-mediated food allergies or food-induced disorders like coeliac disease (see Box 15.2) and food protein-induced enterocolitis syndromes occurring in infants and children. The exact mechanisms of non-IgE-mediated food allergies, including those related to coeliac disease (see Box 15.2), are fairly well known. Type II is antibody-dependent cytotoxic hypersensitivity, Type III is immune-complex-mediated hypersensi-

tivity reactions and Type IV is delayed T-cell-mediated hypersensitivity reactions.

IgE-mediated or *Type I food allergy* is the commonest type of adverse response to food and the mechanisms of the allergic reaction have been clearly worked out. The response is triggered by an antigen which in this case is not an infectious agent or pathogen but a protein in food which contains an IgE epitope recognized by specific lymphocytes. An epitope is a localized region on the surface of an antigen that is capable of eliciting an immune response and combining with a specific antibody. The epitope is the antigenic determinant part of a macromolecule that is recognized by the immune system, specifically by B or T cells and by antibodies.

In an individual with the predisposition to the food allergy, the initial exposure to the food allergen causes the production of IgE antibodies. The

---

Box 15.2. Coeliac Disease.

Coeliac disease, also known as 'gluten-sensitive enteropathy', is a permanent intolerance of ingested gluten that damages the small intestine and that resolves with the removal of gluten from the diet. The manifestations of coeliac disease are the end result of a severe interaction between the human immune system and wheat and its products, the use of which is widespread in present-day diets. The lining of the small intestine is the target of this interaction, which results in both inflammation and damage to the architecture and structure of the small intestinal mucosa. The severe inflammation results in destruction and eventual loss of absorptive surface, with the intestinal villi appearing shortened and flattened and the adjoining crypt layer appearing increased in depth. These changes may be patchy or continuous in the small intestinal mucosa and lead to increased net secretion by the small intestine resulting in malabsorption. Coeliac disease results in loss of fat in the stools and deficiency of micronutrients like iron, folate and fat-soluble vitamins, which results in a syndrome characteristic of severe malabsorption.

Coeliac disease has been reported in both Western and Eastern populations. It affects about 1% of the Western population and is just as common in Latin America and the Middle East. It is hence a global problem. Coeliac disease has a genetic basis as the evidence is quite strong that it occurs in families. It is strongly associated with human leucocyte antigen (HLA) type II genes which are present in chromosome 6. These same HLA types are associated with

increased risk of autoimmune diseases. However, coeliac disease is triggered by environmental factors and specifically the cereal proteins collectively called 'gluten'. These are derived from the commonly consumed cereals wheat, barley and rye. The specific cereal proteins implicated are gliadins and glutenins in wheat and hordeins in barley. These toxic proteins are large and complex molecules. In coeliac disease the consumption of gluten disturbs the homeostasis of the intestinal epithelium, leading to unchecked inflammation of the intestinal mucosa due to a potent immune response which is manifested both as a local cellular response and a humoral response.

Clinically, coeliac disease presents with the signs and symptoms of a malabsorptive syndrome with diarrhoea, steatorrhoea (fatty stools), bloating, flatulence, abdominal pain, weight loss, failure to thrive and multiple deficiency states. Children can present with stunting of growth and intellectual development. The clinical presentation of coeliac disease is often referred to as the 'coeliac iceberg' since only a small proportion manifests the classic signs and symptoms of the disease. Much of coeliac disease may be asymptomatic or silent, or may even be latent gluten sensitivity with the potential to manifest at any time. The earlier methods of confirmatory diagnosis by serial intestinal biopsies before and after ingestion of gluten-free diet or a gluten challenge is now replaced by serological tests for immunoglobulins (IgA and IgG). The mainstay of treatment of coeliac disease is the lifelong adherence to a gluten-free diet.

---

mechanism appears to be as follows. The allergen is processed by APCs and, following its binding to allergen-specific Th cells, these Th cells then proliferate. Sensitization to a food allergen favours the Th2 rather than the Th1 type response and results in the production of cytokines, which in turn promote the differentiation and proliferation of allergen-specific B lymphocytes. These B cells produce allergen-specific IgE antibodies which tend to bind to high-affinity receptors on mast cells and basophils. When exposure to the allergen is repeated by the ingestion of the allergenic food, the food allergen comes into contact with mast cells and basophils bound to the IgE antibody and specific binding of the allergen and the IgE antibody takes place. The binding often occurs through cross-linkages with other IgE antibodies and this cross-linking triggers degranulation of mast cells and basophils, releasing preformed mediators like histamine as well as initiating the synthesis and release of TNF-α, prostaglandins and leucotrienes. It is the release of these mediators that causes the manifestation of the allergic reaction and the adverse response to the ingested food.

The hallmark of IgE-mediated allergic reactions is the generation of allergen-specific CD4+ Th2 lymphocytes and their production of specific cytokines to induce IgE class switching of B lymphocytes. This process along with other interleukins are important growth and activation factors for mast cells, for eosinophil development, as well as for mucus secretion and airway hypersensitivity of the lungs that characterize this allergic reaction. It is now believed that these allergies result from the dysbalance between the protective T regulatory response and a disease-inducing effector Th2 response. The manifestations of IgE-mediated allergic reactions to food in the skin, respiratory, gastrointestinal and other systems, compared with the disorders linked to food due to non-IgE and other cellular mechanisms, are outlined in Table 15.1.

In summary, sensitization of food allergens occurs through the gastrointestinal tract (true food allergens) or via the pulmonary system through cross-reactive aeroallergens. Food allergens enter the mucosal barrier and can be transported throughout the body in an immunologically intact form. Many food allergens are fairly stable to heat, acid and proteases and are resistant to digestion, which plays a critical role in allowing them contact with the intestinal immune system. Ingested food proteins can be transported throughout the body in an

Table 15.1. Types of food allergies and their mechanisms.

Immune mechanism	Disorder(s)
IgE mediated	
Cutaneous	Urticaria
	Angioedema
	Morbilliform rashes
	Flushing/pruritis
Respiratory	Rhinoconjunctivitis
	Laryngospasm
	Wheezing/bronchospasm
Gastrointestinal	Oral allergy syndrome
	Gastrointestinal
	anaphylaxis
Multi-system	Generalized anaphylaxis
	Food- and exercise-induced
	anaphylaxis
Mixed IgE and cell mediated	
Cutaneous	Atopic dermatitis
Respiratory	Asthma
Gastrointestinal	Eosinophilic oesophagitis
	Eosinophilic
	gastroenteritis

immunologically intact form – and would explain why symptoms of food allergies are not restricted to the gastrointestinal tract but cause extra-intestinal symptoms sometimes additionally and at other times exclusively. It is the dysregulated immune response to food allergens consisting of a strong Th2 and IgE response and a low regulatory T-cell and IgG or IgA response that leads to allergic disease due to food. Cross-linking of IgE on tissue mast cells triggers the release of pro-inflammatory mediators and initiates the acute-phase reaction and the recruitment of eosinophils, basophils and lymphocytes. Genetic (i.e. host) and environmental factors influence the individual immune reactions to food allergens.

15.3 Manifestations of Food Allergy

The symptoms and signs that characterize the varied manifestations of an allergic response to food are presented in Table 15.2. They affect a range of different organs: the principal ones affected with manifestations being the skin, respiratory tract, gastrointestinal tract and other systemic manifestations, as well as more severe conditions like non-fatal and fatal anaphylaxis. Anaphylactic reactions to food can be life threatening. Symptoms associated with IgE-mediated reactions, which incidentally are the commonest

Table 15.2. Symptoms of IgE-mediated allergic reactions to food. (Adapted from Opara, 2002.)

Cutaneous reactions	
Urticaria	Appearance of wheals in the skin
Angio-oedema	Swelling of subcutaneous tissue
Atopic dermatitis	Itching and dry skin
Respiratory reactions	
Rhinitis	Inflammation of nasal passages, runny nose
Asthma	Narrowing of airways, wheezing and breathlessness
Laryngeal oedema	Constriction of throat
Gastrointestinal reactions	Abdominal pain, nausea, vomiting, diarrhoea
Systemic reactions	
Anaphylactic reaction	Generalized severe rapid reaction with itching and swelling of oral cavity, and skin, respiratory, gastrointestinal and cardiovascular symptoms. Can be fatal
Oral allergy syndrome	Itching, swelling of lips, tongue and larynx. Other symptoms include urticaria, rhinitis, asthma, laryngeal oedema. May even lead to anaphylaxis

food allergies, occur very quickly within minutes of ingestion of the food concerned. They may also manifest as delayed symptoms or reactions.

15.4 Foods that Cause Allergic Reactions and Their Properties

The major immune-mediated food allergies trigger an IgE-mediated allergic response (Type I allergic response) and a wide range of foods are known to cause this type of food allergy. The most common allergenic foods include:

- cereals – wheat, oats, barley and their products, and also include gluten-induced enteropathy which is strictly not a Type I allergic response;
- crustaceans and other shellfish and their products;
- egg and egg products;
- fish and fish products;
- milk and milk products;

- legumes, peas, peanuts, soybeans and their products;
- tree nuts like brazil nuts, hazelnuts and walnuts, and their products.

The foods which constitute this list are invariably part of the habitual daily diet and the question of why they should elicit an allergic reaction on consumption requires to be addressed.

Immunological characteristics

The allergens present in these foods must possess immunological and biochemical characteristics that permit them to elicit an IgE-mediated immune response. From our understanding of the mechanisms of this immune-mediated reaction, it is evident that the food allergen must selectively bind to a T cell, a B cell or a specific antibody to activate this process. The allergen would need to have the specific epitope that binds to IgE and must be able to cross-link one IgE antibody with another to activate the degranulation of mast cells or basophils to enable manifestation of the response. Thus the basic immunological characteristics of food allergens would include the fact that they possess the IgE epitope and also possess at least two IgE-binding sites to elicit an IgE response. It is now known that even in the absence of the latter ability allergens can initiate adverse reactions by acting as haptens (i.e. small molecules that elicit an immune response when bound to larger molecules), thus enabling cross-linkages. Examination of the biochemical structure of the allergen has hitherto not shown any consistency in the structures of food allergens to account for their behaviour.

Physical and chemical properties

The physical and chemical properties of food allergens indicate that they have molecular weights of between 10 to 70 kDa and that they are glycosylated proteins. However, much smaller molecules can elicit an allergic response and so too can very large molecules of between 200 and 300 kDa as in the case of peanut allergy. But these characteristics are not unique to allergens in food since many other proteins in food fulfil these criteria.

Effects of heat and digestion

Food allergens are generally heat stable and not destroyed at high temperatures. Allergens in cow's milk, fish, soy and peanut are known to be heat resistant. A number of allergens and particularly those in cow's milk, egg, peanut and soybean are also resistant to enzymatic digestion by the gastrointestinal secretions. This feature is not consistent, as peptic digestion of peanut allergen has been shown to eliminate its IgE-binding capacity. Other studies have shown the opposite effect of digestion enhancing the allergenicity of food proteins, with hidden epitopes being unravelled by the process of digestion. Food allergens in fruits and vegetables, on the other hand, are heat labile and more sensitive to the digestive process.

Effects of food processing

Those food allergens that are generally resistant to high temperatures and protein digestion are unlikely to be affected by food processing, which includes thermal processing and enzymatic proteolysis. The allergenicity of the allergens in peanuts, for instance, is enhanced by heating and roasting. Other food processing techniques like phenolic browning diminish the IgE-binding capacities of allergens in apple while lyophilization does the same for fish allergens. Novel foods and novel food processing techniques may have an enormous impact on food allergenicity and is hence a food safety concern.

Cross-reactivity of food allergens

Since different allergens share the same or similar IgE epitopes they may cause cross-reactivity. For instance, individuals with pollen allergies (induced by aeroallergens) such as for birch, oak and mugwort may also suffer food allergy specific to some fruits like apples, pears and kiwi fruits and to vegetables like carrots and celery, as well as to hazelnuts. Cross-reactivity can also occur between allergens present in foods. Cross-reactive allergic responses are known between foods belonging to the legume family and between those belonging to different fish species. The magnitude of the cross-reaction can be highly variable between individuals in the two types of cross-reaction observed clinically, i.e. aeroallergens and food allergens and within-species food allergens. The example of food allergies associated with pollen allergies due to cross-reactivity is a condition called oral allergy syndrome (see Box 15.3).

Box 15.3. Oral Allergy Syndrome.

Oral allergy syndrome (OAS) is one of the most common adverse reactions to food in adults. The foods generally responsible for OAS are fruits and vegetables, but milk, eggs and fish are also known to cause OAS. The symptoms of OAS mainly involve the lips, mouth and cheeks and present as itching and swelling (angio-oedema) of these regions within minutes of chewing or swallowing of the foods implicated. Papulo-vesicular eruptions and laryngeal oedema may follow. Swallowing of the food may lead to gastrointestinal symptoms like nausea, abdominal pain, vomiting and diarrhoea. Life-threatening anaphylaxis can also occur.

Patients with pollen allergies and those with hay fever often present with OAS and complain of oral symptoms when eating fresh fruits and vegetables. This is a good example of cross-reactivity between aeroallergens and food allergens. OAS is an IgE-mediated allergic response and results from cross-reactivity between the pollen, birch most commonly, and a range of botanically related fruits (apple, peach, cherry) and vegetables (carrot, potato, fennel,

celery). The cross-reactivity is due to common allergenic epitopes shared by both the pollens and the fruits and vegetables concerned. Cross-reacting epitopes are weak and are destroyed by cooking or processing of food, and hence usually only raw foods elicit symptoms of OAS. Those with OAS who are allergic to birch react to *Roasaceae* fruits like peach, apple, almond, plum, apricot, pear and strawberry, as well as to potatoes, carrots, hazelnuts, celery and fennel; while those with ragweed allergy react to melons, cantaloupe and honeydew.

Individuals who are allergic to latex (natural rubber) may also present with OAS. This particular type of cross-reactivity is referred to as *latex fruit syndrome*, where sensitization to latex imparts reactivity to fruits, including papaya, banana, avocado, mango, melon, pineapple and peach. This is also an IgE-mediated allergy where the epitopes are common and hence cross-react. *Tree nut allergy syndrome* is another example of cross-reactivity between tree nuts like hazelnut, brazil nut, cashew nuts, etc.

15.5 Factors that Influence Susceptibility to Food Allergies

There are several factors that determine and influence the manifestation of food allergies in individuals. They include genetic predisposition and environmental factors such as early exposure, high consumption and the novelty of foods introduced to the habitual diet. The increasing prevalence of food allergies implies a major role for environmental factors in the development of food allergies in modern societies.

Genetic predisposition

A family history of *atopy* (i.e. a genetic predisposition towards mounting an IgE antibody response) may influence the development of food allergies. Atopic individuals are those who exhibit sensitization to two or more allergens, make IgE constantly and have high levels of circulating IgE. Atopy is associated with allergic diseases like asthma and eczema and increases the risk of food allergies. Children with one atopic parent have a high risk of developing IgE-mediated food allergy, while those with two atopic parents have up to 100% chance of developing a food allergy. Peanut allergy is known to be significantly higher among identical twins than in non-identical twins.

Early exposure to foods

A major cause of the development of food allergy in young children is considered to be early exposure to foods. Since the gut mucosal barrier takes years to mature the gut mucosa exhibits greater permeability in children and thus allows more proteins and allergens to enter the bloodstream. Systemic exposure to these allergens may induce an immune response that may manifest as a food allergy. Thus early introduction of foods may influence the development of IgE-mediated food allergies. Early exposure of young children to peanuts in the USA and to fish in Scandinavia has been implicated as being responsible for the development of allergies to these foods in these countries. However, the development of peanut allergy may also be linked to atopy and the UK government advises that the introduction of peanuts and its products be avoided for infants and children from families with a history of atopy (see Case Study 15.1).

Early introduction of allergens can also occur through the maternal diet transmitted through breast milk to the infant. Allergens to cow's milk and to egg protein have been known to be transmitted via breast milk. Even peanut allergens have been shown to be transmitted through breast milk with risk of potential sensitization of the infant. Sensitization has even been reported to occur *in utero*. Mothers who consume peanuts during pregnancy are more likely to have a child with allergy to peanuts.

Consumption level

High consumption of some foods can result in persistent exposure to the allergen and may lead to IgE-mediated food allergy. The high prevalence of peanut allergy in the USA and fish allergy in Scandinavia has been attributed to the probability of high consumption of these foods in their populations, increasing the risk of these food allergies.

Novelty of foods

Introduction of new or novel foods into the diet may be another reason why food allergies appear. The introduction of soybeans to France and the introduction of kiwi fruits into the USA resulted in increased reports of food allergies related to these foods. The introduction of novel foods and genetically modified foods has the potential to increase a range of new food allergies.

15.6 Diagnosis and Management of Food Allergy

The diagnosis of food allergy depends on a good clinical history followed by a physical examination. Verification of the suspect food can be undertaken by eliminating the food from the diet and then followed by a food challenge. The food challenge has to be double blind and placebo controlled. The other useful investigation for confirmatory diagnosis is a clinical skin test or patch test (see Box 15.4).

Food allergies need to be prevented and treated. The management of food allergies thus includes both preventive measures such as dietary modification during pregnancy, proper infant feeding and use of exclusion diets, as well as novel approaches such as probiotics and gene therapy (see Box 15.4).

Further Reading

Taylor, S.L. and Hefle, S.L. (2006) Food allergy. In: Bowman, B.A. and Russell, R.M. (eds) *Present Knowledge in Nutrition*, 9th edn. International Life Sciences Institute, Washington, DC, pp. 625–634. *A chapter that covers the topic of food allergy comprehensively.*

Case Studies

Case Study 15.1: Recommendations on peanut allergy by the Department of Health, UK.

The Committee on Toxicity of Chemicals in Food, Consumer Products and the Environment of the Department of Health, UK produced a report on peanut allergy in 1998. The Committee was of the opinion that crude peanut oil can contain peanut allergens while refined peanut oil contains no detectable protein by immunoassay and has not caused reaction in peanut-allergic individuals.

The Committee was of the opinion that there was support for the suggestion that peanut allergy in an infant can result from exposure *in utero* or during lactation. However, it concluded that the data on the relationship between peanut consumption by pregnant and lactating women and the incidence of peanut allergy in their offspring were inconclusive and suggested that more research is needed in this area.

The Committee stated that peanut allergy occurs in individuals who have atopy or who have parents or siblings with atopy; and that in common with other atopic diseases, the prevalence of peanut allergy was increasing in the UK.

The Committee issued the following advice regarding peanut allergy.

- Pregnant women who are atopic, or for whom the father or any sibling of the unborn child has an atopic disease, may wish to avoid eating peanuts and peanut products during pregnancy.
- Breastfeeding mothers who are atopic, or those for whom the father or any sibling of the baby has an atopic disease, may wish to avoid eating peanuts and peanut products during lactation.
- In common with the advice given for all children, infants with a parent or sibling with an atopic disease should, if possible, be breastfed exclusively for 4 to 6 months.

- During weaning of these infants, and until they are at least 3 years of age, peanuts and peanut products should be avoided.
- Infants or children who are allergic to peanuts should not consume peanuts or peanut products.

The Committee further recommended that the parents or those charged with the care of peanut-allergic infants and children should also take the following precautions.

- Be vigilant in reading labels on all multi-ingredient foods and avoid any for which doubt exists about the ingredients.
- Be aware that even minute amounts of peanut allergens may result in severe reactions. They should therefore be alert to the possibility of accidental exposure and should ensure that cross-contamination of foodstuffs with peanut allergens does not occur.
- Be aware of the treatment for anaphylaxis should inadvertent exposure occur; for example, at school or the homes of other children.

The Committee stated the need for clear and informative labelling of foodstuffs that contain peanut products and encouraged the labelling of foodstuffs to indicate the presence of any peanuts or peanut products even where this is not specifically required under existing labelling legislation.

Source Material

Chapter 1

Black, R.E., Allen, L.H., Bhutta, Z.A., Caulfield, L.E., deOnis, M., Ezzati, M. and Rivera, J. (2008) Maternal and child undernutrition: global and regional exposures and health consequences. *Lancet* 371, 243–260.

Mata, L. (1979) The malnutrition–infection complex and its environmental factors. *Proceedings of the Nutrition Society* 38, 29–40.

Scrimshaw, N.S. (2003) Historical concepts of the interactions, synergism and antagonism between nutrition and infection. *Journal of Nutrition* 133, 316S–321S.

Scrimshaw, N.S. and SanGiovanni, J.P. (1997) Synergism of nutrition, infection, and immunity: an overview. *American Journal of Clinical Nutrition* 66, 464S–477S.

Scrimshaw, N.S., Gordon, C.E. and Taylor, J.E. (1959) Interactions of nutrition and infection. *American Journal of Medical Sciences* 237, 367–403.

Shetty, P.S. (2009) Food and nutrition. In: Detels, R., Beaglehole, R., Lansang, M.A. and Gulliford, M. (eds) *Oxford Textbook of Public Health*, 5th edn. Oxford University Press, Oxford, UK, pp. 177–197.

Solomons, N.W. (2007) Malnutrition and infection: an update. *British Journal of Nutrition* 98, S5–S10.

Sommer, A., Tarwotjo, I., Djunaedi, E., West, K.P., Loeden, A.A., Tilden, R. and Mele, L. (1986) Impact of vitamin A supplementation on childhood mortality. A randomised controlled community trial. *Lancet* 1, 1169–1173.

World Health Organization (1965) *Report Expert Committee on Nutrition and Infection. WHO Technical Report Series No. 314.* World Health Organization, Geneva, Switzerland.

Chapter 2

Playfair, J.H.L. and Bancroft, G. (2004) *Infection and Immunity*, 2nd edn. Oxford University Press, Oxford, UK.

Wintergerst, E.S., Maggini, S. and Hornig, D.H. (2007) Contribution of selected vitamins and trace elements to immune function. *Annals of Nutrition & Metabolism* 51, 301–323.

Chapter 3

Andrews, F.J. and Griffiths, R.D. (2002) Glutamine: essential for immune nutrition in the critically ill. *British Journal of Nutrition* 87, S3–S8.

Barbul, A. and Dawson, H. (1994) Arginine and immunity. In: Forse, R.A., Bell, S.J., Blackburn, G.L. and Kabbash, L.G. (eds) *Diet, Nutrition and Immunity*. CRC Press, Boca Raton, Florida, pp. 199–216.

Bhaskaram, P. (2002) Micronutrient malnutrition, infection and immunity: an overview. *Nutrition Reviews* 60, S40–S45.

Bogden, J.D. (2004) Influence of zinc on immunity in the elderly. *Journal of Nutrition, Health & Aging* 8, 48–54.

Calder, P.C. (2001) Polyunsaturated fatty acids, inflammation and immunity. *Lipids* 36, 1007–1024.

Calder, P.C. (2004) *n*-3 Fatty acids, inflammation and immunity. *Lipids* 39, 1147–1161.

Chew, B.P. and Park, J.S. (2004) Carotenoid action on immune response. *Journal of Nutrition* 134, 257S–261S.

Dardenne, M. (2002) Zinc and immune function. *European Journal of Clinical Nutrition* 56, S20–S23.

Dudrick, P.S., Alverdy, J.C. and Souba, W.W. (1994) Glutamine and the immune system. In: Forse, R.A., Bell, S.J., Blackburn, G.L. and Kabbash, L.G. (eds) *Diet, Nutrition and Immunity*. CRC Press, Boca Raton, Florida, pp. 217–227.

Erickson, K.L., Medina, E.A. and Hubbard, N.E. (2000) Micronutrients and innate immunity. *Journal of Infectious Diseases* 182, S5–S10.

Failla, M.L. (2003) Trace elements and host defense: recent advances and continuing challenges. *Journal of Nutrition* 133, 1443S–1447S.

Grimble, R.F. (2001) Nutritional modulation of immune function. *Proceedings of the Nutrition Society* 60, 389–397.

Grimble, R.F. (2006) The effects of sulfur amino acid intake on immune function in humans. *Journal of Nutrition* 136, 1660S–1665S.

Ibs, K.H. and Rink, L. (2003) Zinc-altered immune function. *Journal of Nutrition* 133, 1452S–1456S.

Kudsk, K.A. (2002) Current aspects of mucosal immunology and its influence by nutrition. *American Journal of Surgery* 183, 390–398.

Kuvibidila, S. and Baliga, B.S. (2002) Role of iron in immunity and infection. In: Calder, P.C., Field, C.J. and Gill, H.S. (eds) *Nutrition and Immune Function*. CAB International and The Nutrition Society, Wallingford, UK, pp. 209–228.

Li, P., Yin, Y.L., Li, D., Kim, S.W. and Wu, G. (2007) Amino acids and immune function. *British Journal of Nutrition* 98, 237–252.

Maggini, S., Wintergerst, E.S., Beverdige, S. and Horning, D.H. (2007) Selected vitamins and trace elements support immune function by strengthening epithelial barriers and cellular and humoral immune responses. *British Journal of Nutrition* 98, S29–S35.

Popovic, P.J., Zeh, H.J. and Ochoa, J.B. (2007) Arginine and immunity. *Journal of Nutrition* 137, 1681S–1686S.

Prasad, A.S. (1998) Zinc and immunity. *Molecular and Cellular Biochemistry* 188, 63–69.

Prasad, A.S. (2007) Zinc: mechanisms of host defence. *Journal of Nutrition* 137, 1345–1349.

Prasad, A.S. (2008) Clinical, immunological, anti-inflammatory and antioxidant roles of zinc. *Experimental Gerontology* 43, 370–377.

Reifen, R. (2002) Vitamin A as an anti-inflammatory agent. *Proceedings of the Nutrition Society* 61, 397–400.

Rink, L. and Gabriel, P. (2000) Zinc and immune system. *Proceedings of the Nutrition Society* 59, 541–552.

Roth, E. (2007) Immune and cell modulation by amino acids. *Clinical Nutrition* 26, 535–544.

Semba, R.D. (1998) The role of vitamin A and related retinoids in immune function. *Nutrition Reviews* 56, S38–S48.

Semba, R.D. (1999) Vitamin A and immunity to viral, bacterial and protozoan infections. *Proceedings of the Nutrition Society* 58, 719–727.

Semba, R.D. (2002) Vitamin A, infection and immune function. In: Calder, P.C., Field, C.J. and Gill, H.S. (eds) *Nutrition and Immune Function*. CAB International and The Nutrition Society, Wallingford, UK, pp. 151–169.

Shankar, A. (2006) Nutritional modulation of immune function and infectious disease. In: Bowman, B.A. and Russell, R.M. (eds) *Present Knowledge in Nutrition*, 9th edn. International Life Sciences Institute, Washington, DC, pp. 604–624.

Sijben, J.W. and Calder, P.C. (2007) Differential immuno-modulation with long chain-3-PUFA in health and chronic disease. *Proceedings of the Nutrition Society* 66, 237–259.

Stephenson, C.B. (2001) Vitamin A, infection and immunity. *Annual Review of Nutrition* 21, 167–192.

Villamor, E. and Fawzi, W.W. (2005) Effects of vitamin A supplementation on immune responses and correlation with clinical outcomes. *Clinical Microbiological Reviews* 18, 446–464.

Wintergerst, E.S., Maggini, S. and Horning, D.H. (2007) Contribution of selected vitamins and trace elements to immune function. *Annals of Nutrition & Metabolism* 51, 310–323.

Yaqoob, P. (2002) Monounsaturated fatty acids and immune function. *European Journal of Clinical Nutrition* 56, S9–S13.

Yaqoob, P. (2004) Fatty acids and the immune system: from basic science to applications. *Proceedings of the Nutrition Society* 63, 89–104.

Yaqoob, P. and Calder, P.C. (2007) Fatty acids and immune function: new insights into mechanisms. *British Journal of Nutrition* 98, S41–S45.

Chapter 4

Ashworth, A. (2001) Low birth weight infants, infection and immunity. In: Suskind, R.M. and Tontisirin, K. (eds) *Nutrition, Immunity and Infection in Infants and Children. Nestle Nutrition Workshop Series No. 45*. Lippincot, Williams & Wilkins, Philadelphia, Pennsylvania, pp. 121–136.

Bryce, J., Boschi-Pinto, C., Shibuya, K. and Black, R.E. (2005) WHO estimates of the causes of deaths in children. *Lancet* 365, 1147–1152.

Caulfield, L.E., de Onis, M., Blossner, M. and Black, R.E. (2004) Undernutrition as an underlying cause of child death associated with diarrhea, pneumonia, malaria and measles. *American Journal of Clinical Nutrition* 80, 193–198.

Chandra, R.K. (1981a) Immunodeficiency in undernutrition and overnutrition. *Nutrition Reviews* 39, 225–331.

Chandra, R.K. (1981b) Immunocompetence as a functional index of nutritional status. *British Medical Bulletin* 37, 89–94.

Chandra, R.K. (1981c) Immunocompetence. *Clinics in Laboratory Medicine* 1, 631–645.

Chandra, R.K. (1983a) Malnutrition. In: Chandra, R.K. (ed.) *Primary and Secondary Immunodeficiency Disorders*. Churchill Livingstone, London, pp. 187–203.

Chandra, R.K. (1983b) Nutrition, immunity and infection: present knowledge and future directions. *Lancet* 321, 688–691.

Chandra, R.K. (1988) Nutritional regulation of immunity: an introduction. In: Chandra, R.K. (ed.) *Nutrition and Immunology*. Alan Liss Inc., New York, pp. 1–8.

Chandra, R.K. (2000) Foreword. In: Gershwin, M.E., German, J.B. and Keen, C.L. (eds) *Nutrition and Immunology: Principles and Practice*. Humana Press, Totowa, New Jersey, pp. v–vii.

Gross, R.L. and Newberne, P.M. (1980) Role of nutrition in immunologic function. *Physiological Reviews* 60, 188–302.

Jackson, A.A. and Calder, P.C. (2004) Severe undernutrition and immunity. In: Gershwin, M.E., Nestel, P. and Keen, C.L. (eds) *Handbook of Nutrition and Immunity*. Humana Press, Totowa, New Jersey, pp. 71–92.

Scrimshaw, N.S., Gordon, C.E. and Taylor, J.E. (1968) *Interactions of Nutrition and Infection.* World Health Organization, Geneva, Switzerland.

Suskind, R.M., LeWinter-Suskind, L., Murthy, K.K., Suskind, D. and Liu, D. (2001) The malnourished child: an overview. In: Suskind, R.M. and Tontisirin, K. (eds) *Nutrition, Immunity and Infection in Infants and Children. Nestle Nutrition Workshop Series No. 45.* Lippincot, Williams & Wilkins, Philadelphia, Pennsylvania, pp. 23–44.

WHO Multicentre Growth Reference Study Group (2006) WHO Child Growth Standards based on length/height, weight and age. *Acta Paediatrica* 450, 76–85.

Woodward, B. (2001) The effect of protein energy malnutrition on immune competence. In: Suskind, R.M. and Tontisirin, K. (eds) *Nutrition, Immunity and Infection in Infants and Children. Nestle Nutrition Workshop Series No. 45.* Lippincot, Williams & Wilkins, Philadelphia, Pennsylvania, pp. 89–120.

World Health Organization (1995) *Physical Status: The Use and Interpretation of Anthropometry. Technical Report Series No. 854.* World Health Organization, Geneva, Switzerland.

Chapter 5

Farthing, M.J.G. and Ballinger, A.B. (2001) Anorexia and cytokines in the acute phase response to infections. In: Suskind, R.M. and Tontisirin, K. (eds) *Nutrition, Immunity and Infection in Infants and Children. Nestle Nutrition Workshop Series No. 45.* Lippincot, Williams & Wilkins, Philadelphia, Pennsylvania, pp. 303–318.

Jackson, A.A. and Calder, P.C. (2004) Severe undernutrition and immunity. In: Gershwin, M.E., Nestel, P. and Keen, C.L. (eds) *Handbook of Nutrition and Immunity.* Humana Press, Totowa, New Jersey, pp. 71–92.

Katona, P. and Katona-Apte, J. (2008) The interaction between nutrition and infection. *Clinical Practice* 46, 1582–1588.

Keusch, G.T. (2001) Nutrition, immunity, and infectious diseases in infants and children. In: Suskind, R.M. and Tontisirin, K. (eds) *Nutrition, Immunity and Infection in Infants and Children. Nestle Nutrition Workshop Series No. 45.* Lippincot, Williams & Wilkins, Philadelphia, Pennsylvania, pp. 45–54.

Mata, L. (1979) The malnutrition–infection complex and its environmental factors. *Proceedings of the Nutrition Society* 38, 29–40.

Mata, L.J., Urrutia, J.J. and Lechtig, A. (1971) Infection and nutrition of children of a low socioeconomic rural community. *American Journal of Clinical Nutrition* 24, 249–259.

Mata, L.J., Urrutia, J.J., Albertazzi, C., Pellecer, O. and Arellano, E. (1972) Influence of recurrent infections on nutrition and growth in children in Guatemala. *American Journal of Clinical Nutrition* 25, 1267–1275.

Schaible, U.E. and Kaufmann, S.H.E. (2007) Malnutrition and infection: complex mechanisms and global impacts. *PLOS Medicine* 4, e115.doi:10.1371/journal.pmed.0040115.

Scrimshaw, N.S., Gordon, C.E. and Taylor, J.E. (1968) *Interactions of Nutrition and Infection.* World Health Organization, Geneva, Switzerland.

Tomkins, A. and Watson, F. (1989) *Malnutrition and Infection. Nutrition Policy Discussion Paper No. 5.* United Nations Administrative Committee on Coordination, Sub-committee on Nutrition, Geneva, Switzerland.

Chapter 6

Arthur, P., Kirkwood, B., Ross, D., Morris, S., Gyapong, J., Tomkins, A. and Addy, H. (1992) Impact of vitamin A supplementation on childhood mortality in northern Ghana. *Lancet* 339, 361–362.

Chandra, R.K. (1988) Increased bacterial binding to respiratory epithelial cells in vitamin A deficiency. *British Medical Journal* 297, 834–835.

Klemm, R.D., Labrique, A.B., Christian, P., Rashid, M., Shamim, A.A., Katz, J., Sommer, A. and West, K.P. (2008) Newborn vitamin A supplementation reduced infant mortality in rural Bangladesh. *Paediatrics* 122, 242–250.

Rahmathullah, L., Underwood, B.A., Thulasiraj, R.D., Milton, R.C., Ramaswamy, K., Rahmathullah, R. and Babu, G. (1990) Reduced mortality among children in Southern India receiving a small weekly dose of vitamin A. *New England Journal of Medicine* 323, 929–935.

Semba, R.D. (2002) Vitamin A, infection and immune function. In: Calder, P.C., Field, C.J. and Gill, H.S. (eds) *Nutrition and Immune Function.* CAB International and The Nutrition Society, Wallingford, UK, pp. 151–169.

Sommer, A. (1992) Vitamin A deficiency and childhood mortality. *Lancet* 339, 864.

Sommer, A., Hussaini, G., Tarwotjo, I. and Susanto, D. (1983) Increased mortality in children with mild vitamin A deficiency. *Lancet* 2, 585–588.

Sommer, A., Katz, J. and Tarwotjo, I. (1984) Increased risk of respiratory disease and diarrhoea in children with pre-existing mild vitamin A deficiency. *American Journal of Clinical Nutrition* 40, 1090–1095.

Sommer, A., Tarwotjo, I., Djunaedi, E., West, K.P., Loeden, A.A., Tilden, R. and Mele, A. (1986) Impact of vitamin A supplementation on childhood mortality. A randomised controlled community trial. *Lancet* 1, 1169–1173.

Tielsch, J.M., Rahmathullah, L., Thulsiraj, R.D., Katz, J., Coles, C., Sheeladevi, S., John, R. and Prakash, K. (2007) Newborn vitamin A dosing reduces the case fatality but not the incidence of common childhood morbidities in South India. *Journal of Nutrition* 137, 2470–2474.

Villamor, E. and Fawzi, W.W. (2005) Effects of vitamin A supplementation on immune responses and correlation with clinical outcomes. *Clinical Microbiology Reviews* 18, 446–464.

West, K.P., Pokhrel, R.P., Katz, J., LeClerq, S.C., Khatry, S.K., Shreshta, S.R., Pradhan, E.K., Tielsch, J.M. and Pandey, M.R. (1991) Efficacy of vitamin A in reducing preschool mortality in Nepal. *Lancet* 338, 67–71.

Chapter 7

Angeles, I.T., Schluntink, W.J., Matulessi, P., Gross, R. and Sastroamidjojo (1993) Decreased rate of stunting among anaemic preschool children on iron supplementation. *American Journal of Clinical Nutrition* 58, 339–342.

Basta, S.S., Soekirman, M.S., Karyadi, D. and Scrimshaw, N.S. (1979) Iron deficiency anaemia and productivity of adult males in Indonesia. *American Journal of Clinical Nutrition* 32, 916–925.

Chwang, L.C., Soemantri, A.G. and Pollitt, E. (1988) Iron supplementation and physical growth in rural Indonesian children. *American Journal of Clinical Nutrition* 47, 496–501.

Dallman, P.R. (1987) Iron deficiency and the immune response. *American Journal of Clinical Nutrition* 46, 329–334.

Gordeuk, V.R., Thuma, P.E., Brittenham, G., McLaren, C. and Parry, D. (1992) Effect of iron chelation therapy on recovery from deep coma in children with cerebral malaria. *New England Journal of Medicine* 327, 1473–1477.

Harvey, P.W., Heywood, P.F., Nesheim, M.C., Galme, K., Zegan, M., Habicht, J.P., Stephenson, L.S., Radimer, K.L., Brabin, B., Forsyth, K. and Alpers, M.P. (1989) The effect of iron therapy on malarial infection in Papua New Guinean school children. *American Journal of Tropical Medicine and Hygiene* 40, 12–18.

Hershko, C. (1993) Iron, infection and immune function. *Proceedings of the Nutrition Society* 52, 165–174.

Hershko, C., Peto, T.E.A. and Weatherall, D.J. (1988) Iron and infection. *British Medical Journal* 296, 660–664.

Lawless, J.W., Latham, M.E., Stephenson, L.S., Kinoti, S.N. and Pertet, A.N. (1994) Iron supplementation improves appetite and growth in anemic Kenyan primary school children. *Journal of Nutrition* 124, 645–654.

Menendez, C., Kahigwa, E., Hirt, R., Vounatsou, P., Aponte, J.J., Font, F., Acosta, C.J., Schellenberg, D.M., Galindo, C.M., Kimario, J., Urassa, H., Brabin, B., Smith, T.A., Kitua, A.Y., Tanner, M. and Alonso, P.L. (1997) Randomised placebo-controlled trial of iron supplementation and malaria chemoprophylaxis for prevention of severe anaemia and malaria in Tanzanian infants. *Lancet* 350, 844–850.

Mitra, A.K., Akramuzzaman, S.M., Fuchs, G.J., Rahman, M.M. and Mahalnabis, D. (1997) Long term oral supplementation with iron is not harmful for young children in a poor community of Bangladesh. *Journal of Nutrition* 127, 1451–1455.

Murray, M.J., Murray, A.B., Murray, M.B. and Murray, C.J. (1978) The adverse effect of iron repletion on the course of certain infections. *British Medical Journal* ii, 1113–1115.

Prentice, A.M. (2008) Iron metabolism, malaria and other infection: what is all the fuss about? *Journal of Nutrition* 138, 2537–2541.

Prentice, A.M., Ghattas, H. and Cox, S.E. (2007) Host–pathogen interactions: can micronutrients tip the balance? *Journal of Nutrition* 137, 1334–1337.

Oppenheimer, S.J. (1998) Iron and infection in the tropics: paediatric clinical correlates. *Annals of Tropical Paediatrics* 18, S81–S87.

Sazawal, S., Black, R.E., Ramsan, M., Chwaya, H.M., Stoltzfus, R.J., Dutta, A., Dhingra, U., Kabole, I., Deb, S., Othman, M.K. and Kabole, F.M. (2006) Effects of routine prophylactic supplementation with iron and folic acid on the admission to hospital and mortality in preschool children in a high malaria transmission setting: a community-based, randomised, placebo controlled trial. *Lancet* 367, 133–143.

Walter, T., Olivares, M., Pizzaro, F. and Munoz, C. (1997) Iron, anaemia and infection. *Nutrition Reviews* 55, 111–124.

Chapter 8

Bacqui, A.H., Black, R.E., El Arifeen, S., Yunus, M., Zaman, K., Begum, N., Roess, A.A. and Santosham, M. (2004) Zinc therapy for diarrhoea increased the use of oral rehydration therapy and reduced use of antibiotics in Bangladeshi children. *Journal of Health, Population, and Nutrition* 22, 440–442.

Bhandari, N., Mazumder, S., Taneja, S., Dube, B., Agarwal, R.C., Mahalanabis, D., Fontaine, O., Black, R.E. and Bhan, M.K. (2008) Effectiveness of zinc supplementation plus oral rehydration salts compared with oral rehydration salts alone as treatment for acute diarrhoeal diseases in a primary care setting: a cluster randomized trial. *Pediatrics* 121, e1279–e1285.

Bogden, J.D. (2004) Influence of zinc on immunity in the elderly. *Journal of Nutrition, Health & Aging* 8, 48–54.

Cuevas, L.E. and Koyanagi, A.I. (2005) Zinc and infection: a review. *Annals of Tropical Paediatrics* 25, 149–160.

Cunningham-Rundles, S. (1996) Zinc modulation of immune function: specificity and mechanism of interaction. *Journal of Laboratory and Clinical Medicine* 128, 9–11.

Dardenne, M. (2002) Zinc and immune function. *European Journal of Clinical Nutrition* 56, S20–S23.

Haider, B.A. and Bhutta, Z.A. (2009) The effect of therapeutic zinc supplementation among young children with selected infections: a review of the evidence. *Food and Nutrition Bulletin* 30, S41–S59.

Ibs, K.H. and Rink, L. (2003) Zinc-altered immune function. *Journal of Nutrition* 133, 1452S–1456S.

Mahalanabis, D., Lahiri, M., Paul, D., Gupta, S., Gupta, A., Wahed, M.A. and Khaled, M.A. (2004) Randomized double-blind, placebo-controlled clinical trial of the efficacy of treatment with zinc or vitamin A in infants and young children with severe acute lower respiratory infection. *American Journal of Clinical Nutrition* 79, 430–436.

Overbeck, S., Rink, L. and Haase, H. (2008) Modulating the immune response by oral zinc supplementation: a single approach for multiple diseases. *Archivum Immunologiae et Therapiae Experimentalis* 56, 15–30.

Prasad, A.S. (1998) Zinc and immunity. *Molecular and Cellular Biochemistry* 188, 63–69.

Prasad, A.S. (2007) Zinc: mechanisms of host defence. *Journal of Nutrition* 137, 1345–1349.

Prasad, A.S. (2008a) Zinc in human health: effect of zinc on immune cells. *Molecular Medicine* 14, 353–357.

Prasad, A.S. (2008b) Clinical, immunological, anti-inflammatory and antioxidant roles of zinc. *Experimental Gerontology* 43, 370–377.

Rink, L. and Gabriel, P. (2000) Zinc and immune system. *Proceedings of the Nutrition Society* 59, 541–552.

Roy, S.K., Hossain, M.J., Khatun, W., Chakraborty, B., Chowdhury, S., Begum, A., Mah-E-Muneer, S., Shafique, S., Khanam, M. and Chodury, R. (2008) Zinc supplementation in children with cholera in Bangladesh: randomised control trial. *British Medical Journal* 336, 266–268.

Simkin, P.A. (1976) Oral zinc sulphate in rheumatoid arthritis. *Lancet* 2, 539–542.

Chapter 9

Bobat, R., Moodley, D., Coutsoudis, A. and Coovadia, H. (1997) Breastfeeding by HIV-1 infected women and outcomes in their infants: a cohort study from Durban, South Africa. *AIDS* 11, 1627–1633.

Bobat, R., Coovadia, H., Stephen, C., Naidoo, K.L., McKerrow, N., Black, R.E. and Moss, W.J. (2005) Safety and efficacy of zinc supplementation for children with HIV-1 infection in South Africa: a randomised double blind placebo controlled trial. *Lancet* 366, 1862–1867.

Coutsoudis, A., Bobat, R.A., Coovadia, H.M., Kuhn, L., Tsai, W.Y. and Stein, Z.A. (1995) The effects of vitamin A supplementation on the morbidity of children born to HIV infected women. *American Journal of Public Health* 85, 1076–1081.

Dreyfuss, M.L. and Fawzie, W.W. (2002) Micronutrients and vertical transmission of HIV-1. *American Journal of Clinical Nutrition* 75, 959–970.

Fawzi, W.W. (2000) Nutritional factors and vertical transmission of HIV-1: epidemiology and potential mechanisms. *Annals of the New York Academy of Sciences* 918, 99–114.

Fawzi, W. (2003) Micronutrients and human immunodeficiency virus type 1 disease progression among adults and children. *Clinical Infectious Diseases* 37, S112–S116.

Fawzi, W.W., Msamanga, G.I., Spiegelman, D., Urassa, E.J., McGrath, N., Mwakagile, D., Antelman, G., Mbise, R., Herrera, G., Kapiga, S., Willett, W. and Hunter, D.J. (1998) Randomized trial of the effects of vitamin supplements on pregnancy outcomes and T cell counts in HIV-1 infected women in Tanzania. *Lancet* 351, 1477–1482.

Fawzi, W.W., Msamanga, G.I., Hunter, D.J., Urassa, E., Renjifo, B., Mwakagile, D., Hertzmark, E., Coley, J., Garland, M., Kapiga, S., Antelman, G., Essex, M. and Spiegelman, D. (2000) Randomized trial of the effects of vitamin supplements in relation to vertical transmission of HIV-1 in Tanzania. *Journal of Acquired Immune Deficiency Syndromes* 23, 246–254.

Fawzi, W.W., Msamanga, G.I., Spiegelman, D., Wei, R., Kapiga, S., Villamor, E., Mwakagile, D., Mugusi, F., Hertzmark, E., Essex, M. and Hunter, D.J. (2004) A randomized trial of multivitamin supplements and HIV disease progression and mortality. *New England Journal of Medicine* 351, 23–32.

Fawzi, W., Msamanga, G., Spiegelman, D. and Hunter, D.J. (2005) Studies of vitamins and minerals and HIV transmission and disease progression. *Journal of Nutrition* 135, 938–944.

Hickey, M.S. (1994) AIDS: nutrition and immunity. In: Forse, R.A., Bell, S.J., Blackburn, G.L. and Kabbash, L.G. (eds) *Diet, Nutrition and Immunity*. CRC Press, Boca Raton, Florida, pp. 127–146.

Iliff, P.J., Piwoz, E.G., Tavengwa, N.V., Zunguza, C.D., Marinda, E.T., Nathoo, K.J., Moulton, L.H., Ward, B.J., Humphrey, J.H. and ZVITAMBO Group (2005) Early exclusive breastfeeding reduces the risk of postnatal HIV-1 transmission and increases HIV-free survival. *AIDS* 19, 699–708.

Karyadi, E., Schultink, W., Nelwan, R.H., Gross, R., Amin, Z., Dolmans, W.M., van der Meer, J.W., Hautvast, J.G. and West, C.E. (2000) Poor micronutrient status of active pulmonary tuberculosis patients in Indonesia. *Journal of Nutrition* 130, 2953–2958.

Karyadi, E., West, C.E., Schultink, J.W., Nelwan, R.H., Gross, R., Amin, Z., Dolmans, W.M., Schlebusch, H. and van der Meer, J.W. (2002a) A double blind placebo controlled study of vitamin A and zinc supplementation in persons with tuberculosis in Indonesia: effects on clinical response and nutritional status. *American Journal of Clinical Nutrition* 75, 720–727.

Karyadi, E., West, C.E., Nelwan, R.H., Dolmans, W.M., Schultink, J.W. and van der Meer, J.W. (2002b) Social aspects of patients with pulmonary tuberculosis in Indonesia. *Southeast Asian Journal of Tropical Medicine and Public Health* 33, 338–345.

Kiure, A. and Fawzi, W. (2004) HIV. In: Gershwin, M.E., Nestel, P. and Keen, C.L. (eds) *Handbook of Nutrition and Immunity*. Humana Press, Totowa, New Jersey, pp. 303–337.

Kongnyuy, E.J., Wiysonge, C.S. and Shey, M.S. (2009) A systematic review of randomized controlled trials of prenatal and post natal vitamin A supplementation of HIV infected women. *International Journal of Gynaecology and Obstetrics* 104, 5–8.

Kumwenda, N., Miotti, P.G., Taha, T.E., Broadhead, R., Biggar, R.J., Jackson, J.B., Melikian, G. and Semba, R.D. (2002) Antenatal vitamin A supplementation increases birth weight and decreases anemia among infants born to human immunodeficiency virus-infected women in Malawi. *Clinical Infectious Diseases* 35, 618–624.

McMurray, D.N. and Bartow, R.A. (1992) Immunosuppression and alterations of resistance to pulmonary tuberculosis in guinea pigs by protein undernutrition. *Journal of Nutrition* 122, 738–743.

Mangili, A., Murman, D.H., Zampini, A.M. and Wanke, C.A. (2006) Nutrition and HIV infection: review of weight loss and wasting in the era of highly active antiretroviral therapy from the nutrition for healthy living cohort. *Clinical Infectious Diseases* 42, 836–842.

Onwubalili, J.K. (1988) Malnutrition among tuberculosis patients in Harrow, England. *European Journal of Clinical Nutrition* 42, 363–366.

Rwagabwoba, J.M., Fischman, H. and Semba, R.D. (1998) Serum vitamin A levels during tuberculosis and human immunodeficiency virus infections. *International Journal of Tuberculosis and Lung Disease* 2, 771–773.

Scrimshaw, N.S., Gordon, C.E. and Taylor, J.E. (1959) Interactions of nutrition and infection. *American Journal of Medical Sciences* 237, 367–403.

Villamor, E., Msamanga, G.I., Spiegelman, D., Antelman, G., Peterson, K.E. and Hunter, D.J. (2002) Effect of multivitamin and vitamin A supplementation on weight gain during pregnancy in HIV-1 infected women. *American Journal of Clinical Nutrition* 76, 1082–1090.

Wiysonge, C.S., Shey, M.S., Sterne, J.A. and Brocklehurst, P. (2005) Vitamin A supplementation for reducing the risk of mother-to-child transmission of HIV infection. *Cochrane Database of Systematic Reviews* issue 4, CD003648.

Chapter 10

Aggarwal, R., Sentz, J. and Miller, M.A. (2007) Role of zinc administration in prevention of childhood diarrhoea and respiratory illnesses: a meta-analysis. *Pediatrics* 119, 1120–1130.

Allen, L. and Gillespie, S. (2001) *What Works? A Review of the Efficacy and Effectiveness of Nutrition Interventions*. United Nations Administrative Committee on Coordination, Sub-committee on Nutrition, Geneva, Switzerland and Asian Development Bank, Manila.

Bhutta, Z.A., Jackson, A. and Lumbiganon, P. (eds) (2003) Nutrition as a preventative strategy against adverse pregnancy outcomes. *Journal of Nutrition* 133, 1589S–1767S.

Bhutta, Z.A., Ahmed, T., Black, R.E., Cousens, S., Dewey, K., Giugliani, E., Haider, B.A., Kirkwood, B., Morris, S.S., Sachdev, H.P.S. and Shekar, M., for the Maternal and Child Undernutrition Study Group (2008) Maternal and child undernutrition: what works? Interventions for maternal and child undernutrition and survival. *Lancet* 371, 417–440.

Black, R.E., Allen, L.H., Bhutta, Z.A., Caulfield, L.E., de Onis, M., Ezzati, M., Mathers, C. and Rivera, J., for the Maternal and Child Undernutrition Study Group (2008) Maternal and child undernutrition: global and regional exposures and health consequences. *Lancet* 371, 243–269.

Britton, C., McCormick, F.M., Renfrew, M.J., Wade, A. and King, S.E. (2007) Support for breastfeeding mothers. *Cochrane Database of Systematic Reviews* issue 1, CD001141.

Dewey, K.G. and Adu-Afarwuah, S. (2008) Systematic review of the efficacy and effectiveness of complementary feeding interventions in developing countries. *Maternal and Child Nutrition* 4, 24–85.

Dickson, R., Awasthi, S., Williamson, P., Demellweek, C., Paul, G. and Garner, P. (2000) Effects of treatment for intestinal helminth infection on growth and cognitive performance in children; systematic review of randomised trials. *British Medical Journal* 320, 1697–1701.

Engle, P., Bentley, M. and Pelto, G. (2000) The role of care in nutrition programmes. *Proceedings of the Nutrition Society* 59, 25–35.

Gera, T. and Sachdev, H.P.S. (2002) Effect of iron supplementation on the incidence of infectious illness in children: systematic review. *British Medical Journal* 325, 1142–1152.

Gogia, S. and Sachdev, H.S. (2009) Neonatal vitamin A supplementation for prevention of mortality and morbidity in infancy: systematic review of randomised control trials. *British Medical Journal* 338, 919.

Iannotti, L.L., Tielsch, J.M., Black, M.M. and Black, R.E. (2006) Iron supplementation in early childhood; health benefits and risks. *American Journal of Clinical Nutrition* 84, 1261–1276.

Kramer, M.S. and Kakuma, R. (2002) Optimal duration of exclusive breastfeeding. *Cochrane Database of Systematic Reviews* issue 1, CD003517.

Margetts, B.M. and Nelson, M. (1997) *Design Concepts in Nutritional Epidemiology*, 2nd edn. Oxford University Press, Oxford, UK.

Roth, D.E., Caulfield, L.E., Ezzati, M. and Black, R.E. (2008) Acute lower respiratory infections in childhood: opportunities for reducing the global burden through nutritional interventions. *Bulletin of the World Health Organization* 86, 356–364.

Sguassero, Y., de Onis, M. and Carroli, G. (2005) Community based supplementary feeding for promoting the growth of young children in developing countries. *Cochrane Database of Systematic Reviews* issue 4, CD005039.

World Health Organization (1999) *A Critical Link: Interventions for Physical Growth and Psychological Development: A Review*. World Health Organization, Geneva, Switzerland.

Chapter 11

Allen, L. and Gillespie, S. (2001) *What Works? A Review of the Efficacy and Effectiveness of Nutrition Interventions*. United Nations Administrative Committee on Coordination, Sub-committee on Nutrition, Geneva, Switzerland and Asian Development Bank, Manila.

Ashworth, A. (1998) Effects of intrauterine growth retardation on mortality and morbidity in infants and young children. *European Journal of Clinical Nutrition* 52, S34–S42.

Barker, D.J. (2006) Adult consequences of fetal growth restriction. *Clinical Obstetrics and Gynaecology* 49, 270–283.

Bhutta, Z.A., Jackson, A. and Lumbiganon, P. (eds) (2003) Nutrition as a preventative strategy against adverse pregnancy outcomes. *Journal of Nutrition* 133, 1589S–1767S.

Bhutta, Z.A., Ahmed, T., Black, R.E., Cousens, S., Dewey, K., Giugliani, E., Haider, B.A., Kirkwood, B., Morris, S.S., Sachdev, H.P.S. and Shekar, M., for the Maternal and Child Undernutrition Study Group (2008) Maternal and child undernutrition: what works? Interventions for maternal and child undernutrition and survival. *Lancet* 371, 417–440.

Chandra, R.K. (1988) Nutritional regulation of immunity: an introduction. In: Chandra, R.K. (ed.) *Nutrition and Immunology*. Alan Liss Inc., New York, pp. 1–8.

Christian, P. (2003) Micronutrients and reproductive health. *Journal of Nutrition* 133, 1969S–1973S.

Cogswell, M.E., Parvanta, I., Ickes, L., Yip, R. and Brittenham, G.M. (2003) Iron supplementation during pregnancy, anemia, and birth weight: a randomized controlled trial. *American Journal of Clinical Nutrition* 78, 773–781.

Commission on the Nutrition Challenges of the 21st Century (2000) *Ending Malnutrition by 2020: An Agenda for Change in the Millennium*. UN Standing Committee on Nutrition, Geneva, Switzerland.

Kramer, M.S. (1998) Socioeconomic determinants of intrauterine growth retardation. *European Journal of Clinical Nutrition* 52, S29–S33.

Margetts, B.M. and Nelson, M. (1997) *Design Concepts in Nutritional Epidemiology*, 2nd edn. Oxford University Press, Oxford, UK.

Rasmussen, K. (2001) Is there a causal relationship between iron deficiency and iron deficiency anemia and birth weight, length of gestation and perinatal mortality? *Journal of Nutrition* 131, 590S–603S.

Rush, D. (2000) Nutrition and maternal mortality in the developing world. *American Journal of Clinical Nutrition* 72, 212S–240S.

Shetty, P. (2009) Community-based approaches to address childhood undernutrition and obesity in developing countries. In: Kalhan, S.C., Prentice, A.M. and Yajnik, C.S. (eds) *Emerging Societies – Coexistence of Childhood Malnutrition and Obesity*. Nestlé Nutrition Institute, Vevey, Switzerland and Karger, Basel, pp. 227–258.

van den Broek, N. (2003) Anaemia and micronutrient deficiencies. *British Medical Bulletin* 67, 149–160.

World Health Organization (2005) *Make Every Mother and Child Count. World Health Report 2005*. World Health Organization, Geneva. Switzerland.

World Health Organization (2006) *Promoting Optimal Foetal Development. WHO Technical Consultation Report*. World Health Organization, Geneva, Switzerland.

Yajnik, C.S. (2004) Early life origins of insulin resistance and type 2 diabetes in India and other Asian countries. *Journal of Nutrition* 134, 205–210.

Chapter 12

Bogden, J.D., Bendich, A., Kemp, F.W., Bruening, K.S., Shurnick, J.H., Denny, T., Baker, H. and Louria, D.B. (1994) Daily micronutrient supplements enhance delayed-hypersensitivity skin test responses in older people. *American Journal of Clinical Nutrition* 60, 437–447.

Chandra, R.K. (1992) Effect of vitamin and trace-element supplementation on immune responses and infection in elderly subjects. *Lancet* 340, 1124–1127.

Dangour, A.D., Sibson, V.L. and Fletcher, A.E. (2004) Micronutrient supplementation in later life. *Journal of Gerontology* 59, 659–673.

Evans, C. (2005) Malnutrition in the elderly: a multifactorial failure to thrive. *The Permanente Journal* 9, 38–41.

Garry, P.J., Goodwin, J.S., Hunt, W.C. and Gilbert, B.A. (1982) Nutritional status in healthy elderly population: dietary and supplemental intakes. *American Journal of Clinical Nutrition* 36, 319–331.

Goodwin, J.S. (1989) Social, psychological and physical factors affecting the nutritional status of elderly subjects: separating cause and effect. *American Journal of Clinical Nutrition* 50, 120–1209.

Graat, J.M., Schouten, E.G. and Kok, F.J. (2002) Effect of daily vitamin E and multivitamin–mineral supplementation on acute respiratory tract infections in elderly persons. A randomized controlled trial. *Journal of the American Medical Association* 288, 715–721.

Meydani, S.N., Meydani, M., Blumberg, J.B., Leka, L.S., Siber, G., Loszewski, R., Thompson, C., Pedrosa, M.C., Diamond, R.D. and Stollar, B.D. (1997) Vitamin E

---

supplementation and *in vivo* immune response in healthy elderly subjects: a randomized controlled trial. *Journal of the American Medical Association* 277, 1380–1386.

Santos, M.S., Leka, L.S., Ribaya-Mercado, J.D., Russell, R.M., Meydani, M., Hennekens, C.H., Gaziano, J.M. and Meydani, A.N. (1997) Short- and long-term β-carotene supplementation do not influence T cell-mediated immunity in healthy elderly. *American Journal of Clinical Nutrition* 66, 917–924.

Santos, M.S., Gaziano, J.M., Leka, L.S., Beharka, A.A., Hennekens, C.H. and Meydani, A.N. (1998) β-Carotene induced enhancement of natural killer cell activity in elderly men: an investigation of the role of cytokines. *American Journal of Clinical Nutrition* 68, 164–170.

Chapter 13

Baldeon, M.E. and Gaskins, H.R. (2000) Diabetes and immunity. In: Gershwin, M.E., German, J.B. and Keen, C.L. (eds) *Nutrition and Immunology: Principles and Practice*. Humana Press, Totowa, New Jersey, pp. 301–311.

Berbert, A.A., Kondo, C.R.M., Almendra, C.L., Matsuo, T. and Dichi, I. (2005) Supplementation of fish oil and olive oil in patients with rheumatoid arthritis. *Nutrition* 21, 131–136.

Calder, P.C. (2006) *n*-3 Polyunsaturated fatty acids, inflammation, and inflammatory disease. *American Journal of Clinical Nutrition* 83, S1505–1519S.

Clifford, C.K. (2000) Cancer and nutrition. In: Gershwin, M.E., German, J.B. and Keen, C.L. (eds) *Nutrition and Immunology: Principles and Practice*. Humana Press, Totowa, New Jersey, pp. 375–388.

Davis, P.A. and Stern, J.S. (2000) Obesity and immunity. In: Gershwin, M.E., German, J.B. and Keen, C.L. (eds) *Nutrition and Immunology: Principles and Practice*. Humana Press, Totowa, New Jersey, pp. 295–300.

World Cancer Research Fund/American Institute for Cancer Research (2007) *Food, Nutrition, Physical Activity, and the Prevention of Cancer: A Global Perspective*. World Cancer Research Fund International, London.

Chapter 14

Al Faleh, K.M. and Bassier, D. (2008) Probiotics for prevention of necrotizing enterocolitis in preterm infants. *Cochrane Database of Systematic Reviews* issue 1, CD005496.

Allen, S.J., Okoko, B., Marinez, E., Gregorio, G. and Dans, L.F. (2003) Probiotics for treating infectious diarrhoea. *Cochrane Database of Systematic Reviews* issue 2, CD003048.

Basu, S., Chatterjee, M., Ganguly, S. and Chandra, P.K. (2007) Effect of *Lactobacillus rhamnosus* GG in persistent diarrhea in Indian children. A randomized controlled trial. *Journal of Clinical Gastroenterology* 41, 756–760.

Collins, M.D. and Gibson, G.R. (1999) Probiotics, prebiotics and synbiotics: approaches for modulating the microbial ecology of the gut. *American Journal of Clinical Nutrition* 69, 1052S–1057S.

Gibson, G.R. and Roberfroid, M.B. (1995) Dietary modulation of the human colonic microbiota: introducing the concept of prebiotics. *Journal of Nutrition* 125, 1401–1412.

Guarner, F. and Malagelada, J.R. (2003) Gut flora in health and disease. *Lancet* 361, 512–519.

Hickson, M., D'Souza, A.L., Muthu, N., Rogers, T.R., Want, S., Rajkumar, C. and Bulpitt, C.J. (2007) Use of probiotic Lactobacillus preparation to prevent diarrhoea associated with antibiotics: a randomised double blind placebo controlled trial. *British Medical Journal* 335, 80–84.

Lomax, A.R. and Calder, P.C. (2009) Probiotics, immune function, infection and inflammation: a review of the evidence from studies conducted in humans. *Current Pharmaceutical Design* 15, 1428–1518.

van Niel, C.W., Feudtner, C., Garrison, M.M. and Christakis, D.A. (2002) Lactobacillus therapy for acute infectious diarrhoea in children: a meta analysis. *Pediatrics* 109, 678–684.

Chapter 15

Brostoff, J. and Challacombe, S.J. (2002) *Food Allergy and Intolerance*. Elsevier, London.

Chang, C. and Gershwin, M.E. (2000) Nutrition and allergy. In: Gershwin, M.E., German, J.B. and Keen, C.L. (eds) *Nutrition and Immunology: Principles and Practice*. Humana Press, Totowa, New Jersey, pp. 221–231.

Committee on Toxicity of Chemicals in Food, Consumer Products and the Environment (1998) *Peanut Allergy*. Department of Health, London.

Foschi, F.G., Marsigli, L., Ciappeli, F., Kung, M.A., Bernardi, M. and Stefanini, G.F. (2000) Adverse reactions to food. In: Gershwin, M.E., German, J.B. and Keen, C.L. (eds) *Nutrition and Immunology: Principles and Practice*. Humana Press, Totowa, New Jersey, pp. 233–246.

Opara, E. (2002) Food allergy. In: Calder, P.C., Field, C.J. and Gill, H.S. (eds) *Nutrition and Immune Function*. CAB International and The Nutrition Society, Wallingford, UK, pp. 321–346.

Index

Page numbers in **bold** type refer to figures, tables, case studies and boxed text.

HIV/AIDS (*continued*)
  synergism with nutrition 4, 70, 117–118
    benefits of vitamin/mineral supplements
        81, **119**, 121–122, 128, **128**
    micronutrient deficiencies **118**,
        118–121
    wasting and undernutrition 124, **124**
  transmission **115**
    vertical (mother-to-infant) 122–124
    vitamin A supplement effects **129**, 129
hookworms 69, 98, **98**, 147
humoral (B-cell) immunity 15, 17–18
  changes with ageing 156, 160
  effect of vitamin A deficiency 32, 76
  effects of zinc deficiency 105
  undernutrition effects 45–46, 49–50
hygiene hypothesis 177, 181
hyperkeratosis 75, **77**

immunity
  response
    cytokine mediation **12–13**, 20–21
    effects of ageing 154–156, **155**
    effects of dietary fatty acids 30
    hormonal adaptation 62
    macronutrient needs 23, 25, 27–28
    mineral and vitamin redistribution 33, 62–63, 92
    modulation by probiotics 175–176,
        177–178
  suppression, following infection 66, 125–126
  surveillance (against cancer) 167
  system components 8–10, **9**, 21
  tests of function (immunocompetence) 7–8, 51, 53
  see also acquired immunity; innate immunity
immunization
  active (vaccination) 21–22
    effects of zinc supplements 105–106
    influenza vaccination 105, 158, 159
  passive 21
immunoglobulins (Ig)
  activity 19
    IgE, in allergies 183–184, 185
    secretory (IgA) 45, 49–50
  maternal transfer 21, 47, 144
  molecular structure 18, **18**
  responses to vaccines, age-related 156, 161, **162**
  types 18–19, **19**
infants
  complementary feeding **65**, 133, 136
  HIV infection from mother
    effects of micronutrient deficiency **122**,
        122–123
    transmission through breast milk 123–124
    vitamin supplementation trials 123
  mortality, causes 1, 120
  parenteral iron supplements

  increased malaria risk 96
  sepsis incidence 95
  premature, with enterocolitis 176
  small for gestational age (SGA) 143, 147
  see also low birth weight
infection *see* diseases
infectious agents *see* pathogens
inflammation
  acute phase physiology 12, **12–13**
  chronic, and cancer risk 166–167
  response characteristics 11–12
  suppression, due to undernourishment 43
innate immunity 9–10, **10**
  complement system 15
  inflammatory response 11–12, **12–13**
    reactive oxygen and nitrogen species
        (RONS) 166
  phagocytosis 13–15, **14**
insulin-like growth factor (IGF-1) 29, 63–64
intestinal parasites 68–69
  correlation with iron deficiency **98**, 98–99
  treatment of children 138
intrauterine growth restriction/retardation (IUGR)
  causes 143, **143**, 145
  consequences 47, 143–145, **145**
  definition **46**
  see also low birth weight
iodine, as micronutrient **27**, 147
iron nutrition 2, **27**
  deficiency 34, **35**
    global extent 88, 90
    increased infectious disease risk 92–93, **94**
    parasite and diet correlation **98**, 98–99
    reduced infectious disease risk 93, **94**, 95
    stages **91**
  overload 35, **35**, 91, 97
  physiological roles
    immune response function 33–34, 90–92, **92**
    oxygen transport 88, **89**
  regulation and transport **89–90**, 93–94
  sources and absorption **89**
  supplementation
    child growth 99, **99**, 137
    developed countries 92, 93, 95
    developing countries 95–96
    endemic malarial areas 96–97
    interaction with malaria **100**, 100
    in pregnancy 146, 150–152, **151**

kwashiorkor **48**, 49

lactation *see* breastfeeding
Lactobacillus spp. 174, 176, 178
lactose intolerance **182**
leishmaniasis 107, 117

zinc (*continued*)

physiological roles 101, **103**

antioxidant activity 105

as component of metalloenzymes **102**

growth and development **103**

immune response function 35–36, **36**, 104, 104–106, **105**

sources and bioavailability **102–103**

supplementation 101–102

administered during illnesses 109–110, 122

for children and mothers 137, 146–147

in cholera treatment **110–111, 111**

in community health trials **112–113, 113**

effects on disease incidence **107**, 107–108, **108**

for the elderly 159

respiratory infection treatment **111, 111–112, 112**

toxicity, with excess doses 106, 110